Ceramics in Dentistry

Ceramics in Dentistry

Materials, Manufacturing,
and Clinical Applications

Carolyn M. Primus

The American Ceramic Society
ceramics.org

WILEY

Published by John Wiley & Sons, Inc., Hoboken, New Jersey.

Library of Congress Cataloging-in-Publication Data applied for:

Hardback ISBN: 9781119436546

Cover Design: Wiley
Cover Image: Courtesy of Kam Jin and Naomi Deutsch

Set in 9.5/12.5pt STIXTwoText by Straive, Pondicherry, India

Contents

Preface

The contributions of ceramics to our material world are enormous. Ceramics are integral to building large concrete skyscrapers and making minute semiconductor chips; they are seen (dishware) and unseen (glass and most electronics); they range from cheap per kilogram (cement) to costly (glass sculptures or medical devices). Some ceramics look utilitarian (sidewalks), and some are exquisite in appearance (rubies, opals, aquamarine, diamonds, and other gems).

The goal of this text is to illuminate the subtle and apparent contributions of ceramics to our oral health. Other "ceramics in dentistry" texts have focused on dental restoratives, especially alumina, porcelain, glass-ceramic, and zirconia for crowns and bridges. This text is a broader survey of the many dental products that rely on ceramics. Ceramic engineers and material scientists have innovated an expansive choice of industrial ceramics; some have been adapted for medical devices, including dentistry, in a myriad of products and accessories. The ceramics in dentistry include nanoparticles ($<0.1\,\mu m$), micron-sized crystalline or glass powders, and macro-sized single crystals. Some have a temporary use, and others should survive decades of chewing. This wide-ranging description of ceramics in dentistry is meant to inspire readers, both engineers and dentists, to appreciate ceramics and invent better materials and treatments for the oral cavity or bone-related maladies. Innovation requires knowledge of materials, manufacturing processes, and analysis techniques for decision-making and commercialization of dental devices.

Principles of ceramic manufacture and performance are included. Ceramic processing begins with raw materials used to manufacture powders and proceeds to forming techniques and heat treatments to create a useful device. Testing and analysis techniques are essential to ensure the ceramic item performs as intended in vivo. This text combines descriptions of ceramics in general and guide the reader past the hubbub in the dental literature's test results. The whole of the dental literature on ceramics cannot be captured herein. Furthermore, the published dental studies are sometimes conflicting, particularly regarding strength and toughness of ceramics in dentistry. Often, the descriptions of the materials tested are inadequately or erroneously described; many ceramic materials are incompletely understood by the testers and the users (clinicians). Dentists need to refer to the Safety Data Sheet (SDS) at a minimum, for the materials they use or test, like materials engineers do.

I'm indebted to the contributors listed below and to others for their wisdom, guidance, and humanity. My high school chemistry teacher, Mr. Vandercarr, showed me information on space age ceramics and the University of Illinois. This led to my matriculation and a scholarship in ceramic engineering. Professors Alfred Friedman and Clifton Bergeron at the University of Illinois opened the doors of materials science to me with their teaching and kindness in an era when women were not especially welcomed or included. At the University of California, I was lucky enough to study under the guidance of professors Richard Fulrath and Zuhair Munir, who expanded my understanding of materials and laboratory testing for my master's and doctoral studies. From my work at Sandia National Laboratories to my fellowship at Naval Research Laboratory with Dr. Kurt Stern and Dr. David Venezky, I broadened my research to solve engineering problems. I was lucky enough to continue inventing and commercializing products at Gillette. At Dentsply, I recognized the spectrum of ceramics in dentistry, which has delighted and surprised me and sparked this book. Dr. Steven Jefferies trusted my ceramic engineering skills for manufacturing a new, bioactive dental ceramic cement, leading me to the past 30 years of invention and research. My dear dental colleague Professor James Gutmann collaborated with me on ideas, testing, validation, reports, manuscripts, and patents for bioactive cements, materials that help heal the vital tissue in and around teeth. Plus, he was kind enough to treat my own endodontic problems as his patient, and he nominated me to receive an honorary membership with the American Association of Endodontists (2026). Professor Franklin Tay encouraged me to apply for a Small Business Innovative Research (SBIR) grant; Professor James Drummond at the National Institute of Dental and Craniofacial Research, with his impressive combination of dental and ceramic engineering skills and degrees, recognized my ideas for improving oral health and supported my grant. Professors Tay at Augusta University and Lynne Opperman at Texas A&M University orchestrated the research that laid the foundation for commercializing my SBIR ideas, by founding the Avalon Biomed Corporation. Mr. John Bozman provided the manufacturing location and some cheer-leading for the success of the company as we achieved FDA 510(k) clearance and ISO 13485 quality certification that enabled the company to offer a better, economical bioactive cement that we sold on three continents. My husband and I retired from that enterprise, I began this book.

I've been a member of the American Ceramic Society since my undergraduate days, and I'm grateful for the Society's association with Wiley, enabling this book to be published. The team at Wiley has been kind, polite, keen-eyed, patient and helpful; thank you Michael Leventhal, Dimple Philip, Kamalini Christilda, and Elizabeth Rose Amaladoss. I have been heartened to see the evolution of ACerS and its leadership progress from the "Virginia Kyanite pinups" in the Ceramic Bulletin ads to the election of women as the society's leaders, including presidents. Its a joy to be part of the Cement and the Bioceramics divisions, and I'm grateful to be the first recipient of the Larry Hench Lifetime Achievement award.

I'm so appreciative of my friends who have editing skills that have checked and improved the simplicity and clarity of my writing for an audience from dentists to material scientists and engineers. I am especially indebted to Dr. Pamela C. VanBlaricum and Mrs. Susan Spielberg who kindly donated so much of their personal time to overview my writing and make corrections and improvements. Prof. James Gutmann has been a scientific colleague who has also greatly helped me with this text. Ms. Lori Rand, Prof. Sue Holl, Mrs. Heather Whelan, and Ms. Ruthanne Vendy also provided writing/editing support to help me piece together the disparate uses of ceramic in dentistry. Ms. Lori Rand's grammar and writing skills helped me to stay "on topic," adding continuity and readability; I'm so appreciative. The cover artwork was based on the beautiful medical illustrations of teeth by Ms. Naomi Deutsch that are used within this tests rendered, and then artistically rendered by Mr. Kam Jin.

My greatest supporter has been my husband, Gino Primus. I was raised in an era where women were lesser beings; he carried me into the 21st century viewpoint of equality and equal partnership. He also brought his many skills to Avalon Biomed Corporation manufacturing activities, even after he had already retired. No one can be more grateful than I for his loving patience, supporting efforts, and encouragement with my pursuits. He is the partner that my mother, a fervent supporter of women's education, would have wished for me.

Lastly, I am indebted to Dr. H.-S. Chon, Dr. Scott Lunin, APRN Patricia Ciampa-Muske, and Ms. Elizabeth Bornstein whose medical skills enabled me to survive and thrive after ovarian cancer to complete this book.

"Thank you" words cannot convey the heart-felt gratitude I feel for everyone's support though I hope to be able to show my appreciation.

Carolyn M. Primus
Sarasota, Florida

Contributors

- Prof. James L. Drummond, Ph.D., DDS, provided cogent comments on the outline of this book many years ago. He also edited and contributed to the terminology and introduction to teeth and especially the indirect restorations (Chapter 10).
- Bradley D. Craig, Ph.D., of Solventum Corporation (formerly 3M Oral Care Solutions Division) contributed the bulk of Chapter 10 on direct restorations and adhesives and other insights on polymers and properties, in Chapters 4, 6 and 11.
- Dr. David Grossman (formerly of Corning Glass) enhanced the description of glass-ceramics in Chapters 6 and 10 with his deep knowledge and experience with glass-ceramics.
- Dr. Hyungbong Lim of Hass Corporation provided excellent insight into lithium disilicate products for dental use in Chapter 10.
- Dr. Gutmann has been my touchstone for dentistry, endodontics (Chapter 8), dental history, and writing.
- And I thank the Solventum Corporation, NuSmile Ltd., and Hass Corporation for the use of their figures.

1

Introduction

Ceramics include a broad swath of materials in our world and are defined as neither metallic nor organic. Ceramic dental items have been produced from naturally occurring, inorganic minerals and purified chemicals using a bewildering array of formulas and forming methods, often with the aid of heat and sometimes pressure. Ceramic-containing dental products have been used for a vast range of procedures, including esthetic (biomimetic in appearance) replacements of teeth.

This text includes a potpourri of information on dental history, medical device regulation and standards, ceramic manufacturing, and clinical dental uses of ceramics. This text was constructed as an introduction to ceramic technologies that have improved oral public health. The dental ceramics described herein are based on history and praxis; theories for optimizing some property derivations are left to other texts and authors. Dental textbooks and review articles are included in the references for in-depth reading and learning clinical issues. Some morsels from each chapter may be useful for bioengineers of all types, inventors, and dental clinicians for future dental ceramics. Any dental ceramic product begins with an idea and a market need, abbreviated as business, as shown in Figure 1.1; quality and regulatory aspects combine with manufacturing methods to create products; clinical feedback on the products is often the spark for further improvements in this cycle.

Modern dental researchers and companies like to label the evolution of dental materials as "generations" to distinguish improved formulas and products as they become available (1, 2). The differences among generations can be confusing because researchers disagree on the classifications, the generations may overlap, some may not be the distinctions that a materials scientist would use, and others are inaccurate characterizations of materials' distinctions. Therefore, descriptions of the materials were used herein in lieu of labeling the generations of the materials.

Dentistry's progression spans three eras: ancient, 18th to 20th centuries, and the 21st century, as in Figure 1.2. Dental treatments have improved from merely extractions

Ceramics in Dentistry: Materials, Manufacturing, and Clinical Applications,
First Edition. Carolyn M. Primus.

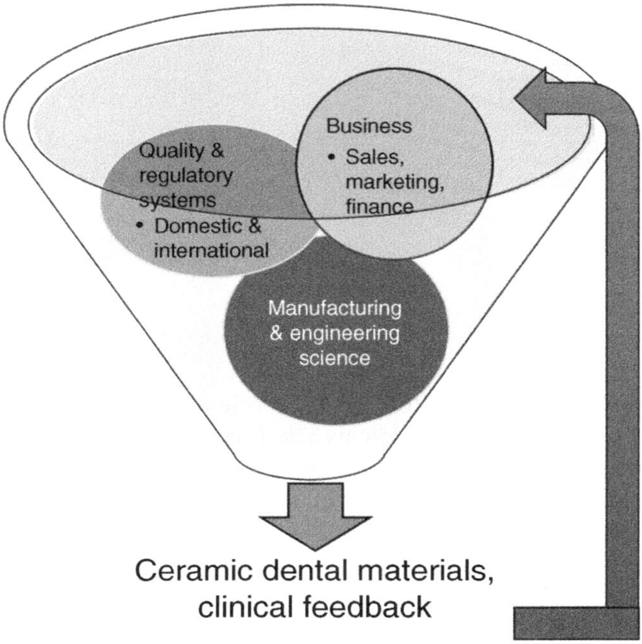

Figure 1.1 This diagram depicts the combination of disciplines required for ceramic dental materials production, and the importance of feedback from their clinical use for improvements.

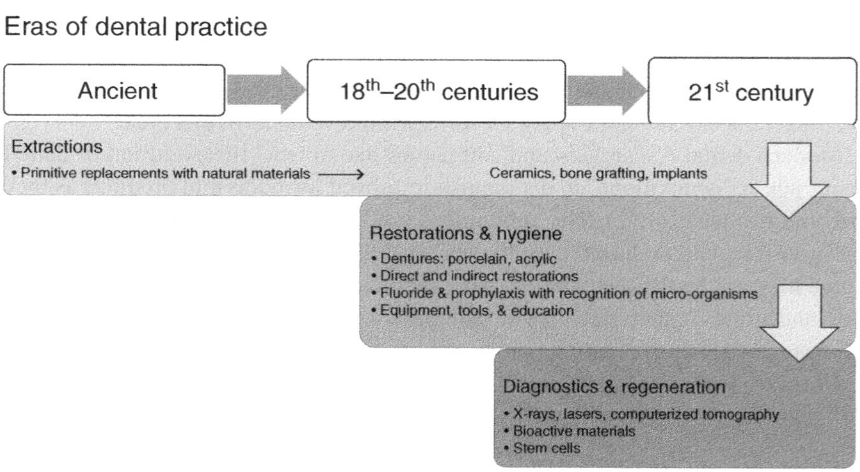

Figure 1.2 This diagram depicts the eras of dentistry over the millennia from primitive to restorative and preservation.

(ancient) to tooth treatments and tooth preservation (18th to 20th centuries), and diagnostics for regeneration (21st century). The emphasis is now on minimally invasive dentistry, supported by evidence-based medicine (EBM) (3): "the conscientious, explicit, and judicious use of current best evidence in making decisions about the care of individual patients ... integrating individual clinical experience with the best available clinical evidence from systematic research."

The goal of this text is to provide an éclaircissement of the intertwined history of ceramic formulas and manufacturing methods, to meet dental needs for all sorts of health problems and health maintenance.

Keywords and Materials in this Text

Alumina
Bioceramic
Bioactive
Biomineralization
Calcium aluminate cement
Calcium phosphate
Calcium silicate cement
Calcium sulfate
Cement
Resin-based composite
Glass
Glass–Ceramic
Glass ionomer cement
Hydroxyapatite
Lithium disilicate
Porcelain
Radiopacity
Silica
Zinc oxide
Zirconia

Terminology

Following is a list of some of the common terms in dentistry used in this text. Other dental-related definitions are in various International Standards Organization Standards listed in Chapter 4 and ISO 1942 or ADA 33 standards on vocabulary.

- American Dental Association (ADA): a professional organization that supports the advancement of public health provided by the dental community, including standards for dentistry.

- Anterior teeth: teeth that are in the front of the mouth.
- Apical: the region at the end of the tooth root(s) in the jaw.
- Alveolar bone: the bone surrounding the tooth roots.
- Bridge: a prosthodontic device that spans more than one tooth.
  - Bridges may be fixed (cemented permanently) or removable (by the patient).
- Buccal: an adjective to describe the side of the tooth facing the cheek.
- Cement: a material used to affix a dental device onto a tooth. Examples of devices are crowns (caps), bridges, and orthodontic brackets.
  - A ceramic powder that reacts with water to form a hard substance; calcium silicate and calcium aluminate ceramic cements are water-setting cements used in some dental procedures but are not used for adhesion of devices unless combined with other materials.
- Cementing: affixing something in the mouth.
- Cementum: the outer layer of teeth below the gum lines, as part of the periodontium that allows attachment of alveolar bone to the teeth.
- Class of restoration: the location on the tooth where a restorative dental material is placed. See Chapter 2 for the locations.
- Compomer: restorative material that combines mainly resin composite with some glass ionomer components.
- Composite (resin-based composite-resin): a monomer with ceramic filler that the dentist cures on the tooth, also known as a resin composite, dental composite, or, colloquially, a "filling."
- Coping: a thin, custom-made covering for the coronal portion of the tooth, as a base for another material used to create the anatomy of a crown or bridge.
- Core: the center coronal portion tooth that is needed to be the foundation for a crown.
  - A core may need to be "rebuilt" with dental materials in some decayed teeth.
- Coronal: the upper, outermost part of a tooth, protruding from the gums tooth.
- Crown: a dental device with tooth anatomy to cover the coronal part of a tooth that is missing.
  - Crowns replace the occlusal anatomy of one tooth, colloquially known as "caps."
- Dental laboratories: a place where dental materials are processed into something for the dentist to use in the operatory where the patient is treated.
- Dentin: partially mineralized (calcium hydroxyapatite) tissue under the enamel, enveloping the dental pulp from the coronal to the apical area.
- Denture: a complete or partial replacement for missing teeth that is removable by the patient.
- Die: replica of one tooth, used in a dental laboratory for making a dental device.
- Direct restoration: a procedure where the dentist directly fashions the restorative material in the patient's mouth, on their teeth.

- Enamel: a thin, translucent, outer covering of a tooth called the crown and is the visible part of the tooth in the mouth composed of hydroxyapatite.
  - Or a glassy coating on a metal or ceramic, also known as porcelain enamel.
- Endodontics: dental specialty that treats the pulp and the roots of teeth.
- Esthetic or cosmetic dentistry: related to imitating or improving the appearance of a patient's original tooth tissues in coloring, form, and texture, which may blend with or imitate surrounding teeth.
  - Use of biomimetic dental materials or methods to create the desired cosmetic results in the oral cavity, which may include teeth, the jaw, or soft tissues.
- Feldspathic porcelain: a misnomer for high thermal expansion porcelain containing leucite crystals in a glass matrix.
- Fixed prosthodontics: the crowns or bridges that are cemented in a patient's mouth, not removable by the patient.
- Furcal: the area under the coronal area of teeth where the roots diverge in multi-rooted teeth.
- Grain size: the size of crystals in a ceramic (or metal); sometimes, the size of powder particles.
- Glass–ceramic: glass items that have intentionally, been partially or fully devitrified (crystallized) under controlled conditions via a special heat treatment.
- Glass-ionomer restorative or cement (GI or GIC): a glass and polycarboxylate/polyacrylic acid material used for affixing dental devices to teeth and for restoring decayed teeth.
- Grain growth: the phenomenon during powder sintering where the particles coalesce and become larger.
- Hydroxyapatite: the calcium phosphate ceramic crystal that is the primary component of teeth and bones.
  - a naturally occurring mineral, $Ca_5(PO_4)_3(OH)$ or $Ca_{10}(PO_4)_6(OH)_2$, abbreviated as HA or HAP; it may be partially carbonated, or partially fluoridated, with partial substitution for the hydroxide.
- Implant: a device that is placed in the alveolar bone that replaces the roots and the crown(s) of missing teeth.
- Indirect restoration: a dental procedure where the dentist shapes the tooth for a restorative material and that device is fashioned outside the mouth; also known as fixed prosthodontics.
- Interproximal: area between the teeth or the tooth structure between teeth.
- International Organization for Standardization (ISO): an independent, non-governmental organization that has developed 24,500 international standards covering almost all aspects of technology and manufacturing, including dentistry.
- Labial: the side of the teeth that is on the front of the anterior teeth, the side of the teeth most apparent when one smiles.

- Lingual: the side of the teeth facing the tongue.
- Luting: the process of cementing a device onto the tooth, usually considered to be mechanical and frictional, not chemical adhesion.
- Mandibular teeth: lower teeth.
- Margins: the edge of a dental restoration or device where it meets the underlying tooth structure.
- Maxillary teeth: upper teeth.
- Microleakage: the ingress of bacteria around the perimeter (margin) of a restoration, or through a root canal from which the pulp has been removed.
- Microstructure or microscopy: structure of a material as revealed by an optical or electron microscope.
  - Optical microscopy requires a flat sample; magnification is less than 1000x.
  - Electron microscopy is used in scanning or transmission modes.
- Mineral trioxide aggregate (MTA): a tricalcium silicate containing cement used for vital pulp therapy and other endodontic indications.
- Model: a replica of several teeth.
- Obturation: the filling of an area, especially the anatomy of the root canal.
- Occlusal: the biting surface of teeth.
- Occlusion: the contact between the upper and lower teeth.
- Odontoblasts: cells that line the pulp cavity of a tooth, from which dentin is formed.
- Operatory: area where the patient is treated and separate from the dental laboratory.
- Organic material: a material containing carbon—carbon (C—C) or carbon—hydrogen (C—H) covalent bonds.
- Orthodontics: dental specialty that moves the position of teeth and the jaws for better occlusion and appearance.
- Pediatric (and adolescent) dentistry: dental specialty that treats the primary teeth or developing permanent teeth.
- Periodontics: dental specialty that treats the tissues surrounding the teeth, including periodic cleaning and diseased tissue.
- Porcelain: a ceramic material consisting of glass and dispersed crystalline particles but not a glass–ceramic.
- Prosthodontics: the aspect or specialty of dentistry that treats missing teeth and extensive tooth anatomy.
  - Fixed prosthodontics: dental devices that are permanently cemented onto one or more teeth to replace missing teeth.
  - Removable prosthodontics: devices that replace missing teeth and may be removed by the patient for cleaning. The device may attach to remaining teeth, e.g., a removable partial denture. Full dentures are also removable prosthodontics.
- Pulp: a living tissue including blood vessels and nerves that circulate and service the teeth's sensations and connects to the body's nerve tissues and blood vessels through the apical foramen of the roots.

- Radiopacity: the quality of absorbing X-rays so that an item can be distinguished in an X-ray image enabling identification of dental materials, decayed teeth, tooth structure, infections, growths around the teeth, bone loss, or other oral health tissues.
- Radiopaque: materials having higher atomic number elements than calcium and phosphorous that absorb X-rays more strongly than dentin or enamel and appear whiter on an X-ray image.
- Resin-modified glass ionomer (RMGI or RMGIC): a combination of a dental resin-based composite material with some glass ionomer cement.
- Restoration or restorative material: a substance used by the dentist to replace the missing anatomy of a tooth.
  - Direct restorations: the material is applied and shaped in the mouth and set (hardened, cured) by a dentist.
  - Indirect restoration: a preformed restoration made outside the mouth that a dentist cements in the mouth.
- Scanning electron microscopy or microscope (SEM): use of an electron beam to create high depth-of-field images of surfaces, usually operated under vacuum.
  - Some SEMs use field emission electron beams, and some operate in air as environmental SEM.
  - Ceramic materials usually need a metallic or graphite coating to create clear images, unless a field electron microscope is used.
  - The images may be low to high magnification (>1000x).
- Sealer: a medium viscosity paste (syrup-like) that endodontists use for filling and sealing root canals after a pulpectomy (removal of the pulp).
- Sealant: a material used to fill the grooves (fissures) and pits of the occlusal part of teeth with the objective of inhibiting bacterial infection in these anatomical details.
- Sintering: the process of consolidating powders, ceramic or otherwise, to reduce the surface area of the powders, usually achieved by heating the powders.
- Transmission electron microscopy (TEM): an imaging technique that uses an electron beam passed through a very thin sample.
- Veneers: thin dental restorations, of ceramic or resin-based composite materials, cemented onto the labial side of anterior teeth to improve the smile's appearance by covering discoloration, restoring anatomy, or creating better alignment.

References

1 Kugel, G. and Ferrari, M. (2000). The science of bonding: from first to sixth generation. *J. Am. Dent. Assoc.* 131 (6): 20S–25S.

2 Camilleri, J. (2017). Will bioceramics be the future root canal filling materials? *Curr. Oral Health Rep.* 4 (3): 228–238.

3 Sackett, D.L., Rosenberg, W.M.C., Gray, J.A.M. et al. (1996). Evidence based medicine: what it is and what it isn't. *BMJ* 312: 71–72.

2

Teeth and Oral Health

Before modern dentistry, dental diseases were frightful! Tooth decay (caries) was prevalent, causing much pain and loss of teeth. The agony of toothaches often led to dire infections (1). Today, dental disease is seldom life-threatening, but dental caries (cavities) remain the most common oral disease affecting 35% of the world's population (2), and is the most common chronic disease among youth aged 6–19 years (3). Dental infections directly impact daily activities and often require iterative dental treatments over a lifetime. Oral disease is manifested in productivity losses due to absenteeism from school and work (indirect costs) as well as the direct cost of treatment. Caries pose a higher burden for poorer and disadvantaged populations (4, 5). Income inequality exacerbates the presence of caries (6) and overall oral health (4, 5). Food insecurity contributes to the caries being untreated (7), affecting 621 million children worldwide (8).

Oral health is a treasured quality-of-life measure supported by dental organizations (9), yet it is often neglected in discussions of global health (10). However, the World Health Organization's (WHO) policies promote oral health as integral to general health and quality of life, including reducing premature mortality (11). Good oral health allows us to function normally to take nourishment, make facial expressions and smile, facilitate phonation (speaking), and have self-esteem to confidently interact with others. The appearance of our teeth has a profound effect on social interactions and professional success. The WHO has resolved that oral health should be promoted worldwide within families, schools, and workplaces, by countries implementing comprehensive and inclusive universal primary healthcare systems. The *Journal of the American Dental Association* presented a narrative review advocating for "coordinated policies and additional resources ... to further improve access to [dental] care, develop dental insurance programs that reduce out-of-pocket costs to lower-income adults, and improve the integration of oral and medical healthcare delivery targeting a common set of patient-centered outcomes" (12).

Ceramics in Dentistry: Materials, Manufacturing, and Clinical Applications,
First Edition. Carolyn M. Primus.

Longer life expectancy makes it ever more important to reduce tooth loss and avoid tooth-related disabilities in the elderly (13).

People take their teeth for granted, but our activities of daily living can injure our teeth and oral tissues with decay, wear, or breakage. A person's lifestyle contributes significantly to oral health, as do societal, environmental, and economic factors. Avoiding sugar, tobacco, and alcohol consumption all contribute to better oral health. Drug abuse and eating disorders are precursors to caries, periodontal problems (gum-related), and erosion of teeth. Some medications can cause oral diseases, such as fungal infections, osteonecrosis, and xerostomia (14). Despite these known risk factors, more than 3.5 billion people worldwide have untreated dental disease, higher than any other non-communicable disease (10). Tooth extractions have declined over the past century, yet 45% of people suffer from decay (caries), periodontal disease, and tooth loss (10, 11). Even with fluoride toothpastes and water fluoridation, caries remain a problem, with one of five Americans having untreated "cavities" (6).

The mouth is the entry point to the oral cavity, the respiratory system, and the digestive system, and correlations of the oral and systemic diseases are becoming elucidated and important (15). Recent studies have correlated oral health with systemic and mental health, including freedom from dementia; however, this does not show causality (16) but indicates risk factors. Periodontal disease co-occurs with poor birth outcomes and some serious systemic diseases such as diabetes, stroke, cardiovascular disease, and respiratory disease (14). Osteoporosis has been correlated with apical periodontitis (lesions in the bone around tooth roots) (17). Tooth loss has been associated with cardiac mortality (18) and mortality from all causes. Fortunately, dental treatment may be a mitigating factor (19). Maintenance, especially tooth brushing with a fluoride-containing dentifrice, and professional teeth cleaning, is required to maintain the health of the gums, chewing muscles, palate, tongue, lips, and salivary glands; without consistent care, tooth loss may occur over a lifetime. Good oral health supports enhanced aging by contributing to better systemic, cognitive, nutritional, and psychological health (20). Dental care professionals need to fully participate in meaningful and system-wide changes to meet the needs of the population equitably (12).

The increase in the world population, human life expectancy, and concerns about our physical appearance have motivated dentists and dental companies to develop better methods, materials, procedures and devices for treating or replacing tooth anatomy or extracted teeth. This text discusses common oral problems and the beneficial contributions of ceramic materials to improving oral health, especially in the past century. The descriptions are a bridge between materials science and dentistry.

Basics of Teeth

Teeth are vital sensory organs contributing to the ease of eating, drinking, speaking, and to our appearance. Humans usually have 32 permanent and 20 primary (deciduous) teeth, as shown in Figures 2.1 and 2.2. The primary teeth begin to form in utero and have entirely emerged by about age three years. After about six years old, the permanent teeth begin to replace the primary ones. The transition of mixed primary and permanent dentition proceeds until age 12 years, except for the third molars, which erupt in young adults. Each tooth may be viewed as an organ, highlighting how special it is for humans to have 52 similar organs in our bodies throughout our lives. Though similar, humans are heterodonts – each tooth has a unique exterior shape depending on its location in the jaw, although variations in anatomy occur among humans.

All teeth have an outer enamel layer in the crown, an inner dentin layer, and a core of dental pulp tissue (Figure 2.3), composing the tooth's crown and root(s).

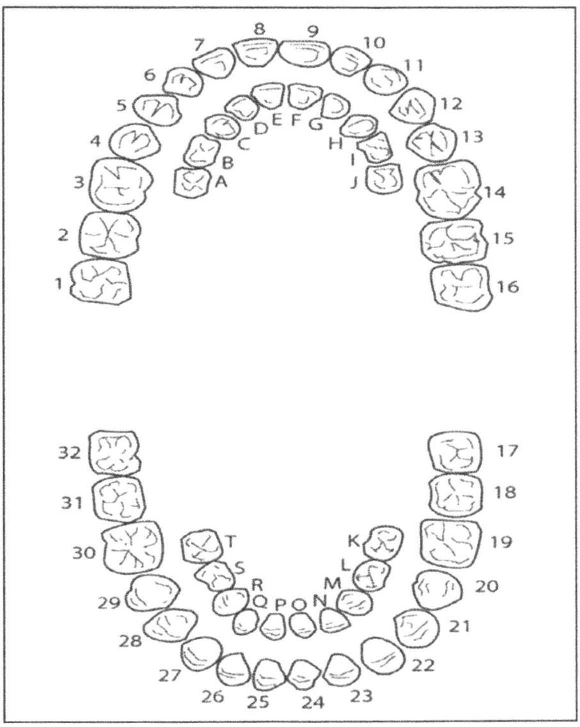

Figure 2.1 Occlusal diagram of primary (inner, lettered) teeth and permanent teeth (outer, numbered) and their designations in the unified numbering system used in the United States.

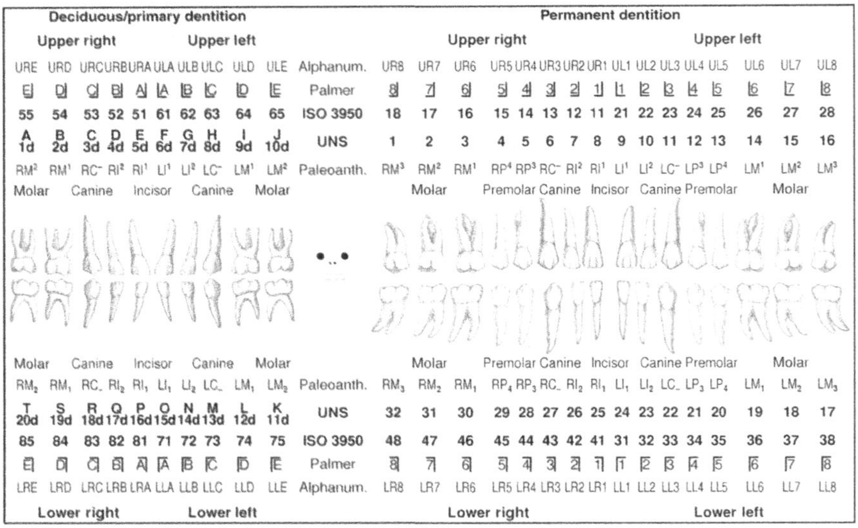

Figure 2.2 Panoramic diagram of primary and permanent teeth in various notation systems: alphanumeric, Palmer, ISO 3950 (FDI), Universal Numbering, and paleoanthropology. *Source:* Henry Vandyke Carter / Wikipedia Commons / https://commons.wikimedia.org/wiki/File:Comparison_of_dental_notations.svg, last accessed on 31 March 2025 / CC BY 4.0." https://en.wikipedia.org/wiki/Dentalnotation#/media/File:Comparisonofdentalnotations.svg / CC BY 4.0.

Table 2.1 Properties of teeth.

Material	Knoop hardness	Fracture toughness (MPa-m$^{1/2}$)	Compressive strength (MPa)	Elastic modulus (GPa)
Dentin (36–38)	68	1.1–2.0	194 ± 31	11–28
Tooth enamel (36–39)	343	0.44–1.55	62 ± 24	52–56, 60–120

These tissues have mechanical properties noted in Table 2.1. Tooth enamel contains about 97% mineral (ceramic) hexagonal hydroxyapatite, $Ca_{10}(PO_4)_6\ (OH)_2$, also written as $Ca_5(PO_4)_3OH$. The crystals are present as prismatic, rod-shaped crystals that overlap like fish scales, about 0.2 μm long by 0.02 μm wide. Dental hydroxyapatite has a partial substitution of carbonate ions (CO_3^{-2}) for the hydroxide ions (OH^-) and small quantities of Na, Cl, F, and Mg substitute in the mineral. The other 3% of the enamel is collagen (fibrous protein connective tissue) and

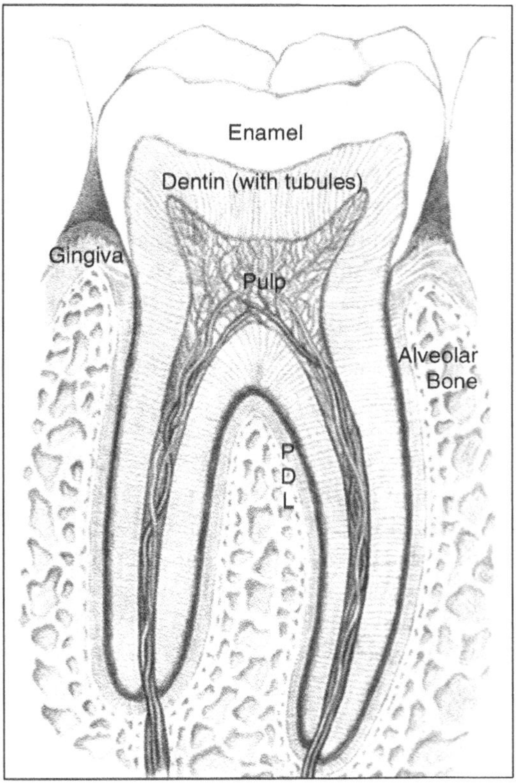

Figure 2.3 Cross section of a molar showing the basic tooth tissues including periodontal ligament (PDL).

water. Enamel is stiff, inelastic, like bones. Dental enamel is more mineralized than bones, which have 60–70% hydroxyapatite. Tooth enamel is the hardest substance in the body, although over 100 causes of enamel defects are known (21).

Dentin underlies the enamel in the crown and composes the walls of the inner cavity around the coronal pulp and the roots. Dentin is less mineralized than enamel, containing about 70% hydroxyapatite and 30% collagen. The mineral portion of dentine is in the form of tubules through which sensory nerves pass, leading from the pulp to the exterior (periodontium) and the alveolar bone. Dentin mineralization increases with age, tending to close the tubules.

Each tooth has a pulpal chamber in the crown that tapers to small foramina in the roots into the bone. This innermost part of the tooth has the pulp, a soft, very sensitive, connective tissue containing blood vessels, nerves, and lymphatic cells. The pulp is the source of tooth pain. Pulp tissue supplies the blood and sensory organs for the health of teeth and limited repair of the dentin.

Teeth are anchored in our jawbones (alveolar bone) via specialized connective tissues of cementum and periodontal ligament. Cementum is a thin, bone-like tissue that coats the roots' surfaces. The collagenous fibers of the periodontal ligament connect the alveolar bone to the cementum to the teeth, creating a "shock-absorbing support system" of fibers (22). The alveolar bone is a living tissue that responds to loading/unloading (biting forces) or muscle strains and gradually "remodels" over time. Gingiva (gum tissue) is connected to the teeth, overlying the bone to protect the tooth's roots and bone from the oral cavity and its vast assortment of microorganisms. This assembly of tissues and anatomy is complex, interactive, and, unfortunately, prone to problems posed by the intake of food and fluids, bacteria, and trauma.

The hard, outer enamel shell of teeth may be broken, dissolved, or eroded. Trauma may cause loss of tooth structure. Tooth enamel is soluble in acids and can be eroded by our dietary acids or the acids secreted by bacteria. With repetitive lifetime stresses, tooth enamel often erodes or develops longitudinal microcracks, as shown in Figure 2.4, a precursor to dental problems such as fractures. Luckily, the underlying dentin, pulp, and the stress-absorbing periodontium support the tooth and make the teeth flaw-tolerant and durable enough for a lifetime of stress.

Unlike bones, enamel is non-living and does not heal (23). When the enamel is breached, it is gone forever because the body cannot regenerate enamel in its original form; a dental treatment is needed to replace the protective enamel with a durable,

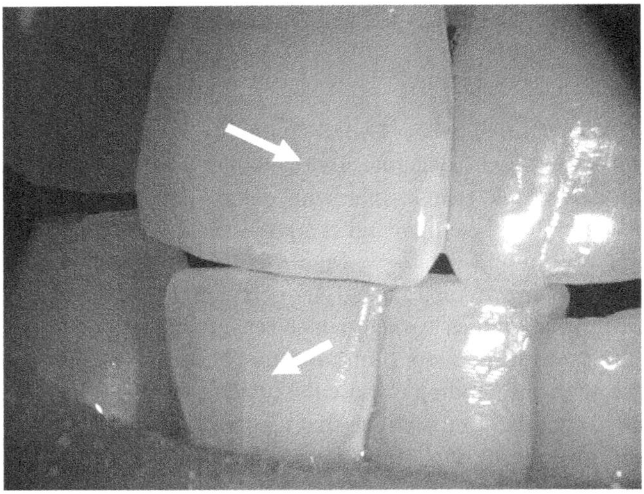

Figure 2.4 Microcracks in teeth. *Source:* National Institute of Standards and Technology/ Public Domain.

adhesive material that mimics the original tooth structure. Many researchers have sought to remineralize enamel and dentin, which has not been achieved except for incipient caries lesions. Nano-sized ceramic particles such as amorphous calcium phosphate nanoparticles, tricalcium silicate cement, porcine amelogenin protein with fluoride, and fluoride ions have been investigated for remineralization with minimal success. To date, the remineralized layers were no thicker than 50 μm (24, 25), much thinner than the usual dental caries attack.

Common Dental Problems

Every day, we expose our oral cavity to acidic foods, bacteria, viruses, and fungi; our oral tissues are prime tissues for communities of microorganisms to inhabit. The oral bacteria species have been estimated to number as many as 700, with any person "accommodating" up to 200 species (26). Bacteria and yeast organisms are ever present, coating our teeth and feeding on food remnants. The species of bacteria change as we mature, and as our dental health changes (27). Some non-oral bacteria may be present; that is, bacteria that commonly reside elsewhere (28) in our bodies, and may be pathogenic. These microbes secrete acids, which can dissolve tooth enamel, as can acidic foods. Salivary secretions are protective because they maintain the oral tissues in a physiologic state (pH ~7) and buffer the acids produced by the bacteria; however, teeth are in a daily battle with these bacterial "homesteaders." The battle can be alleviated with tooth brushing, professional cleaning, and various dental treatments. Fluoride treatments harden the enamel against acids (Chapter 13), and "sealants" (Chapter 9) are a protective coating over pits and fissures on the surface.

Bacteria commonly reproduce on enamel surfaces and asymptomatically start to dissolve the enamel (demineralization). As the bacteria establish larger colonies, their acidic byproducts dissolve/soften the enamel and may establish an irreversible carious lesion. Bacteria may continue to dissolve the enamel and penetrate the dentin. The outer, bacterially infected layer of dentin has an inner layer of reactionary dentin (29), closer to the pulp. See Figure 2.5. The outer layer is highly demineralized, with irreversibly denatured (degraded) collagen fibrils. The inner reactionary dentin layer is partially demineralized, and the collagen remains crosslinked, making it possible to physiologically remineralize the intertubular dentin with some treatments. Removal of the demineralized dentin is standard practice in treating caries. Removal of reactionary dentin is controversial because modern dentistry uses minimally invasive treatments and seeks to remineralize this tissue (30) from within.

If untreated, bacterial infection continues to demineralize the enamel and dentin and reaches the pulp. Pulp infections are also caused by trauma (cracks, breakage, or dislodgement) that may create a bacterial pathway to the pulp. No matter the cause, pulpal inflammation causes pain, and the pulp cells may die. Pulpal healing may

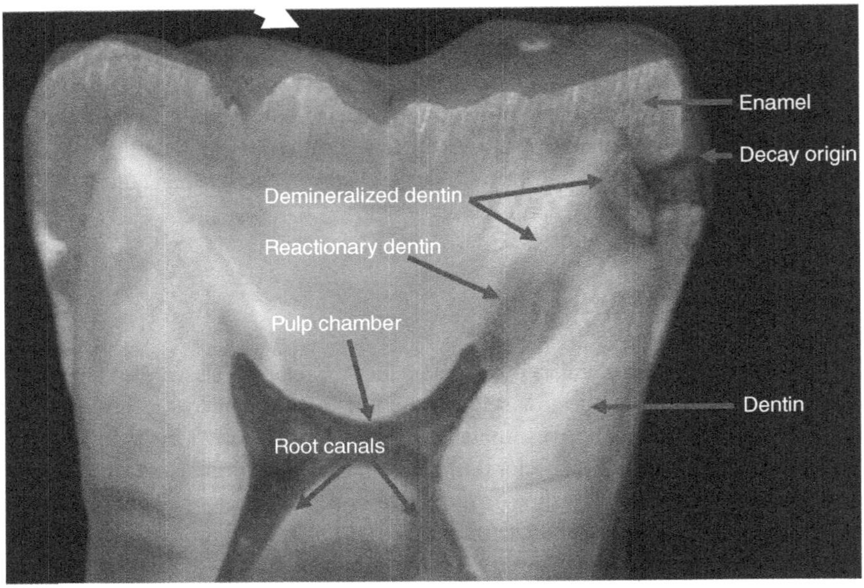

Figure 2.5 Tooth with decay in cross section, showing a common pathway for bacterial progression from enamel inward along the dentinal tubules, dissolving the enamel.

occur by recruiting human dental pulp stem cells (hDPSCs) that hide in perivascular niches; they must differentiate into odontoblast-like cells to form secondary dentin as a barrier to the encroaching infection. Molecular events start the transformation of the stem cells into odontoblasts for reparative dentinogenesis. The odontoblasts can secrete new hard tissue (dentin) as a barrier against further insult and prevent the ingress of disease-causing microbes, which helps the pulp survive. However, if the pulpal damage is severe or untreated, the pulp's response may be insufficient, and disease will progress, killing the pulpal cells – pulp necrosis. Necrosis cannot be reversed; it necessitates the removal of the pulp (pulpectomy) to eliminate pain. Pulpectomy is the first step of root canal treatment (Chapter 8), which is the last dental treatment as a bulwark, to preserve the tooth in the jaw. Without root canal treatment, tooth extraction of teeth with a necrotic pulp is required.

Early childhood caries (ECC), rampant cavities in the primary teeth, is common worldwide; the deciduous teeth are smaller and more vulnerable than the permanent teeth to bacteria. The health of primary teeth should not be overlooked or neglected. Treating caries encourages wellness, reduces pain, and ensures the teeth are in place to support the growth of a child's face. Caries excavation/removal is often performed to treat childhood caries. However, the Hall technique for primary teeth is an alternative; no decay is removed, and the tooth is covered with a stainless steel crown (31). The Hall technique is controversial but cost-effective in school settings and has had success.

Fracture, erosion/wear, tooth sensitivity, and periodontal disease are common problems for adults, even those who have not suffered from caries. Trauma can fracture enamel and dentin, leading to displacement, pulpal infections displacement, or avulsion (forcible removal from the tooth's socket).

Chemical and mechanical erosion/wear occurs over our lifetimes by decades of masticating (chewing) abrasive foods, consuming acidic foods, and inter-tooth contact, which may eventually result in exposure of the underlying dentin, with concomitant tooth sensitivity. Abrasion is also caused by vigorous horizontal tooth brushing with an abrasive dentifrice and a hard toothbrush. Three-body erosion (chemical and mechanical wear) occurs by chewing hard foods (including ice, nuts, and seeds) or non-food foreign objects such as nails, pens, sticks, or pipes. Erosion is the dissolution of the enamel from acid caused by diet, regurgitation, acidic saliva, and idiopathic sources. Dietary sources of erosion include carbonated beverages, fruit juice, and acidic fruit. Regurgitation sources include gastroesophageal reflux disease and eating disorders like anorexia and bulimia. Acidic saliva may be inherent or related to medications. Abfraction is tooth wear from flexural forces, often seen in the upper anterior teeth near the gumline. When teeth touch each other (occlusion), they flex near the gum line on the labial side; V-shaped depressions form when enamel crystals are slowly dislodged under repeated bending; these depressions may expose dentin. Researchers believe enamel, at the cementoenamel junction (CEJ), undergoes this pattern of non-carious destruction with gradual loss of enamel rods (32).

Caries and periodontal disease account for the bulk of dental disease, although a myriad of other problems can affect oral health, from growth defects to cancer. Over a lifetime, a tooth that has had a treatment for caries may need another intervention. The past century has taught us that each dental treatment of a tooth, except prophylaxis, leads to anatomical removal of tooth tissue, enamel, and dentin. Unfortunately, restorations, repairs, or treatments of teeth are subject to failure and need replacement. Each successive treatment on a tooth exacts a cost – removal of soft and hard tissue, – and each restoration can gradually lead to bigger and more expensive treatments, that may culminate in extraction. Tooth extractions leave a person with a disability for the remainder of their life. Implants and dentures may be prescribed to compensate for an extracted tooth, but they are not without problems. Implants may fail to integrate to supply stable bone support (33). Neither dentures nor implants fully replace the masticatory (chewing) strength that teeth have (34). The lifespan (durability) of restorative materials is important. Modern dentistry emphasizes minimally invasive techniques to remove less tooth structure, reducing the likelihood of later problems requiring more treatments, and, hopefully, better long-term outcomes.

Summary of Oral Health

Teeth require care to prevent decay and trauma. Prioritizing preservation means focusing on preventive care, educating patients about oral hygiene habits that protect their natural teeth, and choosing minimally invasive techniques. Ceramics are, and have been, instrumental in dentistry, from prevention of caries to treatment of common maladies, thereby extending each tooth's lifetime. In a classic text (35) on ceramics for dentistry, the author states,

> "It is very probable that the dental profession will be using ... ceramics well into the next century [21st century] for the replacement of lost tooth enamel. Even assuming that the problem of caries is conquered, we must be ever mindful of the effects of natural abrasion on tooth structure, and this problem could likely become of major concern to a longer-living populace demanding the retention of its teeth."

Significant improvements in dental treatments have relied on ceramics. Ceramic materials may appear as biomimetic but truly that has only meant esthetic; only a few bone-graft materials are truly biomimetic. Despite advances in dental techniques and dental products, dental caries remains a worldwide problem along with other oral diseases and dental trauma. Current dental materials are imperfect and may not last a lifetime, although some do. Better, longer-term outcomes are needed with more tooth retention. This text focuses on ceramics used in tooth protection, maintenance, restoration, and replacement and how ceramic materials have contributed.

Ceramics in Chapter 2

The following ceramic materials were mentioned in this chapter:

- hydroxyapatite $Ca_{10}(PO_4)_6(OH)_2$
- carbonated hydroxyapatite, $Ca_5(PO_4,CO_3)3(OH)$
- tricalcium silicate cement

References

1 McLean, J.W. (1989). The quiet revolution in the art and science of dentistry. *RSA J.* 137 (5394): 333–348.

2 Marcenes, W., Kassebaum, N.J., Bernabe, E. et al. (2013). Global burden of oral conditions in 1990–2010: a systematic analysis. *J. Dent. Res.* 92 (7): 592–597.

3 Department of Health and Human Services (2000). *Oral Health in America: A Report of the Surgeon General*. Dept. of HHS, NIDCR, NIH.

4 Hosseinpoor, A.R., Itani, L., and Petersen, P.E. (2012). Socio-economic inequality in oral healthcare coverage: results from the World Health Survey. *J. Dent. Res.* 91 (3): 275–281.

5 Moeller, J., Starkel, R., Quinonez, C., and Vujicic, M. (2017). Income inequality in the United States and its potential effect on oral health. *J. Am. Dent. Assoc.* 148 (6): 361–368.

6 Bashir, N.Z. (2022). Update on the prevalence of untreated caries in the US adult population, 2017–2020. *J Am Dent Assoc.* 153 (4): 300–308.

7 Bahanan, L., Singhal, A., Zhao, Y. et al. (2021). The association between food insecurity, diet quality, and untreated caries among US children. *J. Am. Dent. Assoc.* 152 (8): 613–621.

8 Kassebaum, N.J., Bernabe, E., Dahiya, M. et al. (2015). Global burden of untreated caries: a systematic review and metaregression. *J. Dent. Res.* 94 (5): 650–658.

9 Seeberger, G.K. (2021). Toward vision 2030: building on a 121-year legacy. *J. Am. Dent. Assoc.* 152 (8): 583–585.

10 Varenne, B. (2022). Oral health at the core of the global health agenda. *J. Am. Dent. Assoc.* 153 (5): 393–394.

11 Giannobile, W.V. (2013). Our duty to promote global oral health. *J. Dent. Res.* 92 (7): 573–574.

12 Fellows, J.L., Atchison, K.A., Chaffin, J. et al. (2022). Oral health in America: implications for dental practice. *J. Am. Dent. Assoc.* 153 (7): 601–609. https://doi.org/10.1016/j.adaj.2022.04.002.

13 Liang, L.Y., Tsai, M.C., Shih, K.C. et al. (2022). Tooth life expectancy and burden of tooth loss: two cross-sectional studies in Taiwan. *J Dent Sci.* 17 (3): 1364–1370.

14 Department of Health and Human Services (2021). *Oral health in America: advances and challenges*. Department of Health and Human Services, National Institutes of Health, National Institute of Dental and Craniofacial Research.

15 Cheng, F.-C., Wang, L.-H., Lai, Y.-J., and Chiang, C.-P. (2024). The utility of microbiome (microbiota) and exosomes in dentistry. *D. Dent. Sci* 19 (3): 1313–1319.

16 Abt, E., Kumar, S., and Weyant, R.J. (2022). Periodontal disease and medical maladies: what do we really know? *J. Am. Dent. Assoc.* 153 (1): 9–13.

17 Areal-Quecuty, V., Cantiga-Silva, C., Simon-Soro, A. et al. (2024). Apical periodontitis in osteoporotic postmenopausal women: systematic review and meta-analysis. *Med. Oral Patol. Oral Cir. Bucal.* 29 (5): e711–e718.

18 Aminoshariae, A., Nosrat, A., Jakovljevic, A. et al. (2024). Tooth loss is a risk factor for cardiovascular disease mortality: a systematic review with meta-analyses. *J Endodont* 50 (10): 1370–1380.

19 Liljestrand, J.M., Salminen, A., Lahdentausta, L. et al. (2021). Association between dental factors and mortality. *Int. Endod. J.* 54 (5): 672–681.

20 Chan, A.K.Y., Chu, C.H., Ogawa, H., and Lai, E.H.-H. (2024). Improving oral health of older adults for healthy ageing. *J. Dent. Sci* 19 (1): 1–7.

21 Breuer, M. (1978). *Cosmetic Science*, 355. Academic Press.

22 Liebgott, B. (2011). *The anatomical basis of dentistry*, 3rde, xii, 510. Maryland Heights, MO: Mosby.

23 Newman, M.G., Takei, H.H., and FnA, C. (2012). *Carranza's clinical periodontology*, 11the, xlv, 825. St. Louis, MO: Elsevier/Saunders.

24 Butera, A., Maiorani, C., Gallo, S. et al. (2023). Biomimetic action of zinc hydroxyapatite on remineralization of enamel and dentin: a review. *Biomimetics (Basel)* 8 (1): 1–16.

25 Fan, Y., Sun, Z., and Moradian-Oldak, J. (2009). Controlled remineralization of enamel in the presence of amelogenin and fluoride. *Biomaterials* 30 (4): 478–483.

26 Gutmann, J.L. and Manjarres, V. (2018). Historical and contemporary perspectives on the microbiological aspects of endodontics. *Dent J (Basel)* 6 (4): 1–20.

27 Aas, J.A., Griffen, A.L., Dardis, S.R. et al. (2008). Bacteria of dental caries in primary and permanent teeth in children and young adults. *J. Clin. Microbiol.* 46 (4): 1407–1417.

28 Zaatout, N. (2021). Presence of non-oral bacteria in the oral cavity. *Arch. Microbiol.* 203 (6): 2747–2760.

29 Duncan, H.F. (2022). Present status and future directions-vital pulp treatment and pulp preservation strategies. *Int. Endod. J.* 55 (Suppl 3): 497–511.

30 Lin, L.M. and Rosenberg, P.A. (2011). Repair and regeneration in endodontics. *Int. Endod. J.* 44 (10): 889–906.

31 Tedesco, T.K., Gimenez, T., Floriano, I. et al. (2018). Scientific evidence for the management of dentin caries lesions in pediatric dentistry: a systematic review and network meta-analysis. *PLoS One* 13 (11): e0206296.

32 Nascimento, M.M., Dilbone, D.A., Pereira, P.N. et al. (2016). Abfraction lesions: etiology, diagnosis, and treatment options. *Clin. Cosmet. Investig. Dent.* 8: 79–87.

33 Clark, D. and Levin, L. (2019). In the dental implant era, why do we still bother saving teeth? *Dental Traumatology: Official Publication of International Association for Dental Traumatology* 35 (6): 368–375.

34 Woodmansey, K.F., Ayik, M., Buschang, P.H. et al. (2009). Differences in masticatory function in patients with endodontically treated teeth and single-implant-supported prostheses: a pilot study. *J Endodont* 35 (1): 10–14.

35 McLean, J.W., Hubbard, J.R., and Kedge, M.I. (1979). *The science and art of dental ceramics*, 344. Chicago: Quintessence Pub Co.

36 Iwamoto, N. and Ruse, N.D. (2003). Fracture toughness of human dentin. *J. Biomed. Mater. Res. A* 66 (3): 507–512.

37 Zhang, Y.R., Du, W., Zhou, X.D., and Yu, H.Y. (2014). Review of research on the mechanical properties of the human tooth. *Int J Oral Sci.* 6 (2): 61–69.

38 Chun, K., Choi, H., and Lee, J. (2014). Comparison of mechanical property and role between enamel and dentin in the human teeth. *J. Dent. Biomech.* 5: 1–7.

39 Bechtle, S., Ozcoban, H., Lilleodden, E.T. et al. (2012). Hierarchical flexural strength of enamel: transition from brittle to damage-tolerant behaviour. *J. R. Soc. Interface* 9: 1265–1274.

3

A Synopsis of Dentistry from Antiquity to the Present

Caries and periodontal diseases have always afflicted human teeth, particularly after the adoption of agriculture. Paleopathology has confirmed that periodontal disease and alveolar bone loss afflicted early humans in diverse cultures from ancient Egypt to early pre-Columbian America, and tooth loss was a fact of life.

Pre-Modern Dentistry

Many dental interventions have included ceramics from antiquity. Toothpick-type devices made of wood and bone were used for removing food particles. The earliest known dental "restorative" (a cavity filling) was documented in a third molar at a site in Italy, dating from about 14,000 years ago (1); researchers deduced that flint (microcrystalline silica) tools were used to excavate the tooth, which was filled with beeswax and a carbonate powder; hence, a ceramic instrument and a ceramic powder were part of this original dental intervention! Anthropologists have known that dental mutilation was also performed – definitely not a benefit to oral health – including filing, chipping, drilling, and extraction of teeth. Mayans decorated their anterior teeth with some mineral gemstones (ceramics), having mastered methods to drill and affix (cement) the stones; this was not a tooth treatment of necessity, but it has persisted in cultures even in the 21st century. The periphery (margin) around the ancient inserts was never satisfactory or durable by today's standards.

Egyptians began to develop treatments for toothaches 6000 years ago, but the remedies were not curative. An Egyptian tomb from 2600 BCE identified the occupant as a person who treated teeth, exemplifying the awareness of dentistry. The Sumerians (4100–1750 BCE) recorded their primitive understanding of dentistry in clay texts. Hippocrates and Aristotle studied tooth

Ceramics in Dentistry: Materials, Manufacturing, and Clinical Applications,
First Edition. Carolyn M. Primus.

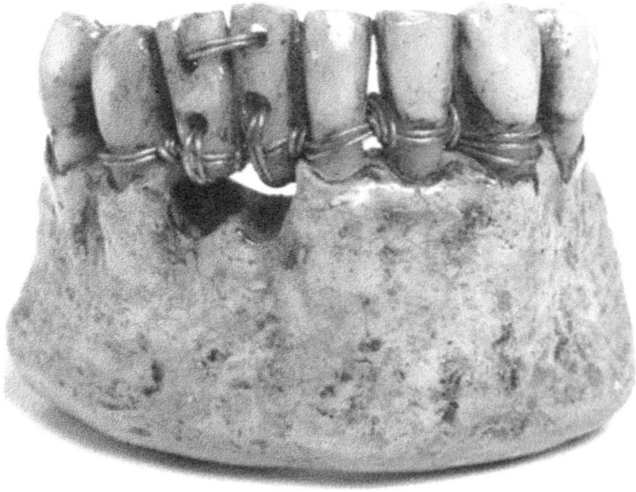

Figure 3.1 A mandible with dental prosthetics made by Etruscans. *Source:* (2) / Springer Nature.

eruption and began to explore methods to stabilize teeth and fractured jaws with wires. In the Common Era, Etruscans began placing "permanent tooth replacements" (fixed prosthodontics) using gold wires and animal (or human) teeth, as shown in Figure 3.1. Sinew and thread secured the replacement teeth to the remaining teeth as a fixed bridge. These methods did not improve much until the 17th century.

Arsenic made its appearance in dentistry before 200 CE. Traditional Chinese medicine texts recorded the use of arsenic sulfide (AsS, also known as As_2S_2 or As_4S_4) to treat toothaches in children. This toxic ceramic compound could kill the pulp cells, but it reduced the pain. Various arsenic-containing recipes continued to be used into the 19th century, including in Western countries, despite the toxicity of AsS and its potential for other oral consequences (3). Chinese texts also mention the use of silver pastes, a predecessor of amalgam, to replace tooth anatomy.

By 1200, dental surgeons and lay barbers in Europe formed guilds, and by the 1500s, the first books devoted to dentistry were written in German and French. Modern dentistry is considered to have begun in the 17th century with writings by Pierre Fauchard on dental anatomy, function, techniques, and dentures (2). Fauchard is credited as the "father of modern dentistry" for his scientific text for dentistry, *Le Chirurgien Dentiste*, published in 1728. However, his text was preceded by others' books regarding dentistry (4) in the 16th century – Zene

Artzney, Bartolomeo Eustachio, Charles Allen, and Madame de Lastrade. Cast metal, gold foil, gold crowns, and amalgam were used at this time, but these materials were not tooth-colored. Posts or anchors in teeth and ceramic coatings on gold (enamel) were being used to replace tooth anatomy.

Artificial teeth began to be developed during the late 1700s. Porcelain dentures were patented in 1789 by Nicolas Dubois de Chemant (5), who used Sevres and Wedgwood porcelains being used for dishes/dinnerware. De Chemant's dentures were entirely porcelain, but they fit poorly over the gums. Individual porcelain teeth with an embedded wire were invented by Guiseppangelo Fonzi in 1807, which could be attached to a denture base that had a better fit over the gums. Polemics erupted over the use of porcelain for dentures rather than "natural" teeth; even the contemporary physicians were initially opposed to the more sanitary and esthetic use of porcelain. Cooler heads eventually prevailed, and famous dental companies made porcelain artificial teeth (Chapter 15), including the England-based Ash company and the US-based SS White company. Claudius Ash improved the porcelain composition over Fonzi's and developed the tube tooth denture design in 1837. The Ash (now part of Dentsply Sirona), SS White, and Justi companies were founded to make porcelain artificial teeth; these companies remain among the manufacturers of dental products.

The first dentifrices were powders mixed with water, starting an enormous leap forward in dental hygiene in the 1700s. The invention of collapsible metal tubes allowed the preparation of paste forms of dentifrice in the 1880s, which were mostly supplanted by plastic tubes for toothpaste. Schools for dental hygienists were formed, and nylon tufted toothbrushes were invented, replacing animal hair in brushes. Dental treatment included prevention.

The 1800s saw significant advances in dental education; schools for dentistry and other dental organizations were founded by the mid-19th century; state licensure became required and dental assistants were accepted in dental practices. Other advances beginning in the 1800s were the introduction of amalgam, a metal alloy composed of silver and mercury; amalgam was remarkably effective and durable, but its dark color was never popular. A durable, tooth-colored material was always a desire of patients. By 1890, microbes were recognized to cause decay rather than "tooth worms" or stomach acid. Around this time, calcium sulfate was used to make dental impressions so that models of the teeth could be created for better-fitting restorative devices. Zinc oxide-based restoratives and cements began to be incorporated into dental practices (see Chapter 11). The fine (small particles) zinc oxide (ceramic) powder was mixed with eugenol, polyacrylic acid, or phosphoric acid; these three cements would self-set into a hard mass in a tooth. Zinc oxide-eugenol remains in use today for a pulp medicament and a temporary cement.

20th Century Dentistry

The 20th century brought other enormous changes in dentistry. Dental laboratories began to provide custom, removable prosthodontics (crowns, bridges, and dentures) for dentists, working in an area separate from the dental operatory. The invention of the "lost wax" metal casting machine enabled dental laboratories to relieve dentists from making metal restorations, such as crowns and partial dentures. Anesthetics, air turbine equipment, and electric handpieces contributed to the growing acceptance of dental treatment. Dental radiographs (X-ray images) and new theories of occlusion (the contact between upper and lower teeth) guided approaches to dental treatment. Acrylic cements and phosphoric acid etching made it possible for metal frameworks to remain affixed on teeth, a significant advancement. Such cements outperformed earlier waxes and water-soluble glues for achieving lasting dental treatments. Fluoride toothpaste became common as a nationwide effort to combat decay along with water fluoridation (NaF) implemented in several cities (Chapter 13) in the 20th century.

Specialties emerged in the 20th century, including orthodontics, pediatrics, and endodontics. The National Institute of Dental and Craniofacial Research (NIDCR, formerly NIDR) was created in 1948, showing the governmental support for oral health research; the impetus was that many prospective soldiers had been disqualified from service in World War II because of their poor oral health (6).

The "Restorative Era" began with the use of ceramic powders. Restoratives, colloquially known as fillings, replace the dentin and enamel of the tooth's crown with substitute materials. The goals were threefold: create ceramic restorations that had the appearance and esthetics of natural teeth; be able to survive in the alternating hot and cold, acidic, and enzymatic oral environment; and withstand the mechanical forces of chewing (mastication) and grinding (7). All restorative materials are customized for a patient's unique dental anatomy. In modern dentistry, the restoratives are divided into direct and indirect. Direct restoratives (Chapter 9) are placed and shaped into the anatomical form by the dentist. The direct restoratives are classified by their location, as shown in Figure 3.2. Silicate restoratives of the 20th century led the way for esthetic "fillings." Manufacturers melted special glass formulas containing fluoride which were ground into powder. The powders were mixed with an acid by the dentist and the mixture hardened (silicate restoratives) in the tooth. The silicate cements were esthetic but not so durable over a lifetime. By mid-century, more durable glass ionomer materials were introduced and are in use today as a restorative and for bonding materials to a tooth.

Most significantly, the "Bowen Restorative Era" began when Dr. Ray Bowen invented bisphenol A-glycidyl methacrylate resin as a direct restorative material in the labs of the American Dental Association. The Bowen-type restoratives were successful because of the inclusion of quartz and glass powders as fillers in a methacrylate-based polymer matrix; the glass particles make these "resin-based

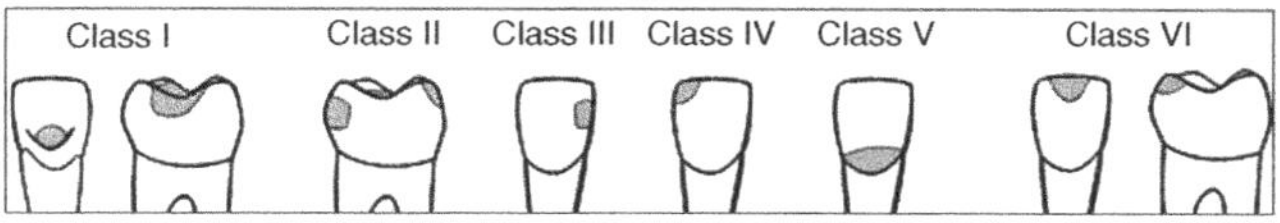

Figure 3.2 Diagrams of five common cavity preparations (locations and shapes) for direct restorations shown in gray.

composites " durable and form the basis for the myriad of today's polymeric direct restorative materials in dentistry. Concomitant with the development of resin composites, phosphoric acid came into dental use. This inorganic acid solution, usually at 37% concentration or less, etches dental enamel by dissolving a little bit of the hydroxyapatite, generating a rough surface to enhance the adhesion of polymeric materials. Etching was the first advance in bonding polymers to teeth, followed by the development of other materials known as "adhesives" and "primers" (Chapter 11). Bowen composites have been developed into resin-based cements, which have largely replaced the zinc oxide-based cements. Resin cements are necessary to support all-ceramic crowns and bridges.

Indirect restorative procedures require dentists to remove carious tissue and shape the problematic tooth with instruments (Chapter 17), followed by forming an impression of the prepared or reshaped tooth. A positive model is made from an intaglio impression, either physically or digitally (Chapter 14). Indirect restorations (Chapter 10) are crafted in a dental laboratory to fit the model; the dentist cements (attaches) the completed indirect restoration onto the tooth. Such restoratives include crowns, bridges, veneers, inlays, and onlays. See Figure 3.3 for examples. Ancillary ceramic powders are necessary for impression materials, model materials, and dental cements (Chapters 14 and 11, respectively).

The ceramic indirect restoration era began with Land's (8) porcelain jacket crowns in the early 1900s, which were stronger than earlier porcelains and more esthetic than metal crowns. Ceramic crowns and bridges of various designs and materials proliferated in the 20th century for their esthetics. Porcelain enamel coatings on dental alloys for crowns and bridges became very successful after the 1950s; special dental alloys were used for enameling, based on noble elements, nickel, or cobalt-chrome; the latter non-precious alloys were used for lower cost. Alumina-reinforced porcelain crowns were promoted in the 1960s (Chapter 10), and high alumina crowns were briefly popular in the late 20th century. Alumina and porcelain-fused-to-metal crowns have given way in the 21st-century marketplace to lithium disilicate and zirconia restorations for crowns and bridges.

The 1980s saw the introduction of the Brånemark invention of implanting a post-like material within the alveolar bone to support a crown, bridge or denture. The successful, complete replacement of a tooth, with the implant as an anchor is considered an enormous advancement in dentistry. Titanium was the original

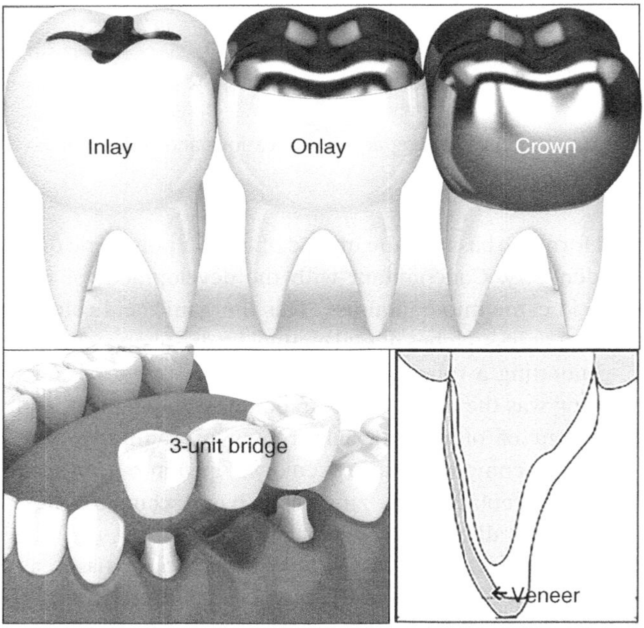

Figure 3.3 Examples of indirect restorations, which are in gray except for the bridge, which is shown in white. The veneer is shown in cross-section on an anterior tooth. *Source (top and bottom left Images):* Aleksandra Gigowska / Adobe Stock Photos.

implant material, but tetragonal zirconia (Chapter 16) is used for some endosseous implants as well as the crowns placed atop the implant. Bioactive ceramic cements, akin to Portland cement, were introduced in the 1990s for endodontic therapy; these cements had a profound impact on endodontic treatments (root-canal procedures) (Chapter 8) and vital pulp therapy for adults and children.

Dentistry has been, and is, replete with inventors who have made the patient more comfortable and the treatments more durable and successful. Some inventions may seem prosaic (dental chairs, lights, curing lights, toothbrushes, floss, lost-wax casting machines, and hand or rotary instruments). Other inventions are key to efficient and effective treatment including anesthetics, X-ray imaging, high and low-speed air-driven or electric handpieces, implants, and bioactive ceramics.

Every modern dental office relies on "dental informatics" – the use of electronics and information science. We have dental informatics because of electronics, which depend on ceramic electronic components (Chapter 18). From this abbreviated recitation, we can begin to appreciate the ingenuity that guided us into 21st-century materials and current dental ceramics.

Summary of Ceramics' Dental Contributions over Time

The versatility of ceramics inevitably led to their use in dentistry, displacing the use of bone and teeth from animals – including human cadavers. Dental ceramics have included glass, porcelain, abrasives, and crystalline materials, including single-crystal ceramics. Today, traditional and modern ceramics are at the forefront of today's dentistry for restoratives, crown/bridge materials, cements, orthodontic brackets, hygiene, bleaches, bioactive materials, abrasives, implants, and bone grafts. Glass formulas have been included in over 3000 patents for dentistry.

Dental procedures have been performed over the millennia but were not as easy or effective as today. Dentistry is now a medical science with a mission to treat oral disease and replace human teeth with alternative materials. The American Dental Association, the International Association for Dental, Oral, and Craniofacial Research, and innumerable dental journals support dentistry; they transformed a trade into a medical science (6).

No modern dental office or dental manufacturer would succeed today without the ceramics present in electronics that make current equipment possible: digital and X-ray imaging, lasers, computerized design and manufacture, batteries, and all the electronic devices enabling efficient offices.

For the student of dental history, the reader is referred to the *Journal of the History of Dentistry*, published by the American Academy of the History of Dentistry (AAHD) at www.apollonia.histden.org, or the Dental Historian from the Lindsay Society at https://lindsaysociety.co.uk/dental-historian-archive/. The AAHD references St. Apollonia as the patroness of dentistry and for those suffering from dental problems. She was a Greek martyr whose teeth were violently extracted or broken by a mob when she did not recant her Christian faith. The Lindsay Society is named after Lilian Lindsay (1871–1960), who was the first woman to qualify as a dentist in the United Kingdom, the president of the British Dental Association, and a leading dental historian.

Ceramics in Chapter 3

The following dental ceramics and inorganic substances were mentioned in this chapter:

- Arsenic sulfide
- Calcium silicate cement (Portland cement)
- Calcium sulfate
- Feldspar
- Glass formulas with fluoride
- Hydroxyapatite

- Kaolin clay
- Lithium disilicate glass–ceramic
- Phosphoric acid
- Porcelain with alumina
- Porcelain denture teeth
- Porcelain enamel
- Silica
  - Amorphous, sand or glass
  - Quartz
- Sodium fluoride
- Zinc oxide
- Zirconia, tetragonal

References

1 Oxilia, G., Peresani, M., Romandini, M. et al. (2015). Earliest evidence of dental caries manipulation in the Late Upper Palaeolithic. *Sci. Rep.* 5: 1–10.

2 Bergmann, C.P. and Stumpf, A. (2013). *Dental ceramics microstructure, properties and degradation*. Springer-Verlag.

3 Cheng, F.-C., Wang, Y.-L., Chang, W.-C., and Chiang, C.-P. (2023). The evolution of arsenic-containing traditional Chinese medicine prescriptions for treatment of toothache due to tooth decay. *J. Dent. Sci.* 19: 1251–1254.

4 Ayroso, J. and Spielman, A.I. (2025). Mademoiselle De Rezé – The first female author on dental remedies – Dissertation Apologétique des Remèdes – 1719. *J. Hist. Dent.* 73 (1): 5–23.

5 Murray, M.D. and Darvell, B.W. (1993). The evolution of the complete denture base. Theories of complete denture retention. A review. Part 1. *Aust. Dent. J.* 38 (3): 216–219.

6 Gutmann, J.L. (2009). The evolution of America's scientific advancements in dentistry in the past 150 years. *J. Am. Dent. Assoc.* 140: 8S–15S.

7 Kohyama, K., Hatakeyama, E., Sasaki, T. et al. (2004). Effects of sample hardness on human chewing force: a model study using silicone rubber. *Arch. Oral Biol.* 49 (10): 805–816.

8 Land, C.H. (1903). Porcelain dental art. *Dent. Cosm.* 45 (6): 437–444. and 615–620.

4

Ceramics in Dental Medical Devices

Medical devices include instruments, machines, implants, and in vitro reagents that are intended for use in the diagnosis, prevention, and treatment of diseases or other medical conditions. The Food and Drug Administration (FDA) government regulations (21CFR, Chapter I, Subchapter H [parts 800–898]) and the ISO 13485 standard "Medical devices – Quality management systems, Requirements for regulatory purposes" have agreed on the definition of medical devices as follows:

- "an instrument, apparatus, implement, machine, contrivance, implant, in vitro reagent, or other similar or related article, including a component part or accessory which is recognized in the official National Formulary, or the United States Pharmacopoeia, or any supplement to them,
- intended for use in the diagnosis of disease or other conditions, or in the cure, mitigation, treatment, or prevention of disease, in man or other animals, or
- intended to affect the structure or any function of the body of man or other animals, and which does not achieve its primary intended purposes through chemical action within or on the body of man or other animals and which is not dependent upon being metabolized for the achievement of any of its primary intended purposes."

In brief, a medical device is an item, not a drug, and is used in the body or for the body. Dental materials, including dental ceramics, are a subset of medical devices. All medical devices should be designed and manufactured following a company's quality system that conforms to ISO 13485. In the United States, the Code of Federal Regulations Part 820[i] outlines the requirements mandated by the Safe Medical Devices Act of 1990. Adherence to the regulations is overseen by the US FDA's Center for Devices and Radiological Health (CDRH). Some medical

i https://www.ecfr.gov/current/title-21/chapter-I/subchapter-H/part-820

Ceramics in Dentistry: Materials, Manufacturing, and Clinical Applications,
First Edition. Carolyn M. Primus.

devices require special clearance or approval from the FDA for use in the United States, that issues many guidance documents to help manufacturers of medical devices comply with these regulations. The FDA web page titled "Medical Device Overview" has guidance for medical devices.[ii] Texts, particularly by ex-FDA experts (1–3), can assist companies in understanding and complying with the regulations, as can consultants.

Medical devices are categorized by the US FDA as Class I, II, or III. In general, Class I devices are low risk and require a company to have an approved quality system but do not require disclosure of the devices to the FDA. Class II devices involve more risk; therefore, safety and efficacy are greater considerations. Class II devices usually require FDA 510(k) clearance. Class III devices undergo a higher level of scrutiny than FDA clearance and need FDA premarket approval (PMA). Many dental devices are Class I; restorative devices are usually Class II, but exceptions exist. The following Class III dental devices are listed in the Code of Federal Regulations for the FDA:

- Karaya and sodium borate with or without acacia denture adhesive containing 12% or more by weight of sodium borate
- Carboxymethylcellulose sodium and cationic polyacrylamide polymer denture adhesive
- Polyacrylamide polymer (modified cationic) denture adhesive
- Polyvinylmethylether maleic anhydride (PVM-MA), acid copolymer denture adhesive, and carboxymethylcellulose sodium (NACMC) denture adhesive
- Root canal filling resin containing chloroform
- Bone grafting materials that contain a drug that is a therapeutic biologic
- Total temporomandibular joint prosthesis – a device intended to be implanted in the human jaw to replace the mandibular condyle and augment the glenoid fossa
- Glenoid fossa prosthesis
- Mandibular condyle prosthesis
- Interarticular disc prosthesis (interpositional implant).

Four of these Class III devices are denture adhesives, which can have a broad, prolonged oral exposure where leaching by saliva may occur. Of these Class III devices, ceramics may be involved as powders, like sodium borate, or structural ceramics for joint implants.

Other governments have also established medical device regulations. The classes of devices are slightly different from the United States in Canada, the

---

ii https://www.fda.gov/industry/regulated-products/medical-device-overview#What%20is%20a%20medical%20device

European Union, and elsewhere. The classifications of risks and requirements for medical device distribution in other countries are mentioned in Table 4.1. Depending on the device's use, that is, its indication, the devices may be subject to certain national or international requirements, as described below. Other countries have equally comprehensive regulations; many are based on the US FDA system although they vary in specifics for compliance. See the partial list of prominent regulatory bodies below.

- The Canadian Medical Devices Regulations (SOR/98-282) are essential to comply with Canada's Food and Drugs Act.[iii]
- Europe has the Medical Device Regulations.[iv]
- The United Kingdom has the Medicines and Healthcare products Regulatory Agency.[v]
- Ministry of Health, Labouré and Welfare of Japan controls medical devices distribution and their regulations.[vi]
- China has the "National Medical Products Administration" for medical devices[vii]; the Chinese FDA.
- India uses the Medical Device Rules 2017 issued by the government and its guidance document is available.[viii]
- Korea's ministry of food and drug safety oversees medical devices.[ix]
- Taiwan has "[Taiwan] FDA's medical device regulations".[x]

Achieving compliance with larger economy countries paves the registration process for companies to sell their products in smaller or less regulated countries although registration papers are always needed. Often, local dental dealers know consultants to help companies gain the necessary approvals for sale in foreign countries. Companies manufacturing medical devices should be compliant with ISO 13485 because most countries require that a device manufacturer be certified by an independent agency that they comply with ISO 13485. Another essential component of medical device manufacture and distribution is risk assessment. This certification

---

iii https://www.canada.ca/en/health-canada/services/drugs-health-products/medical-devices.html

iv https://ec.europa.eu/health/medical-devices-sector/new-regulationsen

v https://www.gov.uk/guidance/regulating-medical-devices-in-the-uk

vi https://www.mhlw.go.jp/english/policy/health-medical/pharmaceuticals/qms.html and https://www.mhlw.go.jp/file/04-Houdouhappyou-11123000-Iyakushokuhinkyoku-Shinsakanrika/regulation_medicaldevices.pdf

vii http://english.nmpa.gov.cn/medicaldevices.html

viii https://www.ipc.gov.in/images/mvpi/GuidanceDocument.pdf

ix https://www.mfds.go.kr/eng/wpge/m39/denofile.do

x https://www.fda.gov.tw/eng/Site.aspx?sid=10168

Table 4.1 Medical device regulation examples.

Country	Classification, risk	Regulatory pathway
United States	I, low	Self-declaration
	II, intermediate	De Novo or 510(k)b
	III, high	Premarket approval (PMA)
Canada	I, low	Health Canada MDEL
	II, medium	
	III, medium to high	Health Canada MDL
	IV, high	
European economic area EFTA (United Kingdom and Turkey)	I, low	Self-declaration
	IIa, medium	
	IIb, medium to high	Notified body approval
	III, high	
Japan	I, general, very low	Self-declaration
	II, controlled, low	Certified body approval
	III, specially controlled, medium	PMDA approval
	IV, specially controlled, high	PMDA approval
Korea	I, very low	Notification
	II, low	Certification, approval
	III, moderate	Approval
	IV, high	
Australia	I, low	Self-declaration
	IIa, medium	
	IIb, medium to high	TGA approval
	III, high	
Brazil	I, low	Notified body approval
	II, medium	
	III, high	Full ANVISA registration
	IV, maximum	
China	I, low	Self-filing
	II, intermediate	China NMPA approval
	III, high	
India	A, low	
	B, low to moderate	CDSCO approval
	C, moderate to high	
	D, high	

is costly and ongoing, with annual audits and inspections to ensure a manufacturer maintains conformance to the quality in the design, production, installation, and servicing of medical devices and related services. Some countries are collaborating on a Medical Device Single Audit Program (MDSAP) for medical device manufacturers to simultaneously satisfy requirements of the many countries[xi].

Standards for Ceramics in Dentistry

Certain national and international standards are pertinent to ceramics used in dentistry. Uniform requirements help dental manufacturers offer better products or services that benefit clinicians and patients. The American Dental Association (ADA) manages dental standards activities in the United States, on behalf of the American National Standards Institute (ANSI), founded in 1918. The ADA uses expert contributions from 600 volunteers in 65 working groups, which include representatives from the dental profession, industry, academia, and government. Table 4.2 has a list of ADA standards where ceramics are directly or indirectly

Table 4.2 ADA & ISO dental products standards, technical specifications, and technical reports.

ADA standard # – title	Corresponding ISO standard #
15 – Dentistry – artificial teeth for dental prostheses	22112
19 – Elastomeric impression materials	4823
25 – Dentistry – gypsum products	6873
27 – Polymer-based restorative materials	4049
30 – Dental zinc oxide – eugenol and zinc oxide – non-eugenol cements	3107
32 – Orthodontic wires	15,841
33 – Dentistry – vocabulary	1942
37 – Dental abrasive powders	20608
38 – Dentistry – compatibility testing for metal-ceramic and ceramic–ceramic systems	9693
39 – Pit and fissure sealants	6874

(*Continued*)

xi https://www.fda.gov/medical-devices/cdrh-international-affairs/medical-device-single-audit-program-mdsap

Table 4.2 (Continued)

ADA standard # – title	Corresponding ISO standard #
41 – Evaluation of biocompatibility of medical devices used in dentistry	7405
48 – Curing lights (powered polymerization activators)	10650
53 – Polymer-based crown and bridge materials	4049
57 – Dentistry – endodontic sealing materials	6876
62 – Dental abrasive pastes	—
69 – Dental ceramic	6872
75 – Resilient lining materials for removable dentures – part 1: short-term materials	10139-1
78 – Dental obturating cone	6877
80 – Dental materials – determination of color stability	7491
89 – Dental operating lights	9680
96 – Dental water-based cements	9917-1 & 2
100 – Dentistry – orthodontic brackets and tubes	27020
111 – Adhesion test methods to tooth structure	11405
116 – Oral rinses	16408
117 – Dentistry – fluoride varnishes	17730
119 – Dentistry – manual toothbrushes	20126
122 – Dental casting and baseplate waxes	15854
126 – Casting investments and refractory die materials	15912
127 – Dynamic loading test for endosseous dental implants	14801
128 – Hydrocolloid impression materials	21563
130 – Dentifrices-requirements, test methods and marking	11609
131 – Dental CAD/CAM machinable zirconia blanks	18675
135 – Denture adhesives	10873
136 – Products for external tooth bleaching	28399
139 – Dental base polymers	20795-1
141 – Dental duplicating material	14356
145 – Interoperability of CAD/CAM systems in dentistry	—
151 – Screening method for erosion potential of oral rinses on dental hard tissues	28888
157 – Powered dental scaler handpieces and tips	18394

Table 4.2 (Continued)

ADA standard # – title	Corresponding ISO standard #
160 – Soft lining materials for removable dentures – materials for long-term use	10139-2
161 – Guidance on color measurement in dentistry	TR 28642
163 – Dental furnace test method for temperature measurement with separate thermocouple	13078
164 – Dental furnace, part 2: test method for evaluation of furnace program via firing glaze	13078-2
171 – Analysis of fluoride concentration in aqueous solutions by use of fluoride ion-selective electrode	19448
172 – Minimal dental implant data set for clinical use	16498
173 – Designation system for dental implants	19429
178 – Orthodontic anchor screws	19023
179 – Shanks for rotary and oscillating instruments	1979
190 – Single-use dental cartridges for local anesthetics	11499
191 – Intra-oral mirrors	9873
206 – Implantable materials for bone filling and augmentation in oral and maxillofacial surgery – contents of a technical file	22794
209 – Dentistry – Test Method for the Evaluation of High Temperature Sintering Furnace Measurement with a Separate Thermocouple	13078
ADA technical report No. 133 – guide to dental lasers and related light-based technologies: technology, science, and safety considerations	—
ADA technical report No. 146 – CAD/CAM abutments in dentistry	—
ADA technical specification No. 150 – method for determination of polymerization shrinkage stress of polymer-based restorative materials	—
ISO – Guidance on testing of wear – part 1: wear by toothbrushing	TR14569-1
ISO – Guidance on testing of wear – part 2: wear by two- and/or three-body contact	TS 14569-2
ISO – Polymer-based luting materials containing adhesive components	TS 16506
Chairside denture base relining materials – part 1: hard type materials	23401-1
Adhesion – Notched-edge shear bond strength test	29022

involved; pertinent technical reports (TR) or specifications (TS) are also listed. Drugs and radiographic film are not included in the ADA's standards purview. The ADA standards are recognized by the Food and Drug Administration for registering new medical devices.

The International Organization for Standardization (ISO), headquartered in Geneva, Switzerland, is the world's largest developer of voluntary international standards, operating independently as a non-governmental organization. Founded in 1947, ISO develops and publishes worldwide technical, industrial, and commercial standards (4) to facilitate international continuity and ensure the safety and reliability of many items for far-flung fields – medical devices, clothing, electronics, metrology, road vehicles, railway and shipbuilding, aerospace, agriculture, rubber, paper, and health care. Safety and efficacy are the goals for dental standards, for the benefit of clinicians and the public (5). Nine ISO subcommittees exist for the codification of the dental standards (Table 4.3). As with the ADA standards committees, the documents are written by expert volunteers who represent national standards organizations from 165 countries. The ISO and the ADA standards committees embrace the principles of openness, balance, lack of dominance, and due process to achieve consensus on test methods and requirements in standards. The ADA's set of standards are often identical adoptions of the ISO standards having the same name.

The ISO's dental materials standards are cross-referenced to the ADA standards in Table 4.2. Quinquennial reviews of standards are required, which helps the methods and criteria to stay current. These national and international standards codify the common terminology, dimensions, labeling, packaging requirements, and test methods for products/devices, and are referenced in later chapters. Some technical reports (TR) or specifications (TS) are also issued by the ISO and the

Table 4.3 International standards organization's subcommittees on dentistry.

Subcommittee (SC)	Committee name
1	Filling and restorative materials
2	Prosthodontic materials
3	Terminology
4	Dental instruments
6	Dental equipment
7	Oral care products
8	Dental implants
9	Dental CAD/CAM systems

ADA. Table 4.2 does not include the ceramics used in dental equipment e.g., lasers, optical glass, and electronic ceramics.

Test methods in the ISO and ADA standards are frequently drawn from other standards issued by ANSI or the American Society for Testing and Materials International (ASTM) for other fields. Other specialized test methods have been developed by the ADA or ISO dental committees, which are validated through inter-laboratory testing by committee members or scientists (6–9). The test methods are particularly useful for manufacturers to perform to be sure that the unified consensus criteria are met (10) as they develop new products. The test methods are meant to be relatively easy for dental researchers or manufacturers to perform. The ISO and ADA standards committees design tests without the most expensive, exclusive, or specialized equipment. For instance, micro-CT is not used for the ISO or ADA tests of dental materials at this time. The ISO or ADA test methods are also frequently used by researchers and dental students whose results are published in scholarly journals (11). Sometimes the methods are not precisely followed by testers, which causes conflicting literature results; however, the publications can be helpful for clinical information and choices. Compliance with specific ADA or ISO standards may be required for regulatory clearance or approval in the United States and internationally. Also, when the test data is disclosed by the manufacturer, informed choices can be made by dental practitioners.

Risk assessments for devices are also imperative for manufacturers to perform for regulatory compliance. The severity and the probability of harm must be estimated/assessed using the guidelines provided in ISO 14971: Application of risk management to medical devices. Risk assessments are written by manufacturers, iteratively reviewed, and maintained over the lifetime of a product to ensure the risk from its use is as low as reasonably possible. From the conception to the end of a product's lifetime (end of sales), manufacturers must re-assess the risks of using their products, incorporating post-market surveillance, published literature, and customer feedback, both direct and indirect.

Biomaterial Basics

Biomaterials include substances that restore function and facilitate the healing for people or animals after injury or disease; examples are bandages, temporary devices, or biosensors. All dental restorative, prosthodontic and temporary materials are biomaterials, which are a subset of all metallic, organic, and ceramic substances, as depicted in Figure 4.1. For this text, bandages and sensors are excluded. Only ceramic-containing biomaterials that support, enhance, or replace damaged tissue or have a biological function are included.

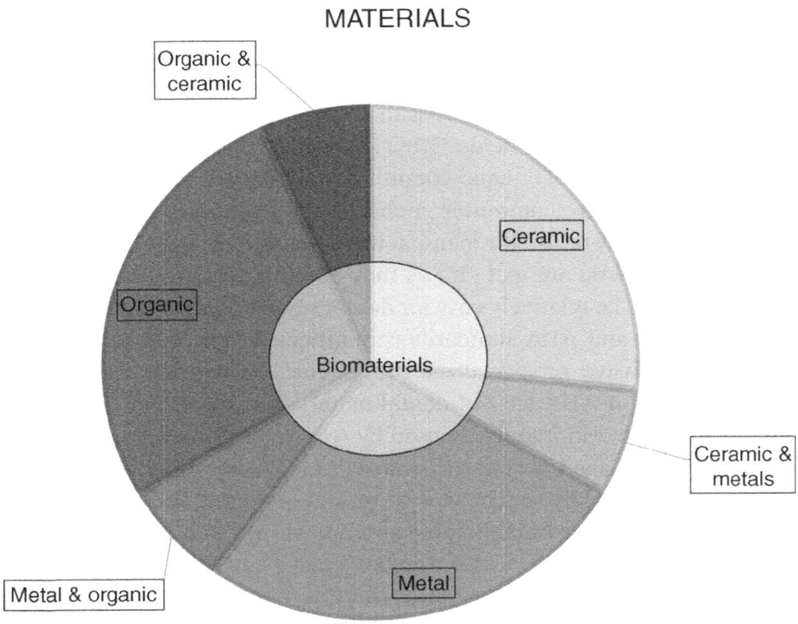

Figure 4.1 Materials classification showing the subset of biomaterials.

Bioceramics are classified as bioinert, bioactive, or bioresorbable (12) as shown in Figure 4.2. Bioinert materials do not elicit a response from the host – they do no harm – a common characteristic among bioceramics that have virtually no solubility in body fluids, water, or lipids. Bioactive ceramics are defined for this text as those that can elicit the formation of a calcium apatite layer, similar to hydroxyapatite, on their surface when tested in vivo, or in synthetic body fluid (SBF), per the ISO 23317 standard "Implants for surgery in vitro evaluation for apatite-forming ability of implant materials." Bioresorbable ceramics are biodegradable, that is, the ceramic is naturally absorbed by the body over time. Such bioceramics may also be bioactive, especially bone grafts. Any of these categories of ceramics may be radiopaque; ordinarily, the bioinert powders are used for this purpose.

Dental bioceramics have been adapted from other industries. Many bioceramic powders are used as fillers for polymers in dentistry. None of the restorative materials duplicate enamel or dentine; they imitate. Zinc oxide has been an important bioceramic for early cements and restoratives. Books (13, 14) and a myriad of articles have described biomimetic materials, including glass, alumina, and zirconia. Other bioceramics facilitate healing such as bioactive glasses and calcium compounds: sulfate, silicate, aluminate, or phosphates. This text includes other unsung bioceramics and inorganic materials that are little-known but have made important contributions to dental practice.

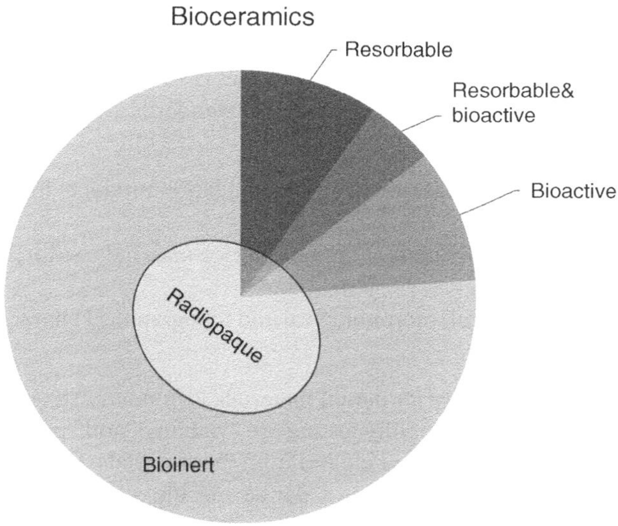

Figure 4.2 Bioceramics classification, primarily inert bioactive and resorbable; some are bioactive and resorbable.

Special Characteristics of Ceramics for Dentistry

Bioceramics for dentistry require special characteristics that may not be needed in other fields. Biocompatibility is always essential while antimicrobial and sterility characterizations can also be useful. Depending on the indication for use, other qualities may be required: radiopacity, color, transparency, fluorescence, and opalescence.

Biocompatibility

Biomedical materials used in dentistry have some common requirements that begin with *primum non nocere (first, do no harm),* a fundamental medical precept attributed to Hippocrates (ca. 460-ca. 377 BCE). Biocompatibility is a universal requirement for medical devices that contact living tissues (15); that is, materials should have an "appropriate" response to the host (body). However, the necessary tests for biocompatibility depend on the use of the materials, such as temporary or permanent use; mucosal contacting or implantation contact with bone. In general, ceramic materials are a natural choice for biomedical uses because they are usually more biocompatible than metals or polymers. Metals may elute ions, and some cause sensitization of teeth. Polymers often react with water and hydrolyze or break down. Monomers are often incompletely polymerized in vivo, leaving reactive residual monomers.

The ISO 10993 set of standards "Biological Evaluation of Medical devices" is used to guide the testing and verification of biocompatibility of materials based on the type and duration of body contact. The first of this series (ISO 10993-1) has a chart for biocompatibility tests, and three other ISO 10993 standards are particularly important for ceramics:

- ISO 10993-14, "Identification and quantification of degradation products from ceramics,"
- ISO 10993-18, "Chemical characterization of medical device materials within a risk management process," and
- ISO/TS 10993-19, "Physico-chemical, morphological and topographical characterization of materials."

A useful summary of biocompatibility for dental materials is in reference (16). Two commonly used terms in biocompatibility testing are "viability" and "proliferation" of cells exposed to medical devices or eluates from the materials. Medical devices encompass far-ranging uses; therefore, a dental-specific standard has been developed for biocompatibility: ISO 7405 "Evaluation of biocompatibility of medical devices used in dentistry," which has been adopted as ADA 41. These standards categorize materials by their tissue contact and duration for suggested biological testing. See Tables 4.4 and 4.5.

Any biomaterial for in vivo use should be compared by a manufacturer to similar medical devices. Assessment includes evaluating and contrasting the compositions and chemical and physical characteristics by testing or finding analyses from the literature to contribute to a risk analysis. The chemical analyses of materials under development should include additives that may have in vivo contact,

Table 4.4 Categories of dental devices by contact from ISO 7405.

Contact type	Tissue contact
Surface	Intact or breached or otherwise compromised oral mucosa. External surfaces of dental hard tissue, including enamel, dentin, and cementum
External communicating	Oral mucosa, dental hard tissues, dental pulp tissue or bone, or any combination of these, and exposure to the oral environment
Implanted	Partially or fully embedded in one or more of the following: • soft tissue, e.g., subperiosteal • bone • pulpodentinal system of the tooth • any combination of these

Table 4.5 Categories of dental devices by duration.

Category	Duration (days)
Limited	<1
Prolonged	1–30
Permanent	>30

Table 4.6 Parameters and tests for analysis of ceramics from ISO 10993-18.

Parameter	Method	Qualitative	Quantitative
Chemical composition and trace substances	X-ray fluorescence*, Inductively coupled plasma	Yes	Yes
Anion measurement	Ion chromatography, pH	Yes	Yes
Valency	Colorimetric analyses	Yes	No
Phases	X-ray diffraction, and microscopy	Yes	No
Microstructure	Microscopy	No	Yes
Extractable leachates	Inductively coupled plasma	Yes	Yes

* Not a measure of esthetic fluorescence.

including sintering aids, mold release, binders, pigments, and coatings. Table 4.6 from ISO 10993-18 includes possible test methods for ceramics; some of these methods are described in Chapter 6. The chemical and physical property information may need to be augmented by biocompatibility testing to determine local, cytotoxic, allergic/sensitizing, systemic, mutagenic, carcinogenic or teratogenic reactions, as discussed in depth in *Biocompatibility of Dental Materials* (15).

Cell culture testing (cytotoxicity) is the first phase for assessing local reactions to materials. The ideal cell culture outcome is that the cells are not affected, harmed, or killed by the material or its leachants. Notably, some materials may be cytotoxic yet suitable for in vivo use. Mitigating factors to consider are the dose (amount), duration, contact location, cytotoxicity diminishing over time, lack of cytotoxicity after setting, and compatibility with diluted leachate. Various cell lines are used; some are specific to the placement of the material: mouse fibroblasts (L929), human gingival fibroblasts, human periodontal ligament (PDLC), and human osteoblast-like MG63 cells. Cell culture tests may require direct contact with the material or extracts (solutions) that have been leached from the test material. The temperature, time, and solvent for extractions, which are commonly 24 hours at 37 °C, are prescribed by the test protocols in the ISO 10993, ADA 41, or ISO 7405 documents. When testing extracts, a specific ratio may be required of the solvent (usually water or cottonseed oil) to the test material by weight or alternatively by surface area.

Molecular toxicology tests assess the response of cells to dental materials via the determination of DNA damage and repair or inflammation mediators. The increase or decrease (upregulation or downregulation) of proteins is also tested, which may indicate a material's impact on healing. These tests are comparatively quick and easy but may not indicate precisely what happens in patients.

Sensitization and irritation tests are the next level of testing, Group II tests in ISO 7405, for dental materials. Genotoxicity and subcutaneous implantation, may be required, depending on the material or its indications for use. Ceramics are highly unlikely to be mutagenic, in contrast to the potential for mutagenicity from polymers. Acute systemic toxicity and subacute systemic toxicity are also tests in Group II. The Group III biocompatibility tests of ISO 7405, the highest level and most costly, are specific to dental implantation sites: pulp, endodontic (root canal and its foramen), and alveolar bone.

If no atoms or ions migrate from the material into the tissue, then no reaction occurs, and the material is inert. Even so, dental materials are foreign bodies, and the corpus may seek to encapsulate the material with fibroblasts if it is implanted (placed subgingivally). Implantation tests are used to see tissue reactions and defenses to a foreign body material over time; inflammation is expected after an implantation surgery but ideally will resolve. Implantation material may be placed subcutaneously, intramuscularly, within bone (including alveolar), or on pulpal tissue. These tests take longer than cell cultures, are much more costly, and require tissue analysis after implantation, which may require several months. Although many ceramic materials are inert, some release ions in water. The ions may cause local reactions, such as cell toxicity, irritation, sensitization, or allergic response. However, when calcium, silicon, or hydroxide ions are eluted, beneficial effects may occur, as described for bioactivity and in Chapter 8.

Antimicrobial

Separate from the biocompatibility tests are the antibacterial and antifungal (antimicrobial) tests. Reduction of virulent bacteria, fungi, and viruses and their biofilms is a benefit for dental treatments, but as a practical matter, microbes cannot be eliminated. Oral bacterial cultures are used for testing materials, although not all oral bacteria can be cultured. The basic antimicrobial testing consists of using planktonic bacterial cultures and measuring colony forming units (CFUs), or live-dead staining for bacteria treated with the test material. The methods of growing biofilms and their diverse microbes can confound comparisons of results. The ISO 22196 standard

"Measurement of antibacterial activity on plastics and other non-porous surfaces" includes some test methods for biofilms. Another test for biofilm removal is under development by an ADA standards committee (ADA 216).

Bacteria and fungi are more vulnerable to antimicrobial agents than mammalian cells, which have thicker cell walls. Bacteria are killed in alkaline (high pH) environments, while most human cells can survive, which is why calcium hydroxide, calcium silicate cement, and calcium aluminate cement are used for their antimicrobial properties in endodontics (Chapter 8). Certain nano-sized ($<0.1\,\mu m$) ceramic particles, such as ceria, are being promoted for antibacterial applications. For this, the unique mechanism against pathogens is via the reversible conversion of the oxidation state between Ce (III) and Ce (IV) – Ce_2O_3 and CeO_2.

Sterility

Sterilization is performed where suitable for medical devices, including some, but not all dental products. Dental instruments, including burrs, are always sterilized. Some of the dental ceramics discussed herein are used in a sterile condition; others are not. For instance, restorative materials that replace tooth anatomy (Chapters 9 and 10) are not required to be sterile because they are placed in the non-sterile environment of the mouth! Dental cements or orthodontic brackets are not sterile; they are also used in the bacteria-lined oral cavity. Materials used below the gumline are sterile, such as bone grafting materials and implants.

Endodontic materials – used in contact with the pulp or in root canals (Chapter 8) – are not all sterile because an infected pulp or root canal system is not truly sterile. The bacterial invasion that necessitates root canal procedure cannot be completely irradiated or inactivated in the root canal system. Aspects of the treatments strive for the elimination of bacteria and biofilms within the tooth. Gutta percha and paper points used in endodontics are usually sterile. Root canal sealers are not sterile, but ideally, they should be antimicrobial.

Sterile or not, all medical devices are manufactured under regulated conditions for cleanliness, denoted in the United States as "Good Manufacturing Practices" (21CFR 808, 812, and 820). The regulations aim to ensure freedom from bioburden, infectious organisms, and extraneous materials. International standards exist for methods of validating and testing sterilization processes: ISO 11137-1, 2 and 3, and ISO 11737-1, 2, and 3.

Bioactivity and Resorption

Bioactive materials have been defined broadly as "having been designed to elicit or modulate biological activity" (17), having a "biological effect" (18), being non-inert, and providing benefits to healing (19). Sometimes bioactivity has been used to describe materials that have antimicrobial effects or modulate biofilms, but these effects may be the result of only chemical interactions of the materials or the materials' toxicity. Biomineralization is a subset of bioactivity where the material forms a layer of hydroxyapatite (HA) on its surface in vivo, the process by which living organisms secrete inorganic minerals (20). This text focuses on the ISO 23317 standard, which has a narrower definition of bioactivity as follows:

> "the property that elicits a specific biological response at the interface of the material, which results in the formation of a bond between tissue and material ... When a bioactive material is implanted in a living body, a thin layer rich in Ca and P forms on its surface. The material then connects to the living tissue through this apatite layer without a distinct boundary. It has been shown that this apatite layer can be reproduced on the surfaces of materials in SBF [synthetic body fluid] as well, and that apatite thus formed is very similar to bone mineral in its composition and structure. As bioactivity increases, apatite forms on the material surface in a shorter time in proportion to this increase. The formation of apatite layers can be detected by thin film x-ray diffraction spectrometry and/or scanning electron microscopy."

In dentistry, bioactivity has customarily been synonymous with biomineralization by materials that elute calcium and hydroxide ions. The elevated pH from the OH ions causes the calcium ions to react with the phosphate ions in body fluids to precipitate a hydroxyapatite-type ($Ca_{10}(PO_4)_6(OH)_2$) layer on the surface of bioactive materials, as expressed in Eq. (4.1):

$$\underset{\text{[calcium ions+phosphate ions+hydroxide ions] in solution}}{10Ca^{+2} \quad +6PO_4^{-4} \quad +2OH^-} \rightarrow \underset{\text{hydroxyapatite precipitate [crystals]}}{Ca_{10}(PO_4)_6(OH)_2} \tag{4.1}$$

The hydroxyapatite layer may begin as an amorphous phase with a ratio of calcium to phosphate lower than the ratio in bone, 1.67. Over time the layer can gain calcium and transform into imperfect crystals of ß-type carbonated pseudo-apatite crystals. The formation of the hydroxyapatite layer is self-limiting as it thickens because the HA layer slows the calcium ion diffusion to the surface to continue the reaction with the body fluids. This precipitation occurs acellularly with simulated body fluid in vitro (21) and in vivo (22).

Certain ceramics cause this biomineralization in vivo or in vitro: "bioglass" silicate glasses, calcium hydroxide, calcium phosphate compounds including hydroxyapatite, calcium silicate cement, and calcium aluminate cements. All these ceramic powders release ions in water to become bioactive.

Some companies have co-opted the term "bioactivity" to describe their restorative materials that elute other ions, such as fluorine, boron, and strontium. These ions do not produce the apatite precipitation of Eq. (4.1). The marketing of these materials as bioactive stems from the broader definition of bioactivity; that is, materials that release ions that interact with the body. Consequently, dentists have become confused about what a bioactive product means and what the benefits are (23). For this text, bioactivity is the formation of surficial hydroxyapatite that occurs in contact with pulpal or periapical tissue, not on the crown of teeth.

Radiopacity

Dentists use X-rays to create images of teeth for diagnosis and confirmation of their treatment for their colleagues and insurance companies. Carious enamel or dentin and pulp tissue appear darker than healthy enamel on X-ray images because these areas have diminished or no hydroxyapatite (calcium phosphate); dentin and enamel appear gray-colored, and pulp is darker. Certain dental materials appear white, having higher radiopacity than tooth structure; these ceramics include higher atomic number metals, higher than calcium and phosphorous present in teeth. Radiopacity is important for all the X-ray procedures performed by dentists; radiopaque ceramics are discussed in Chapter 5.

Color, Opacity, Fluorescence, and Opalescence

As many as 1,173 tooth colors have been reported as unique (24) among people. The transparency decreases from the gingival to the incisal edge of a tooth. Color and transparency of dental materials are critical considerations for esthetic dentistry because teeth are white with tints of red, yellow, and gray. Blue pigments are used to create the illusion of transparency. Therefore, dental materials used to replace coronal anatomy must be available in multiple colors and transparencies to enable restorations to blend with natural teeth. Many ceramic powders are white in color, and other ceramic pigments are used to impart the necessary red, yellow, and gray tints and opacity to a polymer, ceramic restorative material, or cement. Glass phases have been useful in creating translucency.

Color and Dental Shade Guides

Each manufacturer offers a limited selection of shades – colors – for their restorative materials. "Shade guides" are made by manufacturers, which are examples of the color (shade) that the material will create after curing or firing. See examples of shade guides in Figure 4.3. The Vita shade designations have been very popular, using 18 basic shade designations in the following approximate order of decreasing whiteness: OM1, OM2, OM3, A1, B2, D2, A2, C1, C2, D4, A3, D3, B3, A3.5, B4,

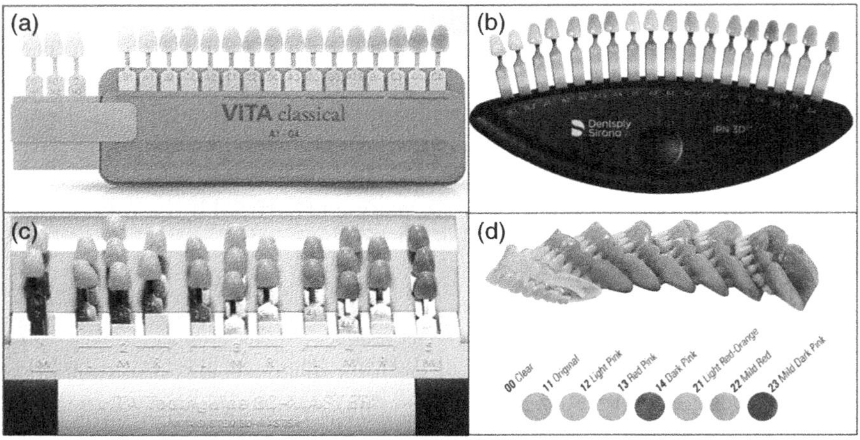

Figure 4.3 Examples of shade guides for dental materials to be used by dentists or dental technicians: (a) Vita classic guide; (b) denture tooth guide; (c) an updated Vita guide; (d) gingival color guide for dentures.

C3, A4, and C4. The color differences from one shade to the next have been arbitrary. Vita Corporation also offers an alternative shade guide more logical in color characteristics; first the lightness (whiteness) is chosen, then the color intensity (chroma), and last, the hue (yellow to red) in this system. Some companies offer shade guides that are made of the same material as the dental material. Other shade guides are made of denture porcelain and may have a variation within the individual shades; it's a guide, not a calibrated standard. The standard Vita shades noted above are not standardized among companies; each manufacturer uses their unique set of pigments they believe is similar to the Vita shades. ISO standard 22598 specifies requirements for tooth-like color representations made of ceramic materials for a dental prosthesis, which are referred to as color tabs in this standard. The shades are, in truth, created at the manufacturers' discretion; shade guides help dentists choose an appropriate shade, which may need "adjustment" after a try-in placement in the mouth.

The original shade guides were formed by hand in molds having the shape of an anterior tooth using several denture porcelain pastes for the gingiva, body, and incisal areas; the chroma and opacity of the pastes decreases from the gingival to the incisal edge. The combination of the colors and the hand forming exemplifies why the term shade guide, not color standard, is used (25). The molded porcelain is vacuum-fired and mounted on flat sticks for the dentist to hold near the patient's teeth for selecting the best shade for a restorative material.

Shade selection (matching) is done visually by dental professionals having good color vision, in their operatory, preferably with a neutral-colored office wall paint and controlled lighting, by placing the shade guide near the adjacent teeth (26). A constant conundrum for dentists and dental technicians has been how to choose a shade to optimize the match to the remaining or adjacent teeth for an esthetic result, which is especially difficult when the color acuity of the dentist is imperfect. The conundrum is worsened because teeth are translucent, and the perceived color of a tooth or restoration depends on color, thickness, and opacity. For instance, the color of thinner translucent restorative devices, such as a porcelain veneer, can be significantly affected by the underlying cement and tooth. Shade selection is complicated because many shade guides, e.g., the Vita shade guide, are made of porcelain, and many restorative materials are resin-based. Metamerism – change in the appearance of materials under different illumination – can lead to discrepancies between ceramics and resin restorative materials. Dehydration of the tooth also contributes to less than perfect choices of restorative material to match the surrounding teeth (27).

Two manufacturers advertise that their resin-based composite material for direct restoration requires only a single shade of resin composite, defying the need for a shade guide. These resin-based composite materials are advertised to contain 260 nm spherical particles that "adapt" (mimic) to the surrounding dentition with the red-yellow hues of teeth, without needing multiple shades.

Special shade guides are also made for the selection of gingival color (Figure 4.3), or for dental technicians to select auxiliary stains to perfect their indirect restorations. Denture teeth have also had their own shade guides and shade designations, which was useful for porcelain denture teeth, but less useful for acrylic artificial teeth.

Opacity

Opacity is the inverse of transparency and "translucency" is just confusing. Opaque ceramics may either have multiple grain boundaries, pores, or a mixture of materials having differing refractive indices, n_d. The latter is very important for polymeric materials with glass fillers described in Chapter 8. The index of refraction is a unitless number representing the ratio of the speed of light in a vacuum divided by the speed of light in the material; the latter is always slower; therefore, any material has an index of refraction greater than 1. The difference in the indices of refraction between two materials (n_1 and, n_2) governs the diversion (refraction) of light at the interface, according to Snell's law, Eq. (4.2),

$$n_1 \cdot \sin(\theta_1) = n_2 \cdot \sin(\theta_2) \tag{4.2}$$

where θ_1 is the angle of incidence of the light and θ_2 is the angle of refraction (diversion) of the light; each is measured from the line perpendicular to the interface shown in Figure 4.4. Every interface in a material alters the passage of light through the material via the differences in indices of refraction and the

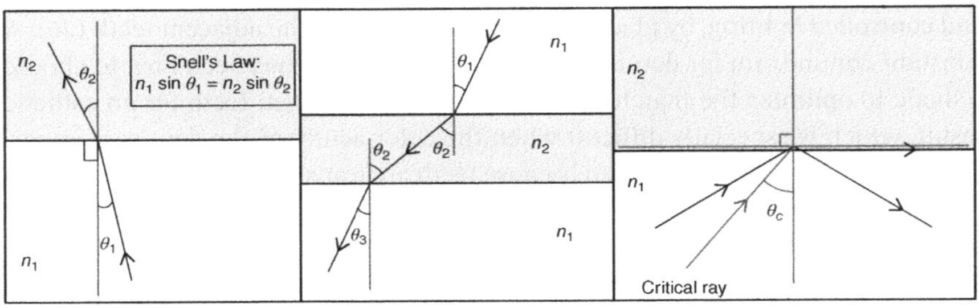

Figure 4.4 Snell's law of refraction where n_1 is the refractive index of the matrix and n_2 is the index of refraction of the particle; θ_1 and θ_2 are the incident and refracted angles showing how the interface diverts the light; θ_3 is the angle of refraction as the diverted light transits a particle back into the matrix; θ_c is the critical angle which, if exceeded, the light cannot pass through the particle; the light is scattered and makes the object opaque.

dispersion between the two phases. At some interfaces, the angle of incidence, θ_1, may be so large (oblique) that the light may not penetrate the material and is reflected. This is the critical angle where $\sin(\theta_2)$ equals 1 (Eq. (4.3), that is, $\sin(\theta_c)$), as depicted in Figure 4.4.

$$n_1 \cdot \sin(\theta_1) / n_2 = 1 = \sin(\theta_c) \tag{4.3}$$

The refractive index of typical dental methacrylate mixtures of resins ranges from 1.46 to 1.65. Silica has an index of refraction of 1.4585, and many common glasses have indices of 1.50–1.51, which are close enough to make non-opaque (translucent) combinations of glass and resin. Special formulas of glass have been developed by manufacturers to match the index of refraction of their resin matrices and achieve translucency. Alumina, zirconia, and titania pigments have higher indices of refraction (1.762–1.778; 2.15–2.18; 2.45–2.85, respectively), which cause scattering at their interfaces and add opacity when added to resins or dental glass. Opacity is controlled by varying the glass, resin, and pigment proportions.

Glass is often transparent but poly-crystalline ceramic restoratives are usually opaque. Light is scattered at the grain boundaries. Very pure alumina, lacking silica and containing only parts per million of magnesia, has been made translucent, but is not used in dentistry. Single-crystal ceramics, such as sapphire orthodontic brackets, are transparent because they lack grain boundaries. Zirconia materials vary in translucency depending on the formula, and the amount and crystal forms present.

Opalescence

Opalescent materials exhibit a remarkable esthetic quality of appearing blue in reflected light or against a dark background, and yellow-orange in transmitted light. Opalescence is present in natural teeth at the incisal edge, giving them a bluish or violet tint, especially in primary teeth or young permanent teeth. To see the opalescence of teeth, an extracted tooth is illuminated from the back side to observe the orange color in the incisal region in tramsitted light.

Opalescence is caused by the preferential scattering of blue/violet light by fine (<0.1 μm) particles; this requires that the particles be about the size of wavelength of blue or violet light (400–500 nm; 0.4–0.5 μm). The particles usually have a higher refractive index for blue light than the longer wavelengths (e.g. yellow or red); this change in the index of refraction is called dispersion. Thus, blue light, with a higher refractive index, will be bent more strongly than red light, leading to scattered blue light, following Snell's law described above. The incisal region of teeth may appear bluish because more blue light is scattered back to the observer, but the longer wavelengths are transmitted through the tooth.

Tooth opalescence is believed to be caused by the presence of fine-grained hydroxyapatite crystals. Fine particles (<200 nm) are used to mimic opalescence in dental materials, such as colloidal silica in resin-based restoratives. Dental porcelains may contain opalescent glass, akin to opal stones, to be biomimetic. Alternatively, a blue stain at the incisal edge may suffice for esthetics.

Fluorescence

Fluorescence is a form of luminescence or light emission; when fluorescent substances are illuminated with light, their metal atoms can be excited with the energy and then relax and emit light of a lower energy (longer wavelength). Human and animal teeth exhibit fluorescence, which imparts a quality of vitality. This quality was not detected until the 20th century when UV lights became common; fluorescence is obvious in UV light which stimulates fluorescent emissions; e.g., nightclub lighting the presence of ambient white light. Some phosphorescence of teeth has been observed lasting up to 30 seconds (28); phosphorescence is light emission that occurs after the energy source is removed. This phenomenon is different from fluorescence, where the light is emitted almost immediately after absorption.

The compounds causing fluorescence in human teeth are mostly organic, particularly the fluorescing molecules of tyrosine, tryptophan, and hydroxypyridine (29). Enamel produces weaker fluorescence than dentin because enamel contains much less organic material. The maxillary and mandibular teeth fluoresce equally, but aging, bleaching, and location within a tooth affect fluorescence. Carious tissue is also less fluorescent; therefore, certain lasers can be used to detect caries by emitting light and revealing dark "spots." Esthetic restorative materials should have fluorescence properties to mimic natural teeth.

Summary of Ceramics for Medical Devices

An assortment of properties and regulatory concerns govern bioceramics in dental devices – when used temporarily or as a permanent addition in our bodies. Governments classify and regulate what dental products can be sold in their countries, often relying on international standards, particularly conformance to ISO 13485.

Special properties of ceramics are needed for some dental bioceramics, particularly biocompatibility, and, often, tooth-like color (translucency, opalescence, and fluorescence) or radiopacity. Some ceramics have unique characteristics of being antimicrobial and bioactive, that find dental utility; some are sterile, and many dental materials are not. Chapter 5 introduces the wide variety of bioceramics used for dental products, including a plethora of glass formulas that span the periodic table. Chapter 6 describes some test methods for verifying and validating dental bioceramic performance.

Ceramics in Chapter 4

Following dental ceramics or inorganic materials were mentioned in this chapter:

- alumina, aluminous porcelains, sapphire, high purity alumina
- calcium aluminate cement
- calcium hydroxide
- calcium silica cement
- calcium phosphates
- ceria
- glass
- "Bioglass"
- hydroxyapatite
- silica
- sodium borate
- titania
- zinc oxide
- zirconia

References

1 Daniel, A., Kimmelman, E., and Trautman, K.A. (2008). *The FDA and worldwide quality system requirements guidebook for medical devices*, 2nd ed., 304. Milwaukee, WI: ASQ Quality Press.

2 Trautman, K.A. (1997). *The FDA and worldwide quality system requirements guide book for medical devices*, 210. Milwaukee, WI: ASQC Quality Press.
3 Whitmore, E. (2012). *Development of FDA-regulated medical products: a translational approach*, 2nd ed., 237. Milwaukee, WI: ASQ Quality Press.
4 Della Bona, A., Wozniak, W.T., and Watts, D.C. (2011). International dental standards–order out of chaos? *Dental Materials*. 27 (7): 619–621.
5 Megremis, S.J. (2022). Assuring the safety of dental materials: the usefulness and application of standards. *Dental Clinics of North America*. 66 (4): 673–689.
6 Kokubo, T. and Takadama, H. (2006). How useful is SBF in predicting in vivo bone bioactivity? *Biomaterials*. 27 (15): 2907–2915.
7 Heintze, S.D. (2006). How to qualify and validate wear simulation devices and methods. *Dental Materials*. 22 (8): 712–734.
8 Spintzyk, S., Geis-Gerstorfer, J., Bourauel, C. et al. (2021). Biaxial flexural strength of zirconia: a round robin test with 12 laboratories. *Dental Materials*. 37 (2): 284–295.
9 Ito, A., Sogo, Y., Yamazaki, A. et al. (2015). Interlaboratory studies on in vitro test methods for estimating in vivo resorption of calcium phosphate ceramics. *Acta Biomaterialia*. 25: 347–355.
10 Darvell, B.W. (2021). Bioactivity – symphony or cacophony? A personal view of a tangled field. *Prosthesis*. 3 (1): 75–84.
11 Darvell, B.W. (2020). Misuse of ISO standards in dental materials research. *Dental Materials*. 36 (12): 1493–1494.
12 Punj, S., Singh, J., and Singh, K. (2021). Ceramic biomaterials: properties, state of the art and future prospectives. *Ceramics International*. 47 (20): 28059–28074.
13 Antoniac, I. (2019). *Bioceramics and biocomposites: from research to clinical practice*. Hoboken, NJ: Wiley, The American Ceramic Society.
14 Kelly, J.R. (2016). *Ceramics in dentistry: principles and practice*, 117. Hanover Park, IL: Quintessence Publishing Co, Inc.
15 Schmalz, G. and Arenholt Bindslev, D. (2009). *Biocompatibility of dental materials*, 1ste, 302. Berlin, Heidelberg: Springer Berlin Heidelberg.
16 Fischer, N.G., de Souza Araujo, I.J., Daghrery, A. et al. (2025). Guidance on biomaterials for periodontal tissue regeneration: Fabrication methods, materials and biological considerations. *Dental Materials*. 41 (3): 283–305.
17 Williams, D.F. (1999). *The Williams dictionary of biomaterials*, 343. Liverpool: Liverpool University Press.
18 Ferracane, J.L., Sidhu, S.K., Melo, M.A.S. et al. (2023). Bioactive dental materials. *JADA Foundational Science*. 2: 1–5.
19 Zhao, X. (2011). Introduction to bioactive materials in medicine. *Bioactive Materials in Medicine*. 1–13.
20 Niu, L.N., Zhang, W., Pashley, D.H. et al. (2014). Biomimetic remineralization of dentin. *Dental Materials*. 30 (1): 77–96.
21 Bozeman, T.B., Lemon, R.R., and Eleazer, P.D. (2006). Elemental analysis of crystal precipitate from gray and white MTA. *Journal of Endodontics*. 32 (5): 425–428.

22 Ricucci, D., Rocas, I.N., Hernandez, S., and Siqueira, J.F. Jr. (2020). “True” versus “Bay” apical cysts: clinical, radiographic, histopathologic, and histobacteriologic features. *Journal of Endodontics.* 46 (9): 1217–1227.
23 Sauro, S., Carvalho, R.M., and Ferracane, J. (2025). The rise of advanced bioactive restorative materials: are they redefining operative dentistry? *Dental Materials.* 41 (11): 1411–1429.
24 Hein, S., Morovic, J., Morovic, P. et al. (2025). How many tooth colors are there? *Dental Materials.* 41: 51–57.
25 O’Brien, W.J., Groh, C.L., and Boenke, K.M. (1989). One-dimensional color order system for dental shade guides. *Dental Materials.* 5 (6): 371–374.
26 O’Brien, W., Oh, W.-S., and Piché, P. (2012). Color parameters of the chromascop shade guide. *Dentistry Journal.* 1 (1): 3–11.
27 Alnusayri, M.O., Sghaireen, M.G., Mathew, M. et al. (2022). Shade selection in esthetic dentistry: a review. *Cureus.* 14 (3): e23331.
28 Lee, Y.K. (2015). Fluorescence properties of human teeth and dental calculus for clinical applications. *Journal of Biomedical Optics.* 20 (4): 1–9.
29 Volpato, C.A.M., Pereira, M.R.C., and Silva, F.S. (2018). Fluorescence of natural teeth and restorative materials, methods for analysis and quantification: a literature review. *Journal of Esthetic and Restorative Dentistry.* 30 (5): 397–407.

5

Ceramics for Dentistry

Ceramics have evolved over the history of civilization. Porous pottery was developed to store food at the dawn of agriculture. With fire, more dense, less porous pots were created – stoneware. Combining raw minerals such as kaolin clay, silica (quartz or sand), and feldspar created the next generation of ceramic objects that were translucent, impermeable, easily cleaned, rigid, chemically resistant, and stronger. An endless variety of ceramics have been created with various combinations of these three minerals and remain in use for manufacturing ceramic items.

Materials science is an engineering discipline that encompasses the development and application of substances, which may be metallic, organic, ceramic, or combinations thereof, as depicted in Figure 4.1. Ceramics are neither metallic nor organic; that is, they are usually compounds, not elements or alloys, and do not contain C—H bonds. Oxides are the most common ceramic compounds, although the carbides, sulfides, iodates, nitrides, fluorides, and borides of metals are also prevalent ceramics. Oxide compounds are often denoted as metals with a suffix that includes "a." For instance, alumina is aluminum oxide (Al_2O_3), silica is silicon dioxide (SiO_2), and zirconia is zirconium dioxide (ZrO_2), the terminology used in this text. The dental literature is often written by non-materials scientists who have occasionally confused silica with silicon and silicone substances. Silicon is an element, a semi-metal; silica is the ceramic oxide of silicon (SiO_2), and silicones are organic polymers containing a silica in a siloxane repeating chain ($-O-R_2$ $Si-O-SiR_2-$), where R is an organic group. The elements of carbon and silicon are "adopted" as ceramics for this text; they are important as abrasives and in electronics, as described in Chapters 17 and 18.

The properties of oxides, including their biocompatibility, are distinct from the metals and polymers; see Table 5.1. Ceramics are usually hard, stiff (high elastic modulus), wear-resistant, acid-resistant, white or translucent, thermally and electrically insulating, and have good compressive strength, with some exceptions to all.

Ceramics in Dentistry: Materials, Manufacturing, and Clinical Applications,
First Edition. Carolyn M. Primus.

Table 5.1 Generalities about materials.

Materials property	Ceramics	Metals	Organics/ polymers
Hardness	High	Low to fairly high	Low
Tensile strength	Low	Low to high	Low to medium
Compressive strength	Medium to high	Medium	Low, often easily compressed
Flexural strength	Often measured	Rarely measured due to plasticity	
Biaxial Strength	Medium	Not measured	Not measured
Fracture toughness	Low to medium	High	Low
Plasticity (inverse of brittleness)	Low, except at higher temperature	Medium to high	Medium to high
Elasticity (inverse of stiffness)	Low	Medium	High
Color	Often white, often opaque, but also other colors. Glass may vary from transparent to opaque and may have color.	Opaque, often gray and lustrous	Milky to clear (unless pigmented)

The flexural strength and tensile strength of ceramics are lower than common metals but usually higher than those of the organic polymers. Ceramic compounds are typically not:

- malleable or ductile at room temperature (no plastic deformation)
- flexible (with exceptions for glass fibers)
- soft (with exceptions for some minerals)
- cytotoxic, mutagenic, or toxic (with exceptions such as lead oxide (PbO), cadmia, chromia, telluria, baria, and arsenic oxide) or
- formable at temperatures below 1000 °C, with exceptions for cement powders that set with water and some new sintering techniques.

Ceramics are frequently described as brittle, which is improperly considered synonymous with low strength. Brittle means a material fails (breaks) without plastic deformation, which is an irreversible change in shape with the formation of internal voids, before fracture and is common for metals. Ceramics usually undergo only elastic deformation before fracture, a reversible change in the shape of a material under stress. The distinction between elastic and plastic deformation is illustrated in Figure 6.3, where samples are illustrated after strength tests. Most ceramics are brittle at room temperature, but many are ductile at high temperatures > 1,000°C. Ceramics are usually stiffer (less flexible) than metals or polymers; therefore, ceramics undergo less deformation before breaking (failure). Ceramics are not necessarily weak because they are brittle.

Ceramics are available as single crystals, polycrystalline, amorphous, and combinations of polycrystalline and amorphous. All four categories are depicted in Figure 5.3. Single crystals are macroscopic in size (>10^{-3} m, >1 mm), whereas polycrystalline ceramics have individual grains ranging from nanometers (10^{-9} m) to a few hundred microns (<10^{-3} m, <1 mm). Crystals are a regular repeating arrangement of atoms in one of seven forms illustrated in Figure 5.1; these crystal forms will be discussed, particularly for zirconia. In contrast, glass is amorphous, non-crystalline, with a random atomic structure depicted in Figure 5.2. This disordered arrangement of atoms contributes to lower stiffness of glasses versus crystalline ceramics.

Polycrystalline ceramics grains or micro-crystals are separated by grain boundaries. The grains may be microscopic single crystals or a combination of ceramic

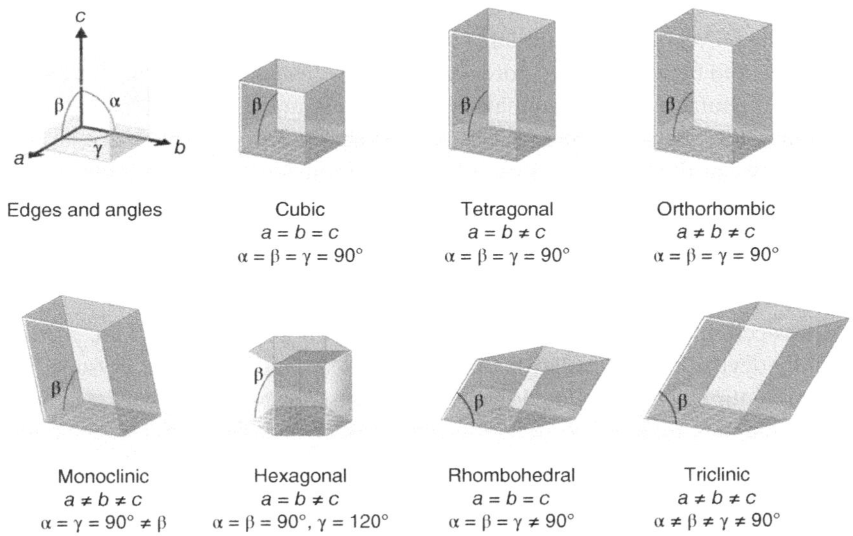

Figure 5.1 The seven crystal forms. *Source:* Ed Vitz et al., 2025 / https://chem.libretexts.org/Bookshelves/General_Chemistry/ChemPRIME_(Moore_et_al.)/10%3A_Solids_Liquids_and_Solutions/10.04%3A_Crystal_Systems, last accessed on 31 March 2025/LibreTexts.

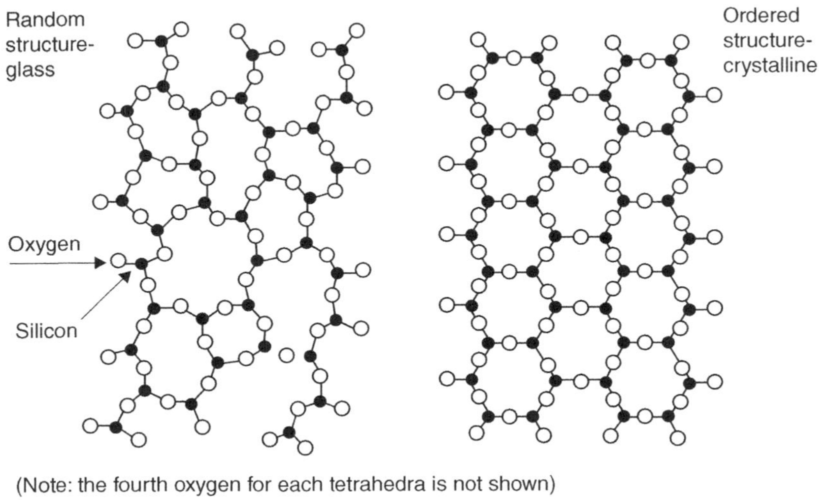

Figure 5.2 Diagram contrasting the atomic arrangement of amorphous silica (glass) on the left and orderly crystalline silica. *Source:* Ashish, 2023 / https://www.scienceabc.com/pure-sciences/is-glass-solid-or-liquid-does-glass-flow-amorphous-crystalline-melting-windows-cathedral.html, last accessed on 31 March 2025 / ScienceABC.

crystal compounds. The grain boundaries are complex and influence the properties of the polycrystalline material (1). Pores (voids) may be present within grains (crystals) and between grains; pores are a source of weakness in ceramics created during manufacturing. Combinations of crystals and glass are "glass-bonded ceramics" or "glass-ceramics." Glass-bonded ceramics have a microscopic glass layer between the crystal grains and are usually made by combining glass and crystalline ceramic powders during manufacturing by sintering, a heating process described in Chapter 7. The glass will commonly deform at a lower temperature than the sintering temperature of the crystals to envelope the crystalline ceramic particles forming an interstitial layer and glassy grain boundaries.

Glass-ceramics are distinctive; they begin as solid glass items and are partially or fully devitrified (crystallized) under controlled conditions. The crystals have been intentionally precipitated in the glass matrix via a special heat treatment. Glass-ceramics are not the random formation of crystals found in polycrystalline glass-bonded ceramics pottery, whitewares, and glazes (glass coatings).

Bioceramics include countless ceramic compounds and glass formulas. They can be grouped based on crystallinity, as illustrated in Figure 5.3, but can alternatively be categorized as bioinert, bioactive, resorbable, or bioactive and resorbable, as shown in Figure 4.2. Some bioceramics are also radiopaque. The breadth of bioceramic formulas is discussed below.

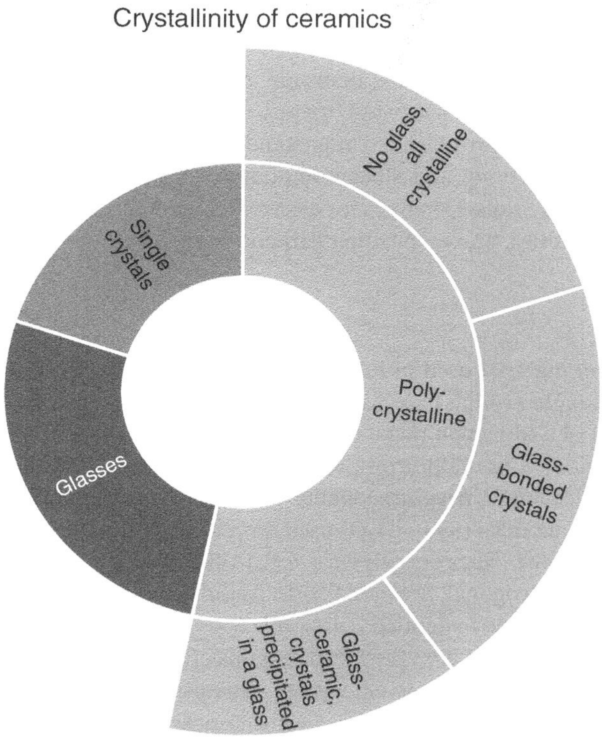

Figure 5.3 Subsets of ceramics based on crystal contents and crystal size. "Single crystals" are macroscopic crystals akin to gemstones. Glasses contain no crystals. Polycrystalline ceramics are categorized as completely crystalline (no glass phase), glass bonded (having an interstitial glass phase between crystals), and glass ceramics. Glass ceramics are cast glass in which crystals are intentionally precipitated via a controlled heat treatment; they may be partially or fully crystalline.

Quotidian Ceramics

Traditional ceramic materials have been divided into eight familiar categories: pottery, tile, terra cotta, bricks, and clay products (e.g. drains), glass, enamels, refractories (for industrial uses), and cements. The traditional ceramics vary in formula to suit the requirements, shapes, and uses but share the use of silica and alumina in their formulas and manufacture. Alumina may be present as a phase or be part of another ceramic compound; examples from this text include spinels, calcium aluminate cements, chrysoberyl, yttrium alumina garnet, and aluminum sulfate. Silicate glasses are common in ceramics, but silica is also present as in some crystalline compounds: steatite/talc, calcium silicate cements, forsterite, and wollastonite. Both silica and alumina are parts of felspar, clays, zeolites, and cordierite, which are mentioned in this text.

Crystalline ceramics and glass (amorphous) items are a reliable and delightful component of our world for buildings, roadways, homes, insulation, dinnerware, food or beverage containers, and art objects. Understanding the properties and manufacturing methods for alumina and silica compounds forms the basis of ceramics, including dental materials. Ceramics for electronics are a modern category that includes alumina, silica, and many other ceramic compounds.

Silica

Silica is the most common material used in human history, both as crystals and glass. Many gemstones (single crystals) are based on large silica crystals, often tinted by a minor amount of a transition metal oxide dissolved in the silica's crystalline matrix (solid solution). Common semi-precious silica jewelry stones are agate, topaz, amethyst, chalcedony, citrine, cristobalite, garnet, and peridot. Opal is a hydrated form of amorphous silica ($SiO_2.nH_2O$) used for jewelry. Crystalline silica is common as quartz, but other silica crystals exist, e.g., tridymite or cristobalite. Silica may have crystal forms of trigonal, hexagonal, orthorhombic, and tetragonal.

Other silica raw minerals are used in dentistry: diatomaceous earth and pumice. Diatomaceous earth powder is the ancient, fossilized remains of the silica exoskeleton of unicellular algae – the tiny, short-lived, aquatic organisms that accumulated in the sediment of rivers, streams, lakes, and oceans. Deposits of diatoms are mined from these areas and used in skin care products, toothpastes, foods, beverages, medicines, rubbers, paints, and filters for water or alcoholic beverages. These powder particles are commonly 10–200 μm in diameter. The powder is fascinating to examine microscopically because of the multitude of honeycomb-like shapes of these exoskeletons, which contain a labyrinth of tiny pores, making it an excellent insulator. The pores allow each particle to absorb liquids and increase the viscosity of a liquid or paste. The sharp edges of the diatoms are mildly abrasive and very drying, making them useful as an insecticide. Diatomaceous rock is light-colored and primarily composed of amorphous silica, but some deposits contain cristobalite (crystalline silica), calcite ($CaCO_3$), and hydrated silica. Impurities include oxides of Na, Mg, Al, Ca, K, Fe, Ti, and P dissolved in the silica.

Pumice is another amorphous silica mineral that is a product of molten lava, released from an underground reservoir under high pressure. When expelled to the surface, the pressure reduction causes the release of dissolved gases within the silica lava, creating a light gray rock with 60–80% porosity. Pumice typically contains more than 55% silica and up to 22% alumina (2). Lesser amounts of potassia, soda, iron oxide, calcia, magnesia, and titania (K_2O, Na_2O, FeO, Fe_2O_3, Fe_3O_4, CaO, MgO, TiO_2) may be present, either dissolved in the silicate glass or as tiny crystals of silicate minerals in the pumice such as feldspar, augite ((Ca,Na)

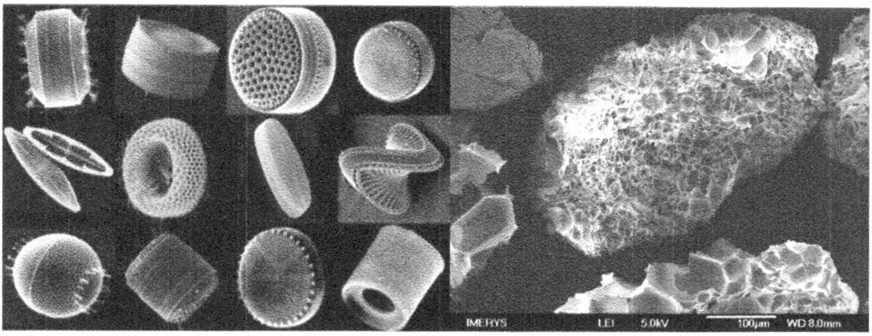

Figure 5.4 Diatoms (left) and perlite (right) micrographs showing porous silica structures that occur in nature.

$(Mg,Fe,Al,Ti)(Si,Al)_2O_6)$, hornblende $((Ca,Na)_{2\text{-}3}(Mg,Fe,Al)_5(Al,Si)_8O_{22}(OH,F)_2)$, or zircon (zirconium silicate, $ZrSiO_4$). Pumice rock is used industrially as a fine powder (flour) that is suitable for use in polishing operations. Perlite, another amorphous volcanic silicate, is more porous than pumice and typically contains 70–75% silica, 12–15% alumina, 3–5% potassia, and 3–4% sodium oxide, with traces of iron oxide, magnesia, and calcia. Images of diatoms and perlite are in Figure 5.4.

Glassmaking and forming (melting, blowing or molding) began about 500 AD in Mesopotamia and Egypt (3). Colored glasses are famously used for stained glass windows because they combine beauty and translucency. The pigments in glass are dissolved metal oxides. The use of pigments evolved from colored Egyptian beads (~2700 BC) to colored glass panes in Assyria (~900 BC) and stained glass windows in Europe after the 11th century (4). For instance, nickel, iron, and sulfur oxides create brown tones when dissolved in glass. Copper oxide produces a green–blue color; iron, chromium, and uranium oxides create other greenish shades. Red glass relies on dissolved gold, copper–tin, selenium– cadmium oxide for color. Blues and purples are created by dissolving these oxides in silicate glass: erbia, neodymium oxide, manganese oxide, cobalt oxide, or copper oxide. Silver makes a clear yellow color in silicate glasses, from pale lemon to deep orange, and may be applied on the glass surface rather than melting into the bulk.

By the 1500s, clear glasses were being melted based on silica and soda (sodium oxide, Na_2O). George Ravenscroft made new, lower melting formulas by melting lead oxide (PbO) with silica, sodium, and potassium carbonate raw materials (SiO_2, Na_2CO_3, or K_2CO_3) in the new coal-fired furnaces. Coal achieved higher temperatures than wood-fired furnaces and improved glass homogenization for better optical and mechanical properties. The development of glass formulas for optical lenses was a remarkable advance in the 17th century based on adding boric and phosphoric oxides to silica to raise the refractive index of the glass. Antoni van

Leeuwenhoek used such glasses to perfect the formation of lenses for the microscope and became the first person to observe bacteria, an essential observation to advance medicine and dentistry. Glass compositions grew more sophisticated in the 19th century as new minerals were incorporated for tailoring the glass properties. The latter half of the 20th century saw a rush of new glass formulas and uses for stovetop glass ovenware, glass fibers for communication, and lasers. Microscopes and magnifying headgear are not essential for dentistry.

Most glasses are silica-based. However, glasses may also be formed based on oxides of boron, phosphorous, and, less commonly, tellurium (TeO_2), in combination with other oxides. Typically, a glass formula will include glass formers (e.g. Si, B, or P oxides), fluxes to lower the forming temperature (e.g. Li, Na, or K oxides), and stabilizers (CaO and SnO_2) to avoid crystal formation and enhance water resistance. The fluxes may be added as oxides or perhaps carbonates for the melting phase. For biocompatibility, PbO-containing glass is not used in dental glasses; neither are those containing antimony, selenium, germanium, or tellurium. Also, cadmia is not used as a pigment. Exotic metallic glasses exist by a rapid quenching technique but are not considered ceramics.

In the mid-1870s, opal glasses were invented that had a milky appearance and streaks of color (5). To create an opaline, glass, a homogeneous glass is heat-treated and two chemically similar glasses separate into two phases that are immiscible; commonly, the matrix is one glass composition and contains microscopic droplets of a second glass, often by the inclusion of phosphate in a silica glass. Figure 5.5 has a transmission electron microscope image of a dental phase-separated glass,

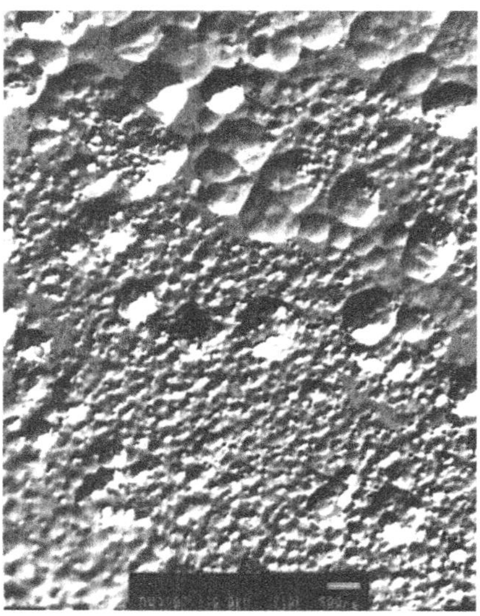

Figure 5.5 Transmission electron microscope image of a phase-separated glass. The droplets of the phase-separated glass are as small as 50 nm and as large as 500 nm.

showing the droplets, ranging in size from 50 to 500 nm. These droplets scatter blue light, as described in Chapter 4. The color and opacity of "opalized" glass is controlled by the difference in the refractive index between the phases and the amount, size, and distribution of each phase. Manufacturing a consistent opalescent appearance in glass is difficult because the temperature and time must be closely controlled throughout the processing.

Contemporary silicate glasses are known to be impervious to water; examples are glass cups and bottles for foods and beverages that do not impart flavor (ions), as well as windows that keep our homes and automobiles dry. Ordinary household glass formulas are also well known for their acid resistance to acids, such as vinegar or orange juice containers, which contain acetic and citric acids. The only acid that corrodes most silica glasses is hydrofluoric acid (HF). Insolubility of a glass is usually essential for dental restorative materials. However, some glass formulas react with water and slowly dissolve, which can be beneficial for the resorbable bioceramics. Some (dental) glass formulas are formulated to be somewhat soluble in phosphoric (H_3PO_4), tartaric ($C_4H_6O_6$), or acrylic ($CH_2{=}CHCOOH$, $C_3H_4O_2$) acids so that a setting reaction can occur to cement the glass particles in a matrix. The interactions of water with glass are complex and include dissociation of water, formation of Si-OH groups, diffusion of water into glass, and diffusion of ions such as sodium out of the glass. Acid-soluble combinations create a hard matrix of dissolved and reacted glass surrounding undissolved glass particles, as described in Chapters 8 and 9.

Thousands of silicate glass formulas have been commercially developed for their unique properties: mechanical, wear resistance, electrical, chemical, optical, or thermal. As described in other chapters, dental glasses vary widely in use, including those for cements, restoratives, glazes, enamel, and especially the glass powders used in combination with polymers. The key dental glass properties, which vary with the required use, are the index of refraction, thermal expansion, melting temperature, and softening point in addition to their capacity to be radiopaque, fluoresce, and show opalescence.

Alumina

Alumina-based and silicate-based minerals are the most common materials in the earth's crust for our everyday and industrial ceramic items. Alumina is the most studied ceramic material because of its abundance and its myriad of practical uses, including those in dentistry. Alumina is an indispensable component of many ceramic materials, including glass, porcelain "whitewares" in our kitchens and restrooms, and polishing compounds. Many silicate glasses contain alumina to achieve special properties, including dental porcelains. Alumina has many crystalline phases, but alpha-alumina (corundum) is the most common phase and is a standard powder for sandblasting, grinding, and polishing surfaces because of its innate hardness. It is also a popular pigment for polymers and porcelains. Single crystals of alpha alumina are called sapphire, valued for their beauty as a gemstone. Sapphires may be colored by minor amounts of transition metals dissolved in the alumina (solid solutions); for example, chromium oxide adds a reddish color (ruby), although other trace metal oxides, such as beryllia, titania, iron oxide, and vanadia, create other colors.

Before WWII, only glass-bonded alumina items were available, also referred to as alumina/aluminous porcelain, made by blending and firing alumina powder with a glass or clay that would vitrify (form a glass) during firing. After sintering, the items had up to 45 weight percent glass between the alumina grains; the glass made it easier to manufacture the alumina items at lower temperatures. These silicate glasses contained calcia or magnesia, often by adding wollastonite or talc ($CaSiO_3$ and $Mg_3Si_4O_{10}[OH]_2$) in the raw materials. Glass-bonded alumina has a plethora of interlocking hexagonal, prismatically-shaped alumina grains; it is hard but weaker than metals.

After WWII, ceramic engineers developed compositions and methods to make stronger alumina products using less silica glass. Higher-purity alumina, up to 99%, was developed, which required higher firing temperatures but was stronger than the earlier glass-bonded alumina formulas. A pure alumina, doped with less than 0.2% MgO, was developed that had very few pores and finer (smaller) alumina grains. This small amount of magnesia prevented the alumina grains from growing during sintering, reducing intergranular stresses. Magnesia-doped alumina has been used to make translucent products, including high-pressure sodium vapor lights for outdoor illumination; these were brighter than low-pressure sodium bulbs (6). High-purity alumina is harder and stronger than many other oxides in bending or tensile strength. Only zirconia, discussed later, has higher strength as a ceramic.

Porcelain and Porcelain Enamel

Porcelain is a ceramic material composed of crystals dispersed in a glass matrix; porcelain is stronger and less opaque than stoneware or earthenware. Its development began in the 6th century for domestic items. Industrially useful porcelain items include spark plugs, electrical insulators for power lines, and domestic items designed for esthetics such as vases, lamps, and dinnerware; these are often glazed, coated with glass.

Quartz (crystalline silica) has been used as a reinforcing, strengthening crystal in a glass matrix. However, quartz crystals expand during heating, especially above the α- to β-transformation temperature of 574 °C; cracks form, weakening the porcelain. Therefore, alumina, not quartz, crystals are used to reinforce (strengthen) porcelain. Alumina powder is combined with glass formulas having a similar thermal expansion (~8 ppm/K); the glasses often contains silica, boron oxide, and small amounts of alumina, soda, and potassia. Such formulas ensure good bonding at the alumina-glass interface and a firing temperature below 1000 °C.

Porcelain enamel is a coating of glass, often containing crystals, fused onto an underlying metal. Enameling has been a decorative art for about five millennia. Gold jewelry and other ornamental objects have been enameled using innovative methods that accommodate the differences in thermal expansion between the gold (14 ppm/K) and the glass (~8 ppm/K). The cloisonné method used small gold wires on the metal, creating small spaces where the ceramic was applied; the gold wires accommodated the stress created by the difference in thermal expansion avoiding cracks in the ceramic. The champlevé technique required that the metal be carved with shallow craters where the ceramic powder was placed to minimize the thermal mismatch stress. Without these clever techniques, the ancient porcelains would have cracked and spalled (lost adhesion to the metal). Also, the porcelain must have a lower fusion temperature than the metal.

In modern times, metal alloys have been enameled, including gold, silver, bronze, iron, steel, and aluminum alloys. The porcelain enamel for each metal alloy requires a glass formula that will bond and have slightly lower thermal expansion, and create a smooth layer after firing without distorting the metal. Familliar uses of enameled base metal alloys include jewelry, water heaters, ovens, stoves, washing machine basins, pots and pans, and barbeque grills. Even enamel road signs have been made. Industrially, the coatings of enamel powder may be sprayed from an emulsion onto the metal before being heated to form a coating. Multiple porcelain layers may be required to create a graded coating that compensates for the disparate thermal expansion of a metal and porcelain coating. In Chapter 10, a dental porcelain formula is described, which has a high thermal expansion, coordinated with those of the dental alloys. Ceramic pigments are used to color the dental porcelain – see Table 5.2.

Glass–Ceramics

Glass-ceramics are a unique group of glass materials that undergo heat treatments after the glass has been shaped. These three steps are required: (1) mixing the ceramic powders for the glass, (2) melting the glass and forming a glass object during cooling, and (3) heat treating the glass article with a specific time–temperature schedule, as described in Chapter 7. The heat treatments cause controlled crystallization (devitrification) and are not just an annealing step to reduce stress. The resulting glass–ceramic objects may be fully or partially crystalline. S. Donald Stookey Corning Glass Works (7) is the first glass–ceramic inventor for his

Table 5.2 Ceramic pigments for dental porcelain or resin-based composites.

Metal pigments present as oxides	Color in porcelain or resin-based composites
Ti, Sn	white
Ce	off white
Bi	yellow
Zr-V	ochre
Zr-V-In	ochre with red tint
Zr-Si-Pr	yellow
Zn-Al-Fe-Cr	light brown
Zr-Si-Fe	red brown
Sn-Si-Ca-Cr	pink
Co-Al	blue

discovery in 1952 of a glass–ceramic containing beta-spodumene solid solution ($Li_2O.Al_2O_3.nSiO_2$) now known as Pyroceram®. This glass–ceramic was remarkable for its excellent heat resistance (thermal shock resistance) due to its low thermal expansion. His later work on glass–ceramics included lithium disilicate, which is now popular in dentistry as described in Chapter 10.

The heat treatments for glass–ceramics are performed to nucleate crystals, then grow the crystals at a higher temperature. Nucleation of tiny crystals occurs when a minor glass component causes the precipitation of the desired crystal phases; the nucleating agent lowers the thermodynamic or kinetic barriers to crystal precipitation, and many nuclei form. The crystal growth phase is performed at a higher temperature where crystals can grow faster; the presence of many nuclei make it easier to create a fine-grained glass–ceramic. A glass–ceramic usually contains more than 50% crystals by volume in a residual glass matrix. Analysis techniques, such as microscopy, differential scanning calorimetry, and X-ray diffraction (Chapter 6), are used to design of the heat treatment schedule.

Well-studied glass–ceramics have contained crystals of beta-quartz, cordierite, mica, lithium disilicate, fluorapatite/hydroxyapatite, and variations with magnesia and silica (8) (Chapters 9 and 10). The potential of lithium disilicate glass–ceramics for indirect restorative dentistry – crowns or inlays – was recognized in 1968 (9) and is important today. Lithium disilicate glass–ceramics have been modified with calcia, alumina, and zinc oxide to improve its properties and ease of manufacture. Some dental literature has misused the term glass–ceramic to refer to any glass with embedded crystals. Herein, the term glass–ceramic is reserved for glasses that are manufactured with a specific, purposeful, two-stage heat treatment to form and grow crystals and achieve unique properties; porcelain or porcelain enamel are used to denote other glass and crystal ceramics combinations.

Bioactive Glasses

Bioactive glasses embrace a range of silicate glass compositions that react in vivo to gradually form mineralized (calcium phosphate) tissue in the physiological body environment while gradually dissolving. Dr. Larry Hench (10, 11) pioneered this field; his 45S5 Bioglass® contained 45% silica, 24.5% each of soda and calcia, and 6% phosphorous pentoxide. Most bioactive glasses are based on glasses containing less than 55 weight percent silica and the other components. Magnesia has been substituted for some of the calcia in bioactive glasses for instance, $55SiO_2$–$26CaO$–$13MgO$–$6P_2O_5$, to decrease the glass solubility and slow the in vivo glass dissolution. However, the leached Mg^{+2} ions reduce the rate of forming the "bioactive" calcium phosphate layer (12). Various examples in the literature have ranges of SiO_2 (45–64%), CaO (10–37%), Na_2O (0–25%), and P_2O_5 (4–9%). Another recent silicate glass formula that promotes bone regeneration includes potassia, phosphorous pentoxide, zinc oxide, calcia, and fluoride (13).

Hench's original work was in bone or hard tissue healing, but the boron-containing bioglasses have also been investigated for soft tissue healing. Boron and fluorine (B and F) exist in the teeth and bones of the human body. Boron is present at less than 6 ppm, and fluorine is present at 21–450 ppm; they are known to be protective factors for dental caries (14). Examples of the formulas for boron-based bioglasses are given below in weight percent:

- 13-93B3: 54 B_2O_3, 6 Na_2O, 22CaO, 8 MgO, $2P_2O_5$, and $8K_2O$ (2% unknown).
- 8A3B: 50.7 B_2O_3, 4.9 Na_2O,16.4 CaO, 4.1 MgO, 3.2 P_2O_5, 9.9 K_2O, and 10.8 Al_2O_3.
- [Kuma's formula]: 8.4 B_2O_3, 45.8 CaO, and 45.8 SiO_2.

Partially crystallized bioactive glasses are available (15) having these formulas:

- Ceravital®: $(40–50)SiO_2$ $(5–10)Na_2O$–(30–35)CaO–(2.5–5.0)MgO–$(10–15)P_2O_5$–$(0.5–3)K_2O$
- Biosilicate®: $48.5SiO_2$–$23.75Na_2O$–23.75CaO–$4P_2O_5$
- Cerabone®: MgO–CaO–SiO_2–P_2O_5, and
- Bioverit®: Na_2O–MgO–CaO–Al_2O_3–SiO_2–P_2O_5–F.

Ceravital has apatite precipitates in a glass matrix. Biosilicate is an apatite-free glass-ceramic with trigonal crystals of $Na_2CaSi_2O_6$. Cerabone contains apatite and wollastonite (monocalcium silicate, $CaSiO_3$) crystals in a MgO–CaO–SiO_2–P_2O_5 glass. Wollastonite does not set with water, unlike tri/dicalcium silicates described later. It will form silanol (Si—OH) groups on its surface with water; the silanol promotes the precipitation and growth of apatite crystals on its surface (16). Bioverit has apatite and mica crystals dispersed in a glass and is "machinable." Mica represents the hydrous potassium and aluminum phyllosilicate minerals, of which there are many. Other glass-ceramic compositions have included the precipitation of fluorocanasite ($Ca_5Na_4K_2Si_{12}O_{30}F_4$) crystals or apatite-canasite for bioactivity (15). All these formulas are less soluble than the original 45S5 Bioglass; solubility influences the resorption rate of a material. In addition to bioactivity, silver and other metals have been incorporated into bioglasses to create antimicrobial characteristics (e.g. $80SiO_2$–15CaO–$5P_2O_5$–[(5–x)Ag–xCuO]) where x ranges from 0 to 5 (17). No one formula for bioactive glasses exists anymore, and bioactive glass-ceramics are undoubtedly suitable for in vivo use for hard and soft tissue healing (18).

Zirconia

Zirconia (ZrO_2), the oxide of zirconium metal (Zr), is a fascinating ceramic because of its high strength and fracture toughness relative to other ceramics. It should not be confused with zircon, which is zirconium silicate ($ZrSiO_4$), a material used in glass formulas, milling/grinding media, and semi-precious gemstone jewelry. The 20th century history of zirconia is interesting; monoclinic, baddeleyite zirconia powder is somewhat rare but is often processed from zircon sand or igneous rocks via chemical processes beginning with fusion with sodium hydroxide, followed by a hydrochloric acid wash (19). Zircon and zirconia were first used industrially as pigments; solid zirconia objects, such as refractory bricks for a furnace, could not be manufactured because pure zirconia would change crystal phases (polymorphs) as it was heated or cooled. The three phases of pure zirconia crystal – monoclinic, tetragonal, and cubic – transform and expand during firing which destroys pure zirconia's integrity. When pure zirconia is melted, it solidifies at 2680 °C and forms cubic crystals, but at 2370 °C, the cubic crystals transform into tetragonal crystals. At 1170 °C, the tetragonal crystals transform into the monoclinic phase. The phase transition from the tetragonal to monoclinic is a martensitic (sudden) phase transformation accompanied by expansion to monoclinic crystals. Monoclinic zirconia has anisotropic thermal expansion, and the transformation causes catastrophic cracking of zirconia objects being fired. This transformation is athermal; that is, the transformation temperature may be changed by the grain size and heating regimen used (20), but phase stability was impossible for pure zirconia. Still, the high (2680 °C) melting point of zirconia was very attractive as a refractory material container for manufacturing lower melting materials.

The problem of zirconia's phase changes was solved when other metal oxides were dissolved in zirconia. Calcia, magnesia, yttria, or ceria (CaO, MgO, Y_2O_3, or CeO_2) readily form solid solutions with zirconia. Less common zirconia dopants are erbia, europia, gadolinia, scandia, lanthana, and ytterbia (Er_2O_3, Eu_2O_3, Gd_2O_3, Sc_2O_3, La_2O_3, and Yb_2O_3). The additions of these stabilizing oxides are often reported in mole percent, which makes it easier to compare the additive oxides rather than weight percentages. Mole percentages are calculated by dividing the weights of the additives by the molecular weight of the stabilizing oxide, calculated with the mole percentage of zirconia (e.g. weight percentage/[123.2(g/mol)]). The stabilizing oxides affect the mechanical properties of zirconia objects. For instance, magnesia-stabilized zirconia is not as strong as yttria-stabilized zirconia in (21) where two dental materials were compared.

Addition of these oxides to zirconia is familiarly denoted as "doping" but is, more accurately, a solid solution of one oxide in another. The doping oxides lower the phase transformation temperature for the cubic to tetragonal and the tetragonal to monoclinic phases (22) because the doping ions are about twice as large in diameter as zirconia, inhibiting the transformation of the tetragonal to the monoclinic phase. For instance, the transformation temperature of tetragonal to monoclinic zirconia is reduced from 1170 °C to about 565 °C for 3-mole percent yttria in zirconia. Phase transformations are slower and less likely to occur at lower temperatures. As a result, the tetragonal phase can be kinetically stabilized, and fine-grained, doped zirconia can be manufactured with tetragonal and cubic phases that persist at room temperature. Formulas that create entirely cubic zirconia are "fully stabilized"; formulas containing cubic crystals with embedded tetragonal crystals are "partially stabilized" (PSZ); formulas with less dopant stabilize 100% tetragonal crystals, tetragonal zirconia. Fully stabilized zirconia requires higher amounts of stabilizing agents, such as 14 weight percent yttria, to achieve the presence of only the cubic phase at room temperature; 3% yttria creates tetragonal zirconia. Partially stabilized zirconia was developed first, and then methods of making purely tetragonal zirconia were developed, which proved to have greater strength and fracture toughness. The finer grains of cubic and tetragonal zirconia, smaller (finer) than 1 μm, are less likely to transform into monoclinic grains.

The phase diagrams for zirconia with three oxides are shown in Figure 5.6 to illustrate how the stabilizing oxides suppress the transformation temperatures. Yttria and ceria in zirconia reduce the transformation temperatures more than magnesia or calcia, and ceria-doped zirconia has a broader compositional range of tetragonal zirconia than yttria. Unfortunately, the ceria-doped zirconia compositions are not as strong as yttria-stabilized tetragonal zirconia. A new approach may be to dope zirconia with ceria (10%) and calcia (0.2%) to lower the firing temperature compared to yttria-stabilized zirconia (26). Also, the benefits of combination of ceria and calcia stabilizers may be higher fracture toughness, slightly lower

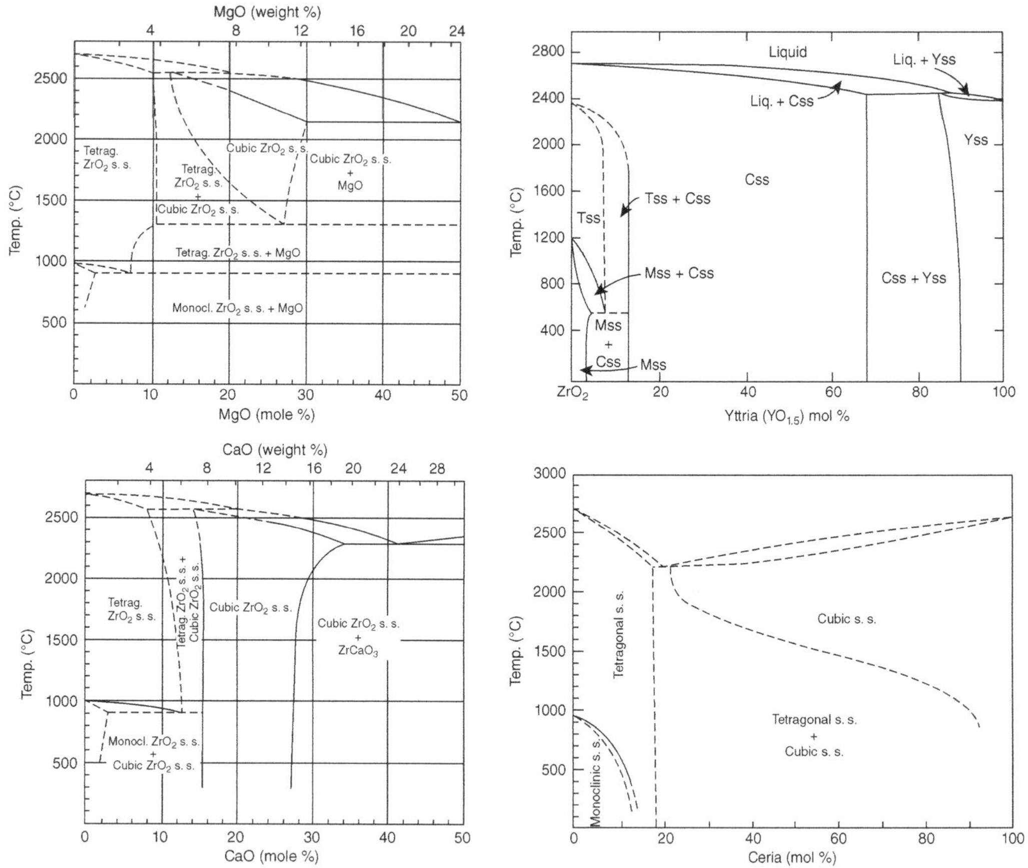

Figure 5.6 Binary phase diagrams for zirconia with four oxide dopants from (23–25). Yttria ($YO_{1.5}$) [https://archive.org/details/basicsolidstatec0000west_k0q9/page/290/mode/2up?q=yttria] reduces the tetragonal to monoclinic transformation temperature more than magnesia, ceria or calcia. Note the difference in scale on the left and the right. SS indicates solid solution; C, M, and T indicate cubic, monoclinic, and tetragonal crystals.

hardness, and greater hydrothermal resistance without loss of flexural strength or translucency. When an excess of the stabilizing oxides is included, the dopant oxides may be present as a separate phase of MgO, CaO, or Y_2O_3 or as mixed metal oxide compounds such as $CaZr_4O_9$; these extra phases are not optimal for strength.

When tetragonal zirconia crystals is stressed, tetragonal grains at a crack tip will transform into the larger monoclinic grains; the larger grains arrest the crack's propagation by compression and close the crack. The propagation of the monoclinic phase is stopped at the grain boundaries, and the crack does not propagate; this is the essence of transformation toughening. The technique of Raman spectroscopy – using a laser to detect characteristic vibrational modes of materials – has provided evidence that this phase transformation does occur on fracture surfaces (27), confirming the theory of the tetragonal zirconia's strength and fracture toughness. Although the monoclinic to tetragonal phase change is reversible (monoclinic to tetragonal) on heating, the near-room temperature uses of zirconia in dentistry or other biomedical uses are unlikely to cause the spontaneous reversal to tetragonal crystals. Small grains do not convert as easily as larger ones; hence, fine-grained ($<5\,\mu m$) tetragonal zirconia is preferred over larger cubic grains.

Yttria has become the favored solute for tetragonal zirconia (YZP) because it lowers the transformation temperature more than the other common stabilizing dopants. Plus, YZP materials have a higher bend strength and fracture toughness than other ceramics. Strength, fracture toughness and appearance have vaulted the YZP material into the pantheon of ceramics for dentistry and other fields. Yttria-stabilized tetragonal zirconia and partially stabilized zirconia enjoy many commercial uses as hip implants and dental restorations (Chapter 10) and dental implants (Chapter 16).

Doped zirconia powders are made by co-precipitation techniques such as mixing yttrium chloride with zirconium oxychloride or zirconium chloride (YCl_3, $ZrOCl_2$, $ZrCl_4$) solutions. The precipitation of the doped powder is completed by heating (acidic) or alkoxide hydrolysis (alkaline) methods. The powders are filtered, dried, pulverized, calcined at about 850 °C, milled, and spray-dried to form flowing porous granules of powder particles for processing into a solid. Granules are dry pressed by manufacturers into a "green body" by uniaxial or cold-isostatic pressing (22). Some zirconia products for dental restoration have layers of 3%, 4%, and 5% yttria (see Chapter 10); successive uniaxial pressing is believed to be used to form the layered powder compacts. These compacted powders are then partially sintered to create ingots or pucks that can be shaped via CAD-CAM designing and milling performed by a dental laboratory. Most zirconia dental restoratives are made by CAD-CAM milling partially sintered zirconia. This clever approach has enabled dental laboratories to easily machine oversized crowns and bridges that undergo final sintering and shrinkage before they are sent to a dentist to be affixed (cemented) in the mouth. The same method is used to make zirconia dental implants or abutments except then the manufacturer performs the final, full sintering for the dentist.

Cubic zirconia is used for coatings, windows, lenses, prisms, and filters. The cubic zirconia phase is rare as a mineral, but large crystals have been made synthetically since the 1960s. Single crystals of cubic zirconia are a popular, lower-cost alternative to diamonds in jewelry because, like diamond, they are cubic, have a similar high index of refraction (2.15–2.18 vs. 2.42) and similar dispersion of wavelength (0.058–0.066 vs. 0.044) contributing to the sparkle of cubic zirconia's gems, making them as pleasing as a diamond. However, the cubic phase of zirconia is slightly less hard than diamond (8–8.5 vs. 10 on the Mohs scale); it can be distinguished from diamond because it is a poorer conductor of heat. Plasma-sprayed zirconia coatings are good thermal barriers (thermally insulating) yet have a high enough thermal expansion to match some metals and not spall (detach). Partially stabilized (tetragonal and cubic) or fully cubic crystals may be present in such coatings. Various other industrial uses are common, including solid electrolytes and oxygen sensors.

Zirconia has been pigmented with trace metal oxides dissolved in the grains, as listed in Table 5.3. These colorant oxides are useful for dental materials and artificial cubic zirconia gemstones.

Table 5.3 Pigments used in zirconia.

Metal present as oxide	Color(s) in zirconia
Cerium	Yellow-orange-red
Chromium	Green
Cobalt	Lilac, violet, blue
Copper	Yellow-aqua
Erbium	Pink
Europium	Pink
Iron	Yellow
Holmium	Pink "champagne"
Manganese	Brown-violet
Neodymium	Purple
Nickel	Yellow brown
Praseodymium	Amber
Thulium	Yellow brown
Titanium	Golden brown
Vanadium	Green

Zircon and zirconia are always accompanied by about 5% hafnia (HfO_2), which is not a phase stabilizer; hafnia is inherent in mineral sources of zirconia. Hafnia is very difficult to segregate from zirconia because, oddly, these two metals have very similar sizes despite the differences in atomic numbers (40 and 72). The heavier hafnia imparts a modicum of greater radiopacity to zirconia. An interesting aspect of the hafnium metal is that it has six isotopes, of which one (^{174}Hf) is a mild alpha-particle emitter (radioactive) (28). Hence, no zirconia is without some radioactivity.

Calcium Compounds

Many calcium compounds are used in dentistry, such as calcium hydroxide, calcium sulfate, calcium silicate cement, calcium aluminate cement, and calcium phosphate cement. Calcium hydroxide is an important antimicrobial material because it has slight solubility in water, where it releases calcium and hydroxide ions, making a solution alkaline (high pH). In the body, the concurrent release of these two ions creates bioactive and antimicrobial reactions beneficial for vital pulp therapy and endodontic procedures, as discussed in Chapter 8. Calcium hydroxide powder is used as a filler in some dental materials; over time, the particles gradually form inert calcium carbonate ($CaCO_3$), which is another filler that has some dental applicability.

Calcium Sulfate

Calcium sulfate ($CaSO_4$) and its related hydrates are minerals with a multitude of important uses in the construction, food, and dental industries. The hemihydrate is known as plaster of Paris or bassanite ($CaSO_4.½H_2O$); its degree of hydration varies somewhat, $CaSO_4.(0.5–0.8)H_2O$. Plaster of Paris is mixed with water to form gypsum, the dihydrate ($CaSO_4.2H_2O$), which has been essential for dental models (Chapter 14), alginate impression material, implantation, and other historical uses. The reversible, partial, and complete dehydration reactions are in Eq. (5.1):

$$\begin{array}{lllll} CaSO_4.2H_2O & \rightarrow CaSO_4.\tfrac{1}{2}H_2O + 1.5H_2O & \rightarrow CaSO_4 & + \tfrac{1}{2}H_2O & \\ \text{Gypsum} & \rightarrow \text{plaster of Paris} + \text{water} & \rightarrow \text{anhydrite} + \text{water} & & (5.1) \\ & 100-150\ ^\circ C & \sim 170\ ^\circ C & & \end{array}$$

The relatively low temperatures (<200 °C) and reversibility of these reactions make calcium sulfate very useful. For instance, calcium sulfate mitigates rapid hardening in other materials, such as alginate, to slow its setting time. All calcium sulfate compounds are poorly soluble in water, which is useful for some dental products discussed in Chapter 14. The γ-anhydrite of $CaSO_4$ is an important desiccant.

Calcium Silica/Aluminate Cements

Calcium silicate cements (Portland cement) are the literal foundation for our modern infrastructure; Portland cement is a multi-component calcium silicate cement for construction of buildings, roads, and industrial facilities. Tricalcium aluminate is a component in calcium silicate cement; other calcium aluminate compounds have important refractory and sanitation purposes. Both calcium silicate and aluminate cements react with water at room temperature to react/harden into a solid mass (set). Such cement products have been called hydrophilic and hydraulic, although neither term is precise. Hydrophilic only connotes the attraction to water or the ability to dissolve in water. Hydraulic has two definitions: needing water to set, and exerting uniform pressure (by a fluid, not necessarily water). Surprisingly, these water-setting calcium cements are bioactive and have become very important in the past three decades for endodontic therapy, including pediatric dentistry – see Chapter 8. Notably, one calcium silicate phase (wollastonite, $CaSiO_3$) is not hydraulic; it does not react with water although it has peripheral uses as a dental bioceramic in a magnesia-based cement containing monopotassium phosphate (KH_2PO_4) and magnesia (MgO) (29).

These calcium cements are composed of multiple ceramic phases (crystal compounds). Calcium silicate cements are primarily powders of tricalcium silicate (alite, $3CaO.SiO_2$, or Ca_3SiO_5) and dicalcium silicate (belite, Ca_2SiO_4, or $2CaO.SiO_2$) with minor amounts of tricalcium aluminate and calcium-alumino-ferrite. Calcium sulfate compounds are a common additive to calcium silicate cements to control the setting time. Calcium aluminate cement powders are mainly composed of calcium monoaluminate ($CaAl_2O_4$ or $CaO.Al_2O_3$). Some calcium such cements contain excess alumina, which is advantageous for refractory (high temperature) furnaces walls and for lining some waste waterlines; minor amounts of other calcium aluminate phases may also be present. The setting reactions with water for the five main phases of the calcium cements are described below. Of the cement phases, tricalcium aluminate sets the fastest, via Eq. (5.2):

$$\begin{array}{ll} 3CaO.Al_2O_3 & +6H_2O \rightarrow 3CaO.Al_2O_3.6H_2O \\ \text{Tricalcium aluminate} + & \text{water} \rightarrow \text{amorphous, hydrated tricalcium aluminate} \end{array} \tag{5.2}$$

The reaction product is a hard, hydrated gel of calcium aluminate. The rapid hydration of the tricalcium aluminate phase accelerates the apparent setting of calcium silicate cement; therefore, some cements intentionally use higher or lower tricalcium aluminate contents (30). When tricalcium aluminate hydrates, it releases heat to cause evaporation of the water needed for hydrating the other phases, which is a reason its presence is controlled in large-scale use of calcium silicate cement. Calcium sulfate is added to react with the tricalcium aluminate and water to form the intermediate products of ettringite ($Ca_3Al_2O_6.3CaSO_4.32H_2O$) or calcium monosulfate ($Ca_3Al_2O_6.CaSO_4.12H_2O$), producing less heat to slows the setting. To transport and pour concrete, the heat of the setting reaction should be minimal. The newer dental cements described in Chapter 8 don't have such constraints and contain rapid-setting cement phases.

The calcium-alumino-ferrite cement phase also undergoes rapid hydration – Eq. (5.3). The reaction products include a hard, hydrated cement product with calcia and alumina and release iron hydroxide into the matrix surrounding the cement particles:

$$\underset{\text{Tetracalcium aluminoferrite + water}}{4CaO.Al_2O_3.Fe_2O_3 + 19H_2O} \rightarrow \underset{\text{amorphous hydrated ferrite}}{2\left[2CaO.Al_2O_3.8H_2O\right]} + \underset{\text{iron oxide hydrate}}{2Fe(OH)_3} \quad (5.3)$$

Calcium sulfate and calcium oxide are added to calcium silicate cements to mitigate the fast setting of the ferrite cement phase in a similar fashion that is used to slow the hydration of tricalcium aluminate. The ferrite cement phase can form several calcium-alumino-ferric-sulfate hydrates, such as $Ca_2(Al,Fe)_2O_5$, $3CaO.(0.5Al_2O_3.0.5Fe_2O_3).3CaSO_4.32H_2O$, or $4CaO.Al_2O_3.Fe_2O_3$ (31). The ferrite cement phase is black, so its use has been limited in dentistry; no benefit has been reported for its presence in endodontic products.

Eqs. (5.4) and (5.5) for tricalcium silicate (alite) and dicalcium silicate (belite) show the hydration setting reactions for the main calcium silicate cement phases:

$$\underset{\text{Tricalcium silicate + water}}{2\left[Ca_3SiO_5\right] + 7H_2O} \rightarrow \underset{\text{amorphous calcium silicate hydrate}}{3CaO.2SiO_2.4H_2O} + \underset{\text{calcium hydroxide}}{3Ca(OH)_2} \quad (5.4)$$

$$\underset{\text{Dicalcium silicate + water}}{2\left[Ca_2SiO_4\right] + 5H_2O} \rightarrow \underset{\text{amorphous calcium silicate hydrate}}{3CaO.2SiO_2.4H_2O} + \underset{\text{calcium hydroxide}}{Ca(OH)_2} \quad (5.5)$$

These calcium silicate particles react to form a hard, amorphous, hydrated calcium silicate matrix, $3CaO.2SiO_2.4H_2O$, concurrently releasing calcium hydroxide into the matrix. Calcium hydroxide is denoted as Portlandite in the cement literature and occasionally in the dental literature (32), which can confuse dentists unfamiliar with the term Portlandite versus calcium hydroxide. Setting times of the calcium silicate cements may vary from minutes to hours, depending on the phases present. After mixing with water and a brief induction period, hydration of tricalcium silicate begins. Dicalcium silicate crystals hydrate more slowly and gradually fill in the porosity of the cement over about four weeks; most of the cement's strength is developed in less than a week.

The two common calcium aluminate cement phases, calcium monoaluminate ($CaO.Al_2O_3$) and monocalcium dialuminate ($CaO.2Al_2O_3$), have interesting hydration reactions that vary with temperature (33). The hydration reactions that occur at body temperature (~37 °C) for the calcium aluminate ($CaO.Al_2O_3$) and monocalcium dialuminate ($CaO.2Al_2O_3$) cement phases are expressed in Eqs. (5.6) and (5.7):

$$\underset{\text{Calcium monoaluminate + water}}{3\left[CaO.Al_2O_3\right] + 12H_2O} \rightarrow \underset{\text{amorphous Ca-aluminate hydrate + aluminum hydroxide}}{3(CaO).Al_2O_3.6(H_2O) + 2\left[Al_2O_3.3H_2O\right]} \tag{5.6}$$

$$\underset{\text{Monocalcium dialuminate + water}}{3\left[CaO(Al_2O_3)_2\right] + 21H_2O} \rightarrow \underset{\text{amorphous Ca-aluminate hydrate + aluminum hydroxide}}{3(CaO).Al_2O_3.6(H_2O) + 5\left[Al_2O_3.3H_2O\right]} \tag{5.7}$$

The hydrated calcium aluminate phases create a high pH matrix with aluminum hydrate during setting, but these reactions are not as exothermic as the tricalcium aluminate hydration.

Pozzolanic cement, known as Roman cement, is based on the reaction of calcium hydroxide or calcia (CaO) with silica and water to harden with a hydrated calcium silicate phase. The hydration (setting) reaction is in Eq. (5.8), where the proportions of the hydrated calcium silicate are indefinite (m, x, and n). The pozzolanic reaction products differ from those of the tri/dicalcium silicates. Alumina, if present, may also participate in hydration:

$$\begin{array}{l} SiO_2 + Ca(OH)_2 + mH_2O \rightarrow (CaO)_x SiO_2.nH_2O \\ \text{Silica + calcium hydroxide + water} \rightarrow \text{hydrated calcium silicate} \end{array} \tag{5.8}$$

Tri/dicalcium silicate cement supplanted pozzolanic cement in the 1800s because Roman cement formulas did not have as high a strength as the calcium silicate cements. However, many pozzolanic cement structures have endured. Pozzolanic cements are being blended in as additives to Portland cements to reduce the production of carbon dioxide, a major contributor worldwide to greenhouse gas emissions. Portland cement is manufactured by blending silica and alumina with calcium carbonate. The powder mixture is heated, and the calcium carbonate decomposes and releases carbon dioxide; at higher temperatures, the calcia and silica/alumina react to form the cement phases described above. When less tri/dicalcium silicate (Portland) content can be used in cements, less carbon dioxide is emitted (34) per kilogram.

All three cements, calcium aluminate, calcium silicate, and pozzolanic, harden by partial dissolution and precipitation of hydrates on the particles' surfaces and have been used in endodontic products (see Chapter 8).

Impurities are present in industrial Portland-type calcium silicate cement for construction (35). Water-setting dental cements are prohibited from being having impurities such as acid-soluble arsenic or lead present at more than 2 or 100 ppm, respectively per ISO 9917-1.

Calcium Phosphates

Calcium phosphate was recognized as the mineral compound in bones in the 18th century (36, 37), and in the 20th century, in vivo mineralization (hydroxyapatite precipitation) was recognized to occur. Many calcium phosphate compounds exist with varied calcium-to-phosphorous atomic ratios and solubilities, as noted in Table 5.4 (39–41). Calcium phosphate compounds have been used as bone grafts (42), in toothpastes (43), and to coat implants (44, 45) – coatings usually made usually by plasma-spraying. Research has been conducted on the suitability of many calcium phosphates for dental materials.

Calcium phosphate cements invented by Lawrence Chow (46) are self-setting bioactive ceramics; the set cement contains hydroxyapatite. His original cement was a reaction of equimolar tetracalcium phosphate (TTCP) and dicalcium phosphate, as in Eq. (5.10):

Table 5.4 Calcium phosphate compounds.

Ca/P	Compound (abbreviation)	Formula	Density (g/cm³)	pH stability range*
0.5	Monocalcium phosphate monohydrate (MCPM)	$Ca(H_2PO_4)_2.H_2O$	2.23	0.0–2.0
0.5	Monocalcium phosphate anhydrate (MCPA)	$Ca(H_2PO_4)_2$	2.58	
1.0	Dicalcium phosphate dihydrate (DCPD, brushite)	$CaHPO_4.H_2O$	2.32	2.0–6.0
1.0	Dicalcium phosphate anhydrate (DCPA, monetite)	$CaHPO_4$	2.89	
1.0	Calcium pyrophosphate (pyro)	$Ca_2P_2O_7$		
1.33	Octacalcium phosphate (OCP)	$Ca_8(HPO_4)_2(PO_4)_4.5H_2O$	2.61	5.5–7.0
1.5	α-tricalcium phosphate (α-TCP)	α -$Ca_3(PO_4)_2$	2.86	
1.5	β-tricalcium phosphate (β-TCP)	β -$Ca_3(PO_4)_2$	3.07	
1.2–2.2	Amorphous calcium phosphate (ACP)	$Ca_x(PO_4)y.nH_2O$		
1.5–1.67	Calcium-deficient hydroxyapatite (CDHA)	$Ca_{10-x}(HPO_4)_x(PO_4)_{6-x}(OH)_{2-x}(0<x<1)$		6.5–9.5
1.67	Hydroxyapatite (HA or HAp)	$Ca_{10}(PO_4)_6(OH)_2$ $Ca_5(PO_4)_3(OH)$	3.15	9.5–12
2.0	Tetracalcium phosphate (TTCP)	$Ca_4(PO_4)_2O$	3.05	

Source: (38) / IntechOpen / CC BY 3.0.
* @ 25 °C.

$$\underset{\text{tetra-Ca phosphate}}{Ca_4(PO_4)_2O} + \underset{\text{dicalcium phosphate}}{CaHPO_4} \rightarrow \underset{\text{hydroxyapatite}}{Ca_5(PO_4)_3OH} \tag{5.9}$$

Dry dicalcium phosphate powders are blended with TTCP, desiccated for storage, and then mixed with water for immediate application; the dicalcium phosphate dihydrate gradually hydrates forming a brushite layer and precipitates amorphous calcium phosphate.

Tetracalcium phosphate powder is created by sintering dicalcium phosphate with calcium carbonate at 1200–1500 °C (Eq. (5.10)), and then pulverized:

$$\underset{\text{dicalcium phosphate}}{2CaHPO_4} + \underset{\text{calcium carbonate}}{2CaCO_3} \rightarrow \underset{\text{tetra-Ca phosphate}}{Ca_4(PO_4)_2O} + \underset{\text{water \& } CO_2}{H_2O + 2CO_2} \tag{5.10}$$

Setting takes about 20 minutes (Eq. (5.9)) but can be accelerated by adding disodium hydrogen phosphate (Na_2HPO_4) or sodium dihydrogen phosphate (NaH_2PO_4) to the water. Like most ceramics, calcium phosphate cement is stronger in compression (~20 MPa) than in tension. Biomineralizing/bioactive magnesium phosphate cements (47–49) are similarly formed; these cements form HA but are generally slow to set and weaker than the equivalent calcium cements.

Radiopaque Ceramics

Radiopaque powders are frequently included to dental materials, so an X-ray image of it will be distinctly whiter than the surrounding soft and hard tissues. Preferably, radiopaque materials contain metals with an atomic number greater than 40 to absorb more X-rays than calcium. Radiopaque materials are frequently bioinert metal compounds, such as barium sulfate ($BaSO_4$); not barium oxide (BaO) which is not biocompatible. Bismuth oxide, urania, terbia, and other rare earth oxides are used for radiopacity, and some are included for fluorescence. Gold and tungsten metal powders and the common radiopaque ceramics listed in Table 5.5 are used for radiopacity. Some glasses are made radiopaque by including strontium oxide or BaO in their formula (50–53) and strontium silicate cements are being tested for using more radiopaque constituents (54–58).

The use of the "heavy metal" compounds can be disturbing to some who assume, erroneously, that all heavy metals are toxic. As mentioned, certain metals are not used in dental glasses; however, lead dioxide is used in polysulfide impression materials (Chapter 14). This highlights the complexity of biocompatibility testing, invention, and medical device product development.

Table 5.5 Radiopaque compounds used in dental materials.

Atomic weight of metals in enamel mineral	Metal	Compounds
31	P, in Hydroxyapatite	$Ca_5(PO_4)_3OH$
40	Ca, in Hydroxyapatite	
Atomic weight of metal	Oxide	Non-oxide radiopaque fillers
48	Titania	
55	Manganese oxide	
56	Iron oxide	
88	Strontia	
89	Yttria	
91	Zirconia	
93	Niobia	
108		Gold
119	Tin oxide	
127		Iodoform, CHI_3
137	—	Barium sulfate
139	Lanthana	
173	—	Ytterbium fluoride
178	Hafnia	
181	Tantalite	
184	Calcium tungstate	Tungsten
209	Bismite	
140	Ceria	

Ceramic Pigments

White, inert ceramic powders are often included in dental products to control their color and opacity and include alumina, titania, tin oxide, ceria, zirconia, and zinc oxide. Yellow and orange pigments are also needed such as iron oxide, iron hydroxide, and praseodymium-zirconia. Pink pigments may contain oxides of manganese, vanadium, or praseodymium. Blue tints are created by oxides of cobalt or vanadium-zirconium. Gray pigments are also needed, which are a combination of oxide powders of zirconium, cobalt, iron, chromium, and vanadium, as well as solid solutions of the spinel compounds – $MgFe_2O_4$, $MnFe_2O_4$,

$CoCr_2O_4$, or $(Mg,Ni)_2MnO_4$, combined with a small amount of tin oxide, SnO_2 (59). The average particle size for pigments is less than 10 μm for these pigments which are dispersed in resins (Chapter 9). Nanoparticles such as silica or silica/zirconia clusters may be added to impart opalescence (US Pat. 8,722,759B2) in composite (resin-based restoratives). Ceramic pigments used in dentistry should have an aggregate content of lead, arsenic, and antimony oxides less than 300 ppm.

These same oxides may be dissolved in ceramic crown and bridge materials of zirconia, lithium disilicate, and dental porcelain (Chapter 10). For instance, in US 2022/0273404 Al, a zirconia or zirconia/alumina dental milling block composition contains minute proportions (less than 1%) of dissolved oxides of these metals: Bi, Ce, Co, Cr, Cu, Er, Eu, Fe, Ho, Mn, Nd, Ni, Pr, Tb, V, Yb, and Zn. Depending on the dopant in the zirconia, the color will change.

Common Ceramic Filler Powders

In addition to pigmentation, ceramic powders are used in a myriad of materials as fillers to thicken liquids or monomers. Fillers are essential for dental resin-based composites, as described in Chapter 9, but many other dental product require ceramic powders. Common fillers are cristobalite (crystalline silica), fumed silica, calcium carbonate, titania (SiO_2, $CaCO_3$, and TiO_2), zeolites and clays are also used. Zeolites are volcanic minerals that have reacted with alkaline groundwater to create microporous, crystalline, aluminosilicate materials of the general formula $M^{n+}{}_{1/n}(AlO_2)^-(SiO_2)_x.yH_2O$, where $M^{n+}{}_{1/n}$ is commonly Na or H; the Si to Al ratio is variable. An example is natrolite, $Na_2Al_2Si_3O_{10}.2H_2O$. Other zeolite minerals are analcime, chabazite, clinoptilolite, heulandite, natrolite, phillipsite, and stilbite. The fine pore size, typically 0.3–0.8 nm, makes zeolites excellent absorbents.

Clay minerals are naturally-occurring, ceramic hydrous aluminum phyllosilicates. A common example is kaolin, $Al_2Si_2O_5(OH)_4$, $Al_2O_3.2SiO_2.2H_2O$. Clays are formed by the deterioration of silicate-bearing minerals – granite – by water, the atmosphere, sunlight, and biological organisms over millions of years. Clays often contain variable amounts of iron, magnesium, alkali metals, and alkaline earths. The clays are classified as kaolinite, montmorillonite-smectite, or illite; all are absorbent, but some clays expand with water. Hydrous kaolin, or "China clay," has fine particles with a plate-like or lamellar shape. Metakaolin is manufactured by calcinating kaolin at 500–700 °C to form a semi-amorphous, layered, whiter powder with pores that will react with calcium hydroxide to harden (set), a pozzolanic reaction. Ball clay, "plastic clay," is a less common mineral composed of 20–80% kaolinite, 10–25% mica, 6–65% quartz, and some organic matter. Halloysite, a subset of kaolin clay, has nanopores in the form of tubes for liquid absorption (60), which can be helpful for thickening and stabilizing liquids and pastes. Bentonite is a soft plastic smectite clay containing montmorillonite, a fine particle hydrous aluminum silicate, which expands with water, creating a gelatinous and viscous substance. The illite clays – hydromica or hydromuscovite – do not expand with water; they are known for their higher potassia content than others: $(K,H_3O)(Al,Mg,Fe)_2(Si,Al)_4O_{10}[(OH)_2.(H_2O)]$. Minor amounts of clays are used in dental materials; their presence is not customarily disclosed because of trade secrets, their minor percentages, and the commonly accepted biocompatibility of clays. Clays' expansion, or lack thereof, can be used to advantage in dental materials during interoral setting.

Zinc Oxide

Zinc oxide (ZnO) powder has age-old and abundant uses in products as a fine, white powder. The economic industrial manufacture of the powder was perfected in the 1800s to exploit its benefits. It is used for cosmetics, rubber, polymers, ceramics, glass, lubricants, paints/pigments, sunscreens, ointments, adhesives, sealing materials, foods, batteries, ferrites, fire retardants, semiconductors, first-aid products, and dental materials, with the benefit of an antibacterial attribute.

Several dental materials were developed based on reactions of zinc oxide with a liquid, where the objective was to create a hard restorative material or to cement a crown on a tooth. Zinc oxychloride dental material was based on the aqueous reaction between ZnO and an acidified $ZnCl_2$ solution as in Eqs. (5.11) or (5.12) (61) that depends on the proportions and reactivity of the ZnO powder. Though insoluble in water, zinc oxide will react with phosphoric acid to form hopeite ($Zn_3(PO_4)_2.4H_2O$) in Eq. (5.13). Zinc oxide powder is sparingly soluble in water, forming zinc hydroxide (Eq. (5.14)); the hydroxide reacts with eugenol ($C_{10}H_{12}O_2$, oil of cloves) to form zinc-eugenolate ($ZnC_{22}H_{24}O_8$) as per Eq. (5.15). The zinc oxide-eugenol materials remain in today's dental armamentarium as a pulp medicament and a popular, inexpensive root canal sealer (Chapter 8). Similar cements can be made with magnesium oxide (62):

$$4ZnO + ZnCl_2 + 5H_2O \rightarrow 4ZnO.ZnCl_2.5H_2O \quad (5.11)$$

$$ZnO + ZnCl_2 + 3H_2O \rightarrow ZnO.ZnCl.3H_2O \quad (5.12)$$

$$3ZnO + 2H_3(PO_4) + H_2O \rightarrow Zn_3(PO_4)_2.4H_2O \quad (5.13)$$

$$ZnO + H_2O \rightarrow Zn(OH)_2 \quad (5.14)$$

$$Zn(OH)_2 + 2C_{10}H_{12}O_2 \rightarrow Zn(C_{10}H_{12}O_2)_2 + H_2O \quad (5.15)$$

Zinc oxide reacts also with polyacrylic acid, forming zinc acrylate, $ZnC_6H_6O_4$; this reaction is the basis for zinc oxide-polycarboxylate cement. Zinc ions have other benefits, such as reducing the enamel's solubility by acting as an inhibitor of matrix metalloproteinases (MMPs). Zinc ions are easily incorporated into apatite, replacing some calcium ions to protect the enamel from acidic carious damage (63).

Miscellaneous Ceramics

Loosely speaking, atomic carbon is a ceramic because it is not part of a methyl group. The graphite form of carbon is a sheet-like insulator used in some furnaces and also available as a powder; the powder has been used in (less popular) toothpastes (Chapter 14) for abrasion of plaque, even though it is dark gray. The graphene films of carbon are a current material of dental interest (64–67) being the thinnest, strongest, and stiffest material known. Graphene, unlike graphite, is a single atomic carbon layer with a honeycomb form, incorporating some carboxylic (COOH) and hydroxide (OH) groups in the layer. Graphene films have been created by liquid phase exfoliation, mechanical exfoliation (higher quality), and most practically by chemical vapor deposition, CVD. These thin coatings have been applied to metals, ceramics, and polymers to enhance mechanical properties, impart greater in vivo mineralization potential, create an antibiofilm and corrosion-resistant layer on metals, or deliver drugs. A prime area for future graphene coatings is titanium implants; implants are integrated in surrounding bone more slowly than desired and have a high potential for deleterious biofilm formation, which graphene may alleviate. Hexagonal borophene nanoparticles or films, similar to graphene, may similarly have a role in implants or instrument coatings (68).

The diamond form of carbon is used as an abrasive in countless industries because of its supreme hardness. Diamond particles are used rotating dental instruments and in some pastes for shaping and polishing teeth and restorations. Tungsten carbide (WC) is another important dental abrasive used for rotating dental instruments and is usually bonded to a mandrel with cobalt metal via liquid phase sintering. Silicon carbide is also a common abrasive for shaping and smoothing in dentistry. Ceramic abrasives for dentistry are discussed in Chapter 17.

Molybdenum disulfide (MoS_2) ceramic has been used as a dry lubricant and as a coating because of its low friction. This sulfide has other uses as a high-temperature heating element for sintering ceramics and in catalysis reactions and electronics, such as switchable transistors and photodetectors.

Diverse inorganic salts are used in dentistry. Some salts are used in water or organic liquid solutions, and others are powders dispersed in resins. They are embraced here because they are inorganic and non-metallic, as ceramics were defined.

Many ceramics are essential for electronic equipment in dentistry. Some oxides offer high electrical resistance and insulation for circuit boards; alumina, beryllium oxide, and aluminum nitride (Al_2O_3, BeO, and AlN) are often used. Ceramics with high dielectric constants are used to create capacitors; the titanates of barium and strontium ($BaTiO_3$, $SrTiO_3$) and lead zirconate titanate (PZT) are necessary. Ferrites (e.g. $BaFe_{12}O_{19}$ and $PbFe_{12}O_{10}$) are magnetic ceramics in high-fidelity speakers and small electric motors, magnetic field detectors, recording devices, computer discs, generators, and video recorders, among other applications. Piezoelectric ceramics are used for transducers, sensors, microphones, and loudspeakers. The titanates demonstrate the piezoelectric behavior. Semiconductors are the backbone of electronics and rely on silicon metal, a semi-metal ceramic. Varistors and thermistors are well-known examples of semiconductor ceramics, as are SiC, $MoSi_2$, and Cu_2O; varistors contain ZnO for temperature sensors, temperature compensators, infrared sensors, switches, and heating systems. All these items are likely to have invisibly located in the electronics of a dental office.

Lasing Ceramics

Dentistry is benefiting from lasers and this section describes laser evolution, with emphasis on ceramics that "lase." Later the dental lasers are discussed (Chapter 18). Laser is an acronym for Light Amplification by Stimulated Emission of Radiation, a phenomenon that occurs when electrons are excited in optical materials like glass, crystal, or gas. Laser light is unlike ambient visible light, which is comprised of multiple wavelengths (colors) and is incoherent; that is, visible light propagates in multiple directions. The light from a laser is coherent meaning the emitted photons have the same (or nearly identical) wavelength and direction. The material determines the wavelength of the laser light. Laser beams stay sharply focused over vast distances, even to the moon and back. Helium–neon gas lasers or liquid dye lasers may operate continuously; others, such as ruby lasers, emit brief pulses of light. No other light-emitting source can generate light pulses as brief as a laser, less than 10^{-16} seconds.

A laser relies on the quantum properties of atoms that absorb energy from an electrical current or a light, causing an electron in the material to be energized and move from a lower-energy atomic orbit to a higher-energy orbit, and then return to its standard orbit and emit photons. Semi-reflective mirrors on the ends of the laser's optical material are usually used to reflect the stimulated photons back and forth in the space between the mirrors, the "cavity." The reflected photons create more photons, moving in the same direction and speed amplifying the photons until enough are present to be transmitted past the mirrors in unison in a focused fashion. An excimer (excited dimer gas) laser may create a beam that passes through the lasing medium with only one pass. Some laser materials can produce more than one wavelength and can be "tuned." Not all lasers emit visible light, infrared lasers being an example.

The first laser was demonstrated in 1960 based on chromium-doped, sapphire crystals, which had been polished to perfection; many more ceramics have since been used to "lase". In 1964, a laser was made from polycrystalline, dysprosium-calcium fluoride, $Dy^{2+}:CaF_2$. This laser was limited because it only "lased" below liquid nitrogen temperature, and CaO scattering centers limited the laser performance. Fluoride ceramic lasers have been based on polycrystalline LiF with submicron grains, hot pressed at 600 °C. In the 1970s, a laser was developed based on Yttralox® ceramic (89% Y_2O_3 – 10% ThO_2 – 1% Nd_2O_3), using submicron powders ($\leq$0.1 μm) co-precipitated from the oxalates of yttrium, thorium, and neodymium. The powder was sintered under hydrogen gas at 2170 °C. The thoria was used to control the grain growth of the yttria; even so, the large grains (~130 μm) and high scattering losses caused by inhomogeneities led to low efficiency. This inefficient yttria-based laser was superseded by the yttrium-aluminum-garnet (YAG) lasers based on $Y_3Al_5O_{12}$, fabricated via the intermediate $Y_4Al_2O_9$ and $YAlO_3$ phases. The YAG ceramic doped with 1.1 at.% neodymia (Nd:YAG) was developed (1995) from pure, submicron oxide powders with low impurities, densified via vacuum sintering. Processing subtleties included using 320 ppm SiO_2 as a sintering aid, ball milling with high-purity alumina balls, spray drying the powders, and sintering at 1700 °C, followed by rapid cooling to get the YAG phase ($Y_3Al_5O_{12}$), not the $Y_4Al_2O_9$ and $YAlO_3$ phases. The efficiency of the Nd:YAG laser was better than that of earlier ones, even single crystals. The polycrystalline YAG ceramic was refined in its manufacture to be almost as powerful as a single crystal laser of the same composition. Pulsed lasers were developed with a Nd:YSAG (yttrium scandium aluminum garnet) ceramic.

High-power lasers need high thermal conductivity. Lutetium oxide, scandia, and yttria sesquioxides (Lu_2O_3, Sc_2O_3, and Y_2O_3) possess higher thermal conductivities than YAG (69); hence, oxide laser compositions have included 10–20% Yb_2O_3; Y_2O_3 with 2.5% Yb_2O_3; and Sc_2O_3 with 1.8% Yb_2O_3. The lutetium and ytterbium ions have very similar ionic radii and bonding forces; therefore, the ytterbium ion can easily substitute for a lutetium ion without the overall thermal conductivity being affected. The power of such lasers has increased from one to one hundred kilowatts. Non-oxide lasers have included Ca/SrF_2 (65/35) with 5% Yb_2O_3 (70).

The early performance of ceramic laser materials was hindered by composition variability, contamination from melting the ceramic in a crucible, phase transitions, and difficulties in dissolving rare earth metals in the ceramic crystals. New ceramic formulas and advances in powder synthesis and sintering methods have contributed to higher-quality lasers. Lower temperature synthesis methods have been useful in making transparent polycrystalline lasing ceramics to replace the difficult-to-cast single crystals. However, the grain boundaries must be free of pores and impurities to create strong, tough, and effective laser materials. Layered lasers have been made in disk shapes or a core with a different cylindrical exterior, to tailor the output (69) based on rare-earth-doped ceramics. Some lasers combine materials to create unique outputs, such as the KTP solid-state laser, which combines a neodymium:yttrium aluminum garnet (Nd: YAG) laser with potassium titanyl phosphate ($K[TiO]PO_4$, KTP) crystal for "frequency doubling" to produce a green laser with a wavelength of 532 nm. Today, lasers are used in industrial manufacturing, microelectronics, and biomedical applications with diverse and unique capabilities including dentistry as discussed in Chapter 18.

The pertinent parameters for lasers are output energy (power), wavelengths, exposure duration, and cross-sectional area of the laser beam at the point of interest. In 2001, the classification standards were substantially revised in Europe (EN) and internationally (IEC). The classes are given below; the higher the classification number, the greater the risk the laser presents.

Class 1: eye-safe under all operating conditions; does not require a laser warning label, such as a laser printer.

Class 1 M: safe for viewing directly with the naked eye, having divergent large-diameter beams, but may be hazardous to view with optical instruments, such as magnifying glasses.

Class 2: visible laser (400–700 nm). The natural aversion to the very bright light will be sufficient to prevent eye damage, although prolonged viewing may be dangerous.

Class 2 M: visible lasers safe for accidental viewing with the naked eye but may be hazardous, as per class 1 M.

Class 3R: continuous-wave laser emitting less than 5 mW visible light, up to five times the emission limit for Class 1 or Class 2 lasers, although the risk of injury is low.

Class 3B: continuous-wave or pulsed laser with light intensity where the hazard of direct beam viewing is serious. Scattered radiation is not hazardous. Continuous emission at wavelengths above 315 nm must be less than 0.5 watts and pulsed lasers' output must be less than 125 mJ in 0.25 seconds.

Class 4: hazardous to view, having sufficient energy to ignite some materials and damage skin. Even diffuse reflections must be avoided. Continuous-wave output levels greater than 500 mW; pulsed systems can produce over 125 mJ in less than 0.25 seconds.

These classifications can be useful for dental personnel and their safe use of laser equipment. Dental applications of lasers are mentioned in most of the remaining chapters, especially Chapter 18.

Nano-sized Ceramic Particles

Some materials mentioned in this chapter are available in powder form. Micron-sized (a millionth of a meter, 10^{-6} m) particles are common in dental materials. Nanoparticles must have at least one dimension smaller than 100 nm ($<10^{-7}$ m), such as the diameter of a fiber, or the mean particle size; therefore, nanoparticles are less than one-tenth the size of conventional, micro-sized ceramic particles. For scale, a human hair is about 40,000 nanometers in diameter. The opportunities for nanoparticles to alter materials arose after 1959 when Nobel Prize-winning physicist Richard Feynman noted that the behavior of atoms on the scale of nanometers is different than on our usual macro-scale of microns or larger; the nanoscale materials experience new forces and create new effects (71).

Silica sols and fumed silica are well-known ceramic nanomaterials. The size of the silica clusters in the sol or fume has been tailored industrially so that innumerable applications are possible industrially and in dentistry, as will be mentioned throughout this text. Zinc oxide is another ceramic that is available as a nano-sized powder; it is familiar as a sunscreen component but is also important in dentistry. Titania nanoparticles are helpful for pigmenting, and calcium carbonate nanoparticles have been used as fillers. Hydroxyapatite nanoparticles have also been made and may have potential for medical devices. The creation of nanoparticles is possible via many reactions, usually via chemical precipitation or a gaseous reaction. However, exploiting the use of nano-sized particles has been difficult because the nano-particles form larger aggregates and agglomerates, bound by chemical or electrostatic forces (72, 73). New methods for redispersion of nanoparticles after drying are needed to fully achieve the potential of the high surface area nano-particles. Other nanomaterials can modify the refractive index in glass for use in mobile phone displays, television displays, and augmented reality. Nanoengineered materials are found in high-power, rechargeable battery systems, thermoelectric materials for temperature control, and tires that improve fuel mileage.

Nanoscale films on glass have made eyeglasses, computer screens, and cameras more water-repellent, anti-reflective, and self-cleaning. Nanostructured ceramic coatings have improved wear resistance for machine parts; nanoscale lubricants and engine oils extend the lifetimes of moving parts in power tools to industrial machinery (71). Graphene, as mentioned earlier, is a nanofilm.

The discriminating dentist needs to ask questions about materials that contain nanoparticles, whether it is a few or 100% nanoparticles and what benefits, or hazards, the nanoparticles impart.

Traditional/Modern and Natural/Synthetic

Traditional ceramics have been formed and fired from mined materials, including clays, feldspars, and silica, in forms from diatoms to flint. The precise compositions of minerals vary worldwide, creating differences in formulas and performance, such as firing behavior, a critical operation for making ceramic articles; these differences lead to product variations among worldwide manufacture of similar products.

Modern ceramics, especially medical devices, are almost exclusively made from refined chemicals and minerals whose compositions are precisely known, with verified purity that leads to reproducibility.

As with foodstuffs, the terms "natural" and "synthetic" are bandied about without much true meaning. Most ceramic articles are synthesized, including glasses. For example, Chapter 10 describes a porcelain that contains leucite crystals. This porcelain can be made from heat-treating potash feldspar, or it can be made by combining various individual ceramic powders constituting the same compositions as potash feldspar. In either case, components are melted, then heat treated for form leucite crystals; the results can be identical with "natural" feldspar or "synthetic" glass. Ceramic dental powders are synthesized and processed to create useful medical devices. Every material, ceramic or otherwise, originates from somewhere in our natural world, so the terms natural and synthetic are too vague to have any significant meaning in dentistry.

Summary of the Variety of Ceramics for Dentistry

Ceramics are distinct from metals and organic materials; like all materials, ceramics have their strengths and weaknesses, literally and figuratively. Ceramics in dentistry have grown out of industrial developments and adapted to treat dental problems. Many dental materials contain quotidian ceramic, aluminates and silicates. Others have components uniquely formulated to have valuable properties, such as strength and esthetics for dental restorations. Zirconia, zinc oxide and calcium compounds – phosphates, sulfates, silicates and aluminates – comprise many dental materials. Scattered throughout this text, the keen reader will note that almost every element with an atomic number less than 92 has been used in dental materials, many as oxides, but also nitrides, sulfates, and salts. Exceptions are these elements – technicum, promethium, thallium, elements with an atomic number higher than 83 with the exception of uranium and thorium, which were mentioned.

The ceramics used in dentistry range from raw materials (e.g. diatoms) to uniquely formulated glasses, for instance, a lanthanum-silicate glass having a low contact angle to infiltrate porous alumina (Chapter 10). Powders of crystalline ceramics are indispensable across the breadth of dental materials: cements, restorations, impression, model materials, and refractories for the dental laboratory, and abrasives.

The diverse ceramics used in dentistry include inorganic salts. Salts are used in solutions, and others are pastes with organic liquids; they are embraced herein as inorganic and non-metallic. Carbon and silicon metals are also incorporated as ceramic for some of their properties. Chapter 6 describes relevant test equipment and methods used by manufacturers, dentists, and dental researchers for examining, testing, and developing bioceramics.

Ceramics in Chapter 5

These ceramic or inorganic materials were mentioned in this chapter.

- alumina
- aluminum hydrate
- aluminum nitride
- aluminum sulfate
- antimony oxide
- arsenic oxide
- augite
- baria
- barium borate
- barium sulfate
- beryllia
- beryllium aluminate, chrysoberyl
- ß quartz
- ß spodumene
- bismite, bismuth oxide
- boron oxide
- cadmia
- calcia
- calcium fluoride, with dysprosium or strontium
- calcium aluminate cement
  - calcium monoaluminate
  - calcium dialuminate
  - tricalcium aluminate - usually present with calcium silicate cement
  - tetracalcium aluminoferrite- usually present with calcium silicate cement

- calcium carbonate, calcite
- calcium phosphates
  - dicalcium phosphate, hydroxyapatite, tetracalcium phosphate, and other phases
- calcium silicate cement, amorphous hydrates
  - alite, tricalcium silicate
  - belite, dicalcium silicate
- calcium sulfate and its hydrates
  - plaster, bassanite, anhydrite, gypsum
- calcium tungstate
- carbon -diamond, graphite, graphene
- ceria
- chromia
- chrysoberyl
- clays
  - bentonite, halloysite, hydromica, hydromuscovite, illite, montmorillonite, smectite
- cobalt oxide
- copper oxide, or copper-tin oxide
- cordierite
- erbia
- feldspar
- ferrites of baria and lead
- fluorapatite
- fluorocanasite
- forsterite
- hafnia
- holmia
- hopeite
- hornblende
- hydrofluoric acid
- hydroxyapatite
- iron oxide, iron oxide hydrate
- lanthana
- lead oxide
- leucite
- lithia
- lithium disilicate
- lithium fluoride
- magnesia
- magnesium phosphate cement

- manganese oxide
- mica
- molybdenum disulfide
- neodymium oxide
- nickel oxide
- niobia
- phosphorous pentoxide, phosphoric acid
- potassia, potassium carbonate
- potassium titanyl phosphate
- praseodymium-zirconia
- semiconductors
  - InGaAs, GaN, GaAs, GaAlAs
- silica glass
  - fumed
  - cristobalite flint, quartz, or tridymite
  - diatomaceous earth, opal, perlite, or pumice
  - with lanthana
- silicon carbide
- selenium-cadmium oxide in glass
- soda, sodium carbonate
- spinels (MX_2O_4) of Mg-Fe, Mn-Fe, Co-Cr, Mg/Ni-Mn
- steatite
- strontia
- sulfur in silicate glass
- talc
- tantalite
- telluria
- tin oxide
- titania
- titanates of baria and strontia
- urania
- vanadia
- wollastonite
- ytterbium fluoride
- yttria with thoria and neodymia
  - yttrium aluminum garnet with lutetia, scandia, ytterbia, erbia
  - yttrium scandium aluminum garnet
- zeolites
  - analcime, chabazite, clinoptilolite, heulandite, natrolite, phillipsite, and stilbite

- zinc oxide
- zirconia, cubic, tetragonal, monoclinic
  - with calcia, ceria, magnesia, yttria
  - with europia, gadolinia, scandia, lanthana, and ytterbia
  - with pigment oxides not mentioned above – bismuth oxide, thulium oxide, ytterbia

References

1 Cantwell, P.R., Tang, M., Dillon, S.J. et al. (2014). Grain boundary complexions. *Acta Mater.* 62: 1–48.

2 Mboya, H.A., Makunza, J., and Mwishwa, Y.H.B. (2011). Assessment of pumice blocks in comparison to cement sand blocks and burnt blocks "the case of Mbeya City – Tanzania". *J Civ Eng Res Prac.* 8 (1): 43–56.

3 Gnesin, G.G. (2016). Revisiting the history of materials science glass, glaze, and enamel over the millennia. I. Glass. *Powder Metall. Met. Ceram.* 54 (9–10): 624–630.

4 Raguin, V.C. and Higgins, M.C. (2003). *Stained glass: from its origins to the present*, 288. New York: H.N. Abrams.

5 Pye LD, Stevens HJ, LaCourse WC. Introduction to glass science: proceedings of a Tutorial Symposium held at the State University of New York, College of Ceramics at Alfred University, Alfred, New York, June 8–19, 1970. Available from: https://ezaccess.libraries.psu.edu/login?url=http://dx.doi.org/10.1007/978-1-4757-0328-3.

6 Burke, J.E. (2013). Lucalox alumina: the ceramic that revolutionized outdoor lighting. *MRS Bull.* 6: 61–68. https://doi.org/10.1557/s0883769400046133.

7 DeCeanne, A.V., Fry, A.L., Wilkinson, C.J. et al. (2021). Examining the phase evolution of lithium disilicate glass-ceramics with lithium tantalate as a secondary phase. *J. Am. Ceram. Soc.* 105 (1): 268–278.

8 Grossman, D.G. (1988). The science of castable glass ceramics. In: *Proceedings of the Fourth International Symposium on Ceramics Perspectives in dental ceramics*, Perspectives in dental ceramics (ed. J.D. Preston), 117–133. Quintessence.

9 MacCulloch, W.T. (1968). Advances in dental ceramics. *Brit Dent J.* 124 (8): 361–365.

10 Cannio, M., Bellucci, D., Roether, J.A. et al. (2021). Bioactive glass applications: a literature review of human clinical trials. *Materials.* 14 (18): 1–25.

11 Hench, L.L. (2011). Glass and glass-ceramic technologies to transform the world. *Inter J App Gl Sci.* 2 (3): 162–176.

12 Diba, M., Tapia, F., Boccaccini, A.R., and Strobel, L.A. (2012). Magnesium-containing bioactive glasses for biomedical applications. *Int J App Gl Sci.* 3 (3): 221–253.

13 Kondo, T., Otake, K., Kakinuma, H. et al. (2024). Zinc- and fluoride-releasing bioactive glass as a novel bone substitute. *J. Dent. Res.* 103 (5): 526–535.

14 Saeed, F., Muhammad, N., Khan, A.S. et al. (2020). Prosthodontics dental materials: from conventional to unconventional. *Mater. Sci. Eng. C Mater. Biol. Appl.* 106: 110167.

15 Montazerian, M. and Dutra, Z.E. (2016). History and trends of bioactive glass-ceramics. *J. Biomed. Mater. Res. A* 104 (5): 1231–1249.

16 Abd El-Hamid, H.K., Fayad, A.M., and Elwan, R.L. (2024). Evaluation of bioactivity, biocompatibility, and antibacterial properties of tricalcium silicate bone cement modified with wollastonite/ fluorapatite glass and glass-ceramic. *Ceram. Int.* 50 (14): 25322–25332.

17 Wong, K.-W., Li, Y.-J., Yang, H.-C. et al. (2024). Antimicrobial properties of bimetallic-containing mesoporous bioglass against Enterococcus faecalis. *J Dent Sci.* 1–12.

18 Kaou, M.H., Furko, M., Balazsi, K., and Balazsi, C. (2023). Advanced bioactive glasses: the newest achievements and breakthroughs in the area. *Nanomaterials (Basel).* 13 (16): 2287.

19 Cyriac, B. (2023). Zirconia: synthesis and characterization. In: *Zirconia – new advances, structure, fabrication and applications* (ed. U.B. Al-Naib), 168. Rijeka: IntechOpen.

20 Heuer, A.H. and Hobbs, L.W. (1981). *Case Institute of Technology. Ceramics Group., American Ceramic Society. Science and technology of zirconia*, vol. ix, 479. Columbus, Ohio: American Ceramic Society.

21 Sundh, A. and Sjogren, G. (2006). Fracture resistance of all-ceramic zirconia bridges with differing phase stabilizers and quality of sintering. *Dent. Mater.*: official publication of the Academy of Dental Materials 22 (8): 778–784.

22 Cesar, P.F., Miranda, R.B.P., Santos, K.F. et al. (2024). Recent advances in dental zirconia: 15 years of material and processing evolution. *Dent. Mater.*: official publication of the Academy of Dental Materials 40 (5): 824–836.

23 Duwez, P.O.L. and Odell, F. (2006). Phase relationships in the system zirconia – ceria. *J Amer Cer Soc.* 33 (9): 274–283.

24 Duwez, P.O.L., Odell, F., and Brown, F.H. (2006). Stabilization of zirconia with calcia and magnesia. *J Amer Cer Soc.* 35 (5): 107–113.

25 West, A.R. (1999). *Basic solid state chemistry*, 2nde, xvi, 480. New York: John Wiley & Sons.

26 Li, M., Cokic, S., Van Meerbeek, B. et al. (2025). Novel zirconia ceramics for dental implant materials. *J. Mater. Sci. Technol.* 210: 97–108.

27 Liao, Y., Gruber, M., Lukic, H. et al. (2020). Fracture toughness of zirconia with a nanometer size notch fabricated using focused ion beam milling. *J Biomed Mater Res B Appl Biomater* 108 (8): 3323–3330.

28 Emsley, J. (2001). *Nature's building blocks: an A–Z guide to the elements*, 538. Oxford; New York: Oxford University Press.

29 Tay, K.C., Loushine, B.A., Oxford, C. et al. (2007). In vitro evaluation of a ceramicrete-based root-end filling material. *J Endodont* 33 (12): 1438–1443.

30 Liu, W.N., Chang, J., Zhu, Y.Q., and Zhang, M. (2011). Effect of tricalcium aluminate on the properties of tricalcium silicate-tricalcium aluminate mixtures: setting time, mechanical strength and biocompatibility. *Int. Endod. J.* 44 (1): 41–50.

31 Collepardi, M., Monosi, S., Moriconi, G., and Corradi, M. (1979). Tetracalcium aluminoferrite hydration in the presence of lime and gypsum. *Cem. Concr. Res.* 9 (4): 431–437.

32 Gandolfi, M.G., Taddei, P., Tinti, A., and Prati, C. (2010). Apatite-forming ability (bioactivity) of ProRoot MTA. *Int. Endod. J.* 43 (10): 917–929.

33 Lothenbach, B., Pelletier-Chaignat, L., and Winnefeld, F. (2012). Stability in the system CaO–Al2O3–H2O. *Cem. Concr. Res.* 42 (12): 1621–1634.

34 Dembovska, L., Bajare, D., Pundiene, I., and Vitola, L. (2017). Effect of pozzolanic additives on the strength development of high performance concrete. *Procedia Engineering.* 172: 202–210.

35 Primus, C.M. (2006). Comments on "arsenic release provided by MTA and Portland cement" by Duarte MA, et al. *Oral Surg. Oral Med. Oral Pathol. Oral Radiol. Endod.* 101 (4): 416–417. author reply 7–8.

36 Dorozhkin, S.V. (2012). Calcium orthophosphates and human beings: a historical perspective from the 1770s until 1940. *Biomatter.* 2 (2): 53–70.

37 Dorozhkin, S.V. (2010). Calcium orthophosphates as bioceramics: state of the art. *J. Funct. Biomater.* 1 (1): 22–107.

38 Khalil, I., Abdulaziz, A., Khalid, A.A. et al. (2022). Chapter 7. Brushite: synthesis, properties, and biomedical applications. In: *Crystallization and applications* (ed. S. Youssef Ben and M. Riadh), 188. Rijeka: IntechOpen.

39 Dorozhkin, S.V. (2017). *Hydroxyapatite and other calcium orthophosphates: bioceramics, coatings and dental applications*, 470. New York: Nova Science Publishers.

40 Dorozhkin, S.V. (2017). *Hydroxyapatite and other calcium orthophosphates: biocomposites, self-setting formulations and dissolution*, 379. New York: Nova Science Publishers.

41 Dorozhkin, S. (2013). Self-setting calcium orthophosphate formulations. *J. Funct. Biomater.* 4 (4): 209–311.

42 Zhou, H., Yang, L., Gbureck, U. et al. (2021). Monetite, an important calcium phosphate compound-its synthesis, properties and applications in orthopedics. *Acta Biomater.* 127: 41–55.

43 Medvecky, L., Stulajterova, R., Giretova, M. et al. (2018). Effect of tetracalcium phosphate/monetite toothpaste on dentin remineralization and tubule occlusion in vitro. *Dent. Mater.*: official publication of the Academy of Dental Materials 34 (3): 442–451.

44 Moseke, C. and Gbureck, U. (2010). Tetracalcium phosphate: synthesis, properties and biomedical applications. *Acta Biomater.* 6 (10): 3815–3823.

45 Jung, J.H., Kim, S.Y., Yi, Y.J. et al. (2018). Hydroxyapatite-coated implant: Clinical prognosis assessment via a retrospective follow-up study for the average of 3 years. *J Adv Prosthodont.* 10 (2): 85–92.

46 Xu, H.H., Wang, P., Wang, L. et al. (2017). Calcium phosphate cements for bone engineering and their biological properties. *Bone Res.* 5: 1–19.

47 Mestres, G., Aguilera, F.S., Manzanares, N. et al. (2014). Magnesium phosphate cements for endodontic applications with improved long-term sealing ability. *Int. Endod. J.* 47 (2): 127–139.

48 Kaiser, F., Schroter, L., Stein, S. et al. (2022). Accelerated bone regeneration through rational design of magnesium phosphate cements. *Acta Biomater.* 145: 358–371.

49 Schroter, L., Kaiser, F., Kuppers, O. et al. (2024). Improving bone defect healing using magnesium phosphate granules with tailored degradation characteristics. *Dent. Mater.*: official publication of the Academy of Dental Materials 40 (3): 508–519.

50 Tanaka, C.B., Lopes, D.P., Kikuchi, L.N.T. et al. (2020). Development of novel dental restorative composites with dibasic calcium phosphate loaded chitosan fillers. *Dent. Mater.*: official publication of the Academy of Dental Materials 36 (4): 551–559.

51 Kikuchi, L.N.T., Freitas, S.R.M., Amorim, A.F. et al. (2022). Effects of the crosslinking of chitosan/DCPA particles in the antimicrobial and mechanical properties of dental restorative composites. Dental materials: official publication of the Academy of. *Dent. Mater.* 38 (9): 1482–1491.

52 Khvostenko, D., Hilton, T.J., Ferracane, J.L. et al. (2016). Bioactive glass fillers reduce bacterial penetration into marginal gaps for composite restorations. *Dent. Mater.* 32 (1): 73–81.

53 Jang, J.H., Lee, M.G., Ferracane, J.L. et al. (2018). Effect of bioactive glass-containing resin composite on dentin remineralization. *J. Dent.* 75: 58–64.

54 Adel, S., Hashimoto, K., Kawashima, N. et al. (2022). Biocompatibility and pro-mineralization effect of tristrontium aluminate cement for endodontic use. *J Dent Sci.* 17 (3): 1193–1200.

55 Pelepenko, L.E., Marciano, M.A., Francati, T.M. et al. (2022). Can strontium replace calcium in bioactive materials for dental applications? *J. Biomed. Mater. Res. A* 110 (12): 1892–1911.

56 Dumrongvute, K., Adel, S., Wada, T. et al. (2021). Distrontium cerate as a radiopaque component of hydraulic endodontic cement. *Materials (Basel).* 15 (1): 1–10.

57 Wu, T., Lu, T., Shi, H. et al. (2023). Enhanced osteogenesis, angiogenesis and inhibited osteoclastogenesis of a calcium phosphate cement incorporated with strontium doped calcium silicate bioceramic. *Ceram. Int.* 49 (4): 6630–6645.

58 Feng, S., He, F., Fang, X. et al. (2021). Enhancement of mechanical strength and osteogenesis, and inhibition of osteoclastic activity for β-tricalcium phosphate bioceramics by incorporating calcium silicate and magnesium-strontium phosphate. *Ceram. Int.* 47 (17): 24191–24197.

59 Zaichuk, A.V. and Belyi, Y.I. (2013). Improvement of the compositions and properties of gray ceramic pigments. *Glas. Ceram.* 70 (5–6): 5.

60 Vergaro, V., Abdullayev, E., Lvov, Y.M. et al. (2010). Halloysite clay nanotubes: characterization, biocompatibility and use as drug carriers. *NSTI-Nanotech.* 3: 395–396.

61 Sorrell, C.A. (2006). Suggested chemistry of zinc oxychloride cements. *J Amer Cer Soc.* 60 (5–6): 217–220.

62 Walling, S.A. and Provis, J.L. (2016). Magnesia-based cements: a journey of 150 years, and cements for the future? *Chem. Rev.* 116 (7): 4170–4204.

63 Ziyati, O., Abou-Obeida, S., Mtalai, N., and Boussiri, K.E. (2024). Zinc and oral health: literature review. *OALib.* 11 (07): 1–23.

64 Zhang, O.L., Niu, J.Y., Yin, I.X. et al. (2023). Bioactive materials for caries management: a literature review. *Dent J (Basel).* 11 (3): –59.

65 Somaie, R.A., El-Banna, A., and El-Korashy, D.I. (2023). Effect of incorporation of nano-graphene oxide on physicochemical, mechanical, and biological properties of tricalcium silicate cement. *J. Mech. Behav. Biomed. Mater.* 146: 106078.

66 Radunovic, M., Pavic, A., Ivanovic, V. et al. (2022). Biocompatibility and antibiofilm activity of graphene-oxide functionalized titanium discs and collagen membranes. *Dent. Mater.* 38 (7): 1117–1127.

67 Nizami, M.Z.I., Yin, I.X., Lung, C.Y.K. et al. (2022). In vitro studies of graphene for management of dental caries and periodontal disease: a concise review. *Pharmaceutics.* 14 (10): 1997.

68 Asaduzzaman Chowdhury, M., Kamal Uddin, M.M., Masud Rana, M. et al. (2023). Synthesis and characterization of borophene for future applications. *Results in Chemistry.* 6:101071.

69 Sanghera, J., Kim, W., Villalobos, G. et al. (2012). Ceramic laser materials. *Materials (Basel).* 5 (2): 258–277.

70 Sanghera, J., Kim, W., Villalobos, G. et al. (2013). Ceramic laser materials: past and present. *Opt. Mater.* 35 (4): 693–699.

71 Holthaus, D. (2024). When smaller is better: the promise of nanomaterials. *Cer Glass Mfg.* 5: 4–7.

72 Endres, S.C., Ciacchi, L.C., and Mädler, L. (2021). A review of contact force models between nanoparticles in agglomerates, aggregates, and films. *J. Aerosol Sci.* 153: 105719.

73 Shrestha, S., Wang, B., and Dutta, P. (2020). Nanoparticle processing: understanding and controlling aggregation. *Adv. Colloid Interf. Sci.* 279: 1–16.

6

Testing of Ceramics

Manufacturers of dental materials verify the utility of their products for their intended use via tests such as those described in this chapter. Each dental material balances multiple properties required for its desired indication for use and needs, such as tooth-like color and transparency, radiopacity, insolubility in water and acid, wear and erosion resistance, thermal insulation, high elastic moduli (elasticity), good compressive strength, fair flexural strength, and biocompatibility. Macroscopic properties are often tested – hardness, strength (compressive, bend, or tensile), elasticity, fracture toughness, radiopacity, solubility, wear resistance, thermal expansion, setting time, adhesion, fluidity (before setting), transparency, color, wear resistance, and bioactivity. The required or pertinent testing depends on the material's intended use. Ceramics for restorative uses are limited by their lower tensile strength and fracture toughness compared to common metals.

A key point for discussing materials properties is that a specific, irrefutable value for properties is rarely known. Ranges for properties' values should be accepted as an inevitable part of testing. The variations are easily seen in the literature, especially among dental publications. Test results of materials depend on the formula, microstructure, and sample preparation; the details of each test's execution, its reproducibility, and precision; the equipment, software, and its maintenance/calibration used in analysis; and the operator skill (1). Some of the tests described here have been used in the ISO and ADA standards for testing dental materials; however, most tests do not have a well-known correlation with clinical success or failure, which is the ultimate test. The results are used for comparisons and as benchmarks based on materials that are known to perform well clinically.

Strength measurements of ceramics are very common for dental ceramics because of the emphasis on ceramic-containing restoratives. Table 6.1 has a collection of some measured values for tooth enamel, dentin, and various all-ceramic restoratives mentioned in this text. The strength increases from leucite porcelains

Ceramics in Dentistry: Materials, Manufacturing, and Clinical Applications,
First Edition. Carolyn M. Primus.

Table 6.1 Properties of teeth and selected ceramics for dentistry.

Material	Thermal expansion coefficient (ppm/K)	Hardness (GPa)	Knoop hardness	Fracture toughness ($MPa\text{-}m^{1/2}$)	Flexural strength* (MPa)	Compressive strength (MPa)	Elastic modulus (GPa)
Tooth enamel (2–10)	7.8–17	~4	260–343	0.5–2.1	478–493	62–386	54–120
Dentin (2, 3, 5, 6, 8, 11, 12)	8.3–11	1.3	50–68	1.1–3.1	10, 164	194–340	11–28
Gypsum (13, 14)			10–65	0.2	1–20	6–40	0.5–2.5
Quartz	8.6		820			<2070	37
Fused silica	0.5	5		0.65	198–220	1522–1678	71–75
Silicate restoratives (15)	7.6		70		<170	140–186	~21
Alumina w/ 10% glass	7.0	4.5–5.0			337	2480	275
Alumina – high purity	7.4	~22	1800	3.3–5.0	551	2550	366–393
Sapphire	8.0	15		2.2–4.3 (16)	634		434
Spinel $MgO.Al_2O_3$	7.6–8.8	12.5–13 (17) (18)		1.9 (17)	110–245 (17)	988–1918 (19)	240–260
Cerestore (20)	5.6				172.4	1048	12.3
Dicor (21)	7.2	3.8–5.7		1.25–1.45	64–122		69 (22)
Leucite porcelain	13.5–14.5	5.9–6.2		0.86–1.02 (23)	85–122 (22)	350–550 (24)	20
Lithium disilicate (25)	9.4–10.5 (26)	5.7–6.9 (27)		1.4–2.5 2.1–2.3 (27)	210–420	275–341 (28)	70–103
Zirconia- tetragonal	10–11	12–13		7–12	800–1500	>2900	200–210

Material	Thermal expansion coefficient (ppm/K)	Hardness (GPa)	Knoop hardness	Fracture toughness (MPa-m$^{1/2}$)	Flexural strength* (MPa)	Compressive strength (MPa)	Elastic modulus (GPa)
Resin composites	16–94 (6)	0.8–1.2		1.0–2.3	60–200	320–400	2–20 (30)
Indirect Comp (29)	16–21				77–150	136–500	
Glass ionomers	10.2–11.4	0.4–0.8 (31)		0.4–1.0	40–50 (32)	60–300	15–20
Resin-modified glass ionomers		40–124 (33)		0.3–1.5 (34)	20–70		3–5
Silicon carbide	7.9	0.6–3.8	2480	3.5–9.8	310–655	3900	370–420
Tungsten carbide- 6% cobalt	4.3				1.790–2210	5170–5930	614–648
Silicon nitride	2.9	14.7–18.6		6–10	150–1200	75–800	120–330
Diamond	1.5–3.8	54–131	7000	6.0–10.7	800–1400	4500–5800	800–925

* May be 3- or 4-point bending or biaxial flexural strength tests.
Source: From reference (35), Chapter on Crystallography and Engineering Properties of Ceramics, or (36, 37) unless noted.

to glass-ceramics to tetragonal zirconia. Certain generalizations can be made about materials' strengths from surveying the data in Table 6.1. Zirconia materials are profoundly stronger in flexural and compressive strength and are tougher than earlier ceramics for restorations. The thermal expansions of porcelains are essential for matching their underlying metal or ceramic. Thermal expansion match to teeth is less important to the durability of crowns (Chapter 10) but should be considered for direct restoratives (Chapter 9). Strength and toughness are predictive of durability. Abrasives require high hardness for shaping or grinding of materials (Chapter 17). For example, alumina and silicon carbide are used to shape resin-based composite resins, lithium disilicate, or teeth. Diamond-coated instruments are needed to abrade and shape alumina or zirconia. Generic materials testing methods follow.

Strength Tests

Ceramics fracture because they contain microscopic flaws, pores, or cracks, but their overall performance is also influenced by inherent fracture toughness, as discussed below. The strength of ceramics is measured in many ways: three- or four-point bending (flexural), biaxial flexural, uniaxial compressive or tensile, and bonding. Tests and equipment have been devised to measure flexural strength, as depicted in Figure 6.1.

Flexural strengths are often measured using the 3- or 4-point bend test with small, beam-shaped samples supported by 3 or 4 loading pins; the formulas in Eqs. (6.1) and (6.2) are used to calculate flexural strength by measuring the sample's dimensions and the load at which fracture occurs:

$$\text{3-point flexural, strength}, \sigma = 3 * \text{Load} * \text{span} / (2\,\text{width} * (\text{thickness})^2) \quad (6.1)$$

$$\text{4-point flexural, strength}, \sigma = 3 * \text{Load} * \text{span} / (4 * \text{width} * (\text{thickness})^2) \quad (6.2)$$

The 4-point bend test distributes the load over a larger area and makes the test less sensitive to small cracks and setup errors.

Biaxial flexure tests are an alternative flexural method using disc-shaped samples; several modes are used – ring or ball supports with ring or piston pressure (38). The biaxial test method is included in three ISO standards for ceramics: ISO 6474 (alumina ceramics for surgery), ISO 13356 (zirconia ceramics for surgery), and ISO 6872/ADA 69 (Dentistry – Ceramic materials). Biaxial tests require a knowledge of Poisson's ratio (ν) related to deformation [expansion or contraction] perpendicular to the specific direction of loading. The strength calculation

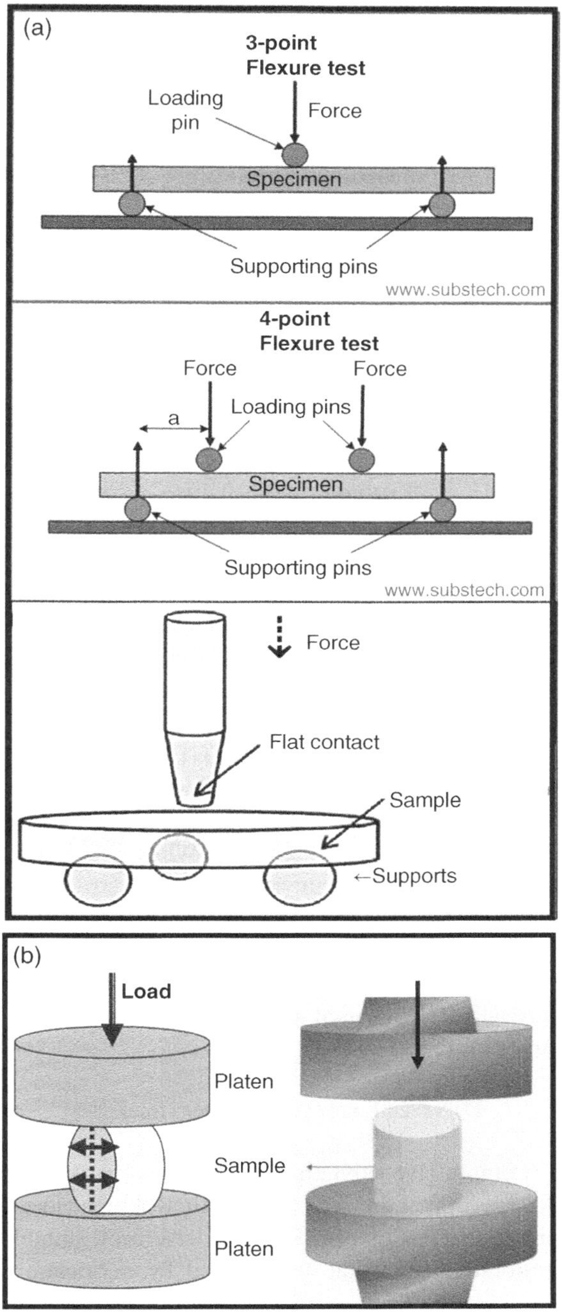

Figure 6.1 (a) Strength test configurations: 3-point, 4-point, and biaxial flexural tests (top to bottom). The 4-point bend test usually uses a span where "a" is 1/4 of the distance between the lower supporting pins. The biaxial test configuration shown is a piston non 3 balls. (b) Diametral (left) and compressive (right) strength test configuration.

in Eq. (6.3) requires calculations of the X and Y parameters via Eqs. (6.4) and (6.5), where ν is Poisson's ratio (e.g. 0.31 for zirconia), r_1 is the radius of the support circle, r_2 is the radius of the loaded area (pushing in the center), and r_3 is the radius of the specimen:

$$\text{Biaxial strength on 3-supports}, \sigma = -0.2387 \times \text{Load} \times (X - Y) / (\text{thickness})^2 \quad (6.3)$$

$$X = (1+\nu)\ln(r_2/r_3)^2 + [(1-\nu)/2](r_2/r_3)^2 \quad (6.4)$$

$$Y = (1+\nu)\left[1 + \ln(r_1/r_3)^2\right] + (1-\nu)(r_1/r_3)^2 \quad (6.5)$$

Material strengths must be compared using the same standard test technique and with similar sample preparation and size; different test methods have disparate strength values. In one study, the mean values decreased from 4-point bending to 3-point bending to biaxial flexure (39); differences in stress distributions and other test details create differences among test values.

The elastic modulus indicates how much bending – stiff (high value) or flexible (low value) – a material undergoes when stressed. Elasticity, E or Young's modulus, can be calculated from the deflection of a sample while being bent, that is, the slope of the linear portion of a stress–strain curve recorded during uniaxial and flexural tests. Nano-indentation is another method (40) to determine the elastic modulus.

The ultimate tensile strength (UTS) is the maximum stress a material can withstand before failing (breaking) while being stretched or pulled. Ductile materials, such as most metals and polymers, experience plastic deformation before tensile failure, as depicted in Figure 6.2. When a tensile (stretching) stress is placed on a ceramic material, its unyielding atomic structure prevents the redistribution or relief of stress. As shown in Figure 6.2, the elongation (stretchability) of ceramics before brittle fracture is less than 1%, in contrast to the 20% elongation of some stainless steels at ductile failure. Rather than this UTS test, the diametral tensile strength (DTS) is used and calculated as in Eq. (6.6) for cylindrical samples that are compressed on their side:

$$\text{DTS} = 2 * \text{Load} / (\pi * \text{diameter} * \text{thickness}) \quad (6.6)$$

Compressive strength (CS) is the ability of a material to withstand a pressure load, as opposed to tensile strength, where the load is elongating the sample (pulling it apart). Compression tests have been suitable for comparing materials for restorative uses that are stressed by mastication forces. The performance of

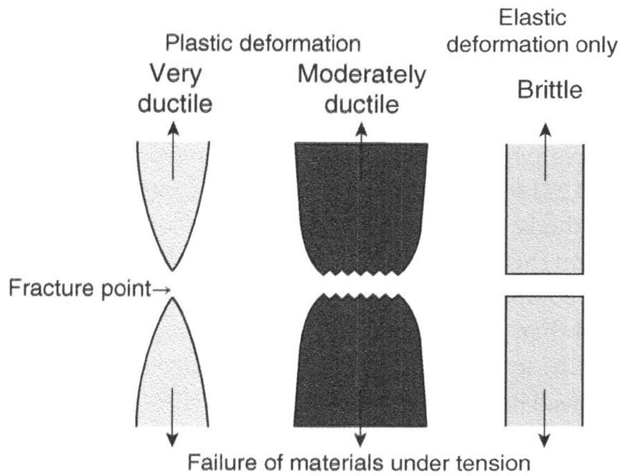

Figure 6.2 Illustration of ductility or brittle fracture.

compressive tests requires that the faces and load platens are accurately parallel and normal to the long axis to avoid stress concentrations, as depicted in Figure 6.1b. The length-to-diameter ratio affects the values and should be twice as long as the sample diameter for calculating the strength as per Eq. (6.7):

$$\text{CS} = \text{Load} / (\text{cross-sectional area}) \tag{6.7}$$

Making ceramic samples for CS testing requires experience with the material; obviously flawed samples must be rejected. Another problem exists: ceramics can abrade the testing platens, but if a pad is placed thereon, “parasitic” stresses can distort the results. This method, though widely used, is not as relevant as it appears (1).

Fracture Toughness

Fracture toughness is a property that describes the ability of a material containing a crack to resist fracture (41). The higher the fracture toughness, the more difficult it is to propagate a crack in that material. It’s an important property since imperfections, such as microscopic scratches, cracks, voids, and pores, cannot be avoided entirely during the fabrication of ceramics. Generally, ceramics have lower fracture toughness than metals (<10 vs. 20–100 $\text{MPa-m}^{1/2}$).

Fracture toughness is calculated from linear elastic fracture mechanics (LEFM). The crack propagation is monitored, and fracture toughness is calculated. Fracture toughness testing is performed using samples having a tiny, partial crack with a notch-tip radius less than the grain diameter in a polycrystalline material. Several toughness test methods rely on a sharp “pre-crack” (notch) to achieve reliable results. These tests are not as simple as the strength tests above; methods for the tests (42, 43) are in ASTM C1421 (Standard Test Methods for Determination of Fracture Toughness of Advanced Ceramics at Ambient Temperature); ISO 21113 "Fine ceramics (advanced ceramics, advanced technical ceramics – Test method for fracture toughness of monolithic ceramic thin plates at room temperature)"; and ISO 23146 "Fine ceramics (advanced ceramics, advanced technical ceramics) – Test methods for fracture toughness of monolithic ceramics – Single-edge V-notch beam (SEVNB) method." The single-edge notch beam (SENB) test, also known as the compact tension test, requires the ceramic sample to have a notch in the center, and then a bending stress is applied to cause failure. The double-cantilever beam (DCB) test is another test design with a sample having a partial crack bending stress. The chevron notched beam (CNB) test modifies the 3-point bend test method using a notch that is V-shaped. The focused ion beam (FIB) milling method has been used to make nanometer-sized notch tips smaller than 100 nm, even smaller than the grain size of fine-grained zirconia (41). The CNB and SENB tests are widely accepted for fracture toughness measurement of ceramics.

The fracture toughness tests are based on the energy required to propagate a crack through a new grain. Extra energy is required to fracture a grain; more energy is required than diversion of the crack along a grain boundary. Cracks that encounter glass at a grain boundary – in a glass-bonded ceramic – proceed much more easily than in a fully crystalline material without a glassy intergranular layer. Hence, highly pure alumina is stronger and tougher than glass-bonded alumina. For a similar reason, the fracture toughness of polycrystalline alumina is higher than the fracture toughness of single-crystal alumina (sapphire); crack propagation is easier through sapphire (alumina) orthodontic brackets than polycrystalline alumina brackets (Chapter 12). Polycrystalline ceramics have higher fracture toughness than single-crystal ceramics because cracks are diverted at grain (crystal) boundaries (GBs), requiring a longer fracture path and more energy to traverse the sample.

ISO 6876 for dental ceramics recommends a fracture toughness of restorative materials higher than 3.5 MPa-m$^{1/2}$ for three-unit bridges and higher than 5 MPa-m$^{1/2}$ for longer bridges. The values for fracture toughness of porcelains or glass-ceramics are much less than those of yttrium tetragonal zirconia, which has been reported to have a fracture toughness of 5.6–8.9 MPa-m$^{1/2}$ (41); hence the utility of zirconia for all-ceramic restorations (Chapter 10).

Microindentation (Microhardness)

Hardness is the resistance of a material to localized plastic deformation induced by either mechanical indentation or abrasion; many test methods are used. Mohs's hardness testing is a relative hardness measurement using a scratch test for

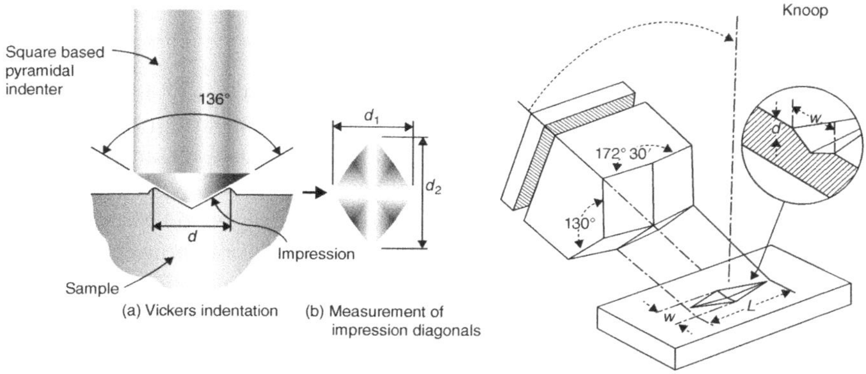

Figure 6.3 Vickers (left) and Knoop (right) micro-indentations on a ceramic. Note the differences in the shape and angles of the diamond indenter used for each.

minerals. Spherical (Brinell) and conical (Rockwell) indenters are used for materials other than ceramics, which are tested for their hardness on a micro, not macroscale. The popular ceramic hardness tests are Vickers or Knoop tests performed with diamond indenters, which are the hardest naturally occurring material and suitable for indenting hard ceramics. Both tests are performed on polished ceramic surfaces to obtain measurable indentations, such as those shown in Figure 6.3.

The Vickers diamond indenter has the shape of a small diamond pyramid; a Knoop indenter's shape is an elongated pyramid. These indenters are slowly lowered under a specified load, from 10 to 1000 g, and then lifted. The indentation size is measured to determine a hardness value, calculated including the indentation force. The Vickers hardness number is computed from the average of the two diagonals of the indentation, as in Eq. (6.8); the Knoop hardness is calculated using Eq. (6.9) where Load is in grams of force, and the measured lengths of the diagonals are in microns:

$$H_V = 1854.4 * \text{Load} / (\text{average diagonal})^2 \tag{6.8}$$

$$H_K = 14{,}229 * \text{Load} / (\text{long diagonal})^2 \tag{6.9}$$

The Vickers microhardness values are expressed in Gigapascals, unlike the dimensionless Knoop values. Generally, ceramics are quite hard, certain metals are rather hard, and materials with polymers are the least hard materials. Hardness values are pertinent to comparing restorative materials, cleaning materials, and abrasive ceramics for shaping teeth and restorations.

Adhesion

Good bond strength is essential when materials are attached to a tooth. Many bond strength test setups are used and are classified as macro- or microscopic: microtensile, tensile, microshear, shear, micropush-out, push-out, and interfacial fracture toughness. Microscopic bond tests may be more reliable values because they test a more uniform interfacial stress field (44). Shear bond tests are important for assessing the joining of dissimilar dental materials or joining dental materials to teeth, especially direct restoratives. The American National Standards Institute (ANSI)/ADA 111 standard (Adhesion Test Methods to Tooth Structure) has helpful guidance for testing. All adhesion tests have their difficulties in execution and comparison of materials (45, 46).

Dimensional Change/Stability

The dimensional stability of dental materials, during setting and over time, is very important for the restorative materials that are custom-fit to teeth; microns of change can matter, particularly at the margins and on the occlusal surfaces. A few dental standards have tests and some requirements: endodontic sealers (Chapter 8), polymer restorations (Chapter 9), CAD-CAM ceramic fixed prosthodontics (Chapter 10), and impression and model materials used for creating precise dental replicas (Chapter 14). Neither expansion nor shrinkage is desired for root canal sealers, direct restorative materials, or impression materials.

Monomeric materials are common for direct restorations (Chapter 9), and the polymerization process commonly causes shrinkage of these materials. The ISO 17304 document "Dentistry – Polymerization shrinkage: Method for determination of polymerization shrinkage of polymer-based restorative materials" is applied for such determinations. No requirements exist, but shrinkage during curing is known to cause stresses within the tooth, and dentists should be aware. The elastomeric impression materials have a test and requirement on dimensional stability: <1.5% linear change after 24 hours – in ISO 4823 "Elastomeric impression and bite registration materials" of ADA 19 although other methods are used (47–49). Some polymers may swell with water to counteract polymerization shrinkage.

A test method has been developed for ISO 6873/ADA 25 for gypsum-based products used to create dental models. The change in the length of a 100 mm (10 cm) long sample is determined before and after setting. Depending on the type of gypsum, the setting expansion should be less than 0.3% after two hours. The ADA 57:2021 standard for endodontic sealers has a test method for the linear change in the length of right circular cylinders that are soaked in water for 30 days; the change in length must be less than 1%.

Shrinkage of ceramics commonly occurs during the sintering (firing) process for making dense ceramic objects such as crowns. The shrinkage factor is crucial for the computer-aided design of crowns; the shrinkage must be known when creating an oversized computer-aided design of a crown or bridge for computer-aided machining. After machining, the material is sintered in a dental laboratory furnace, and the shrinkage occurs; hence, the shrinkage factor is very important for making crowns that fit. The ISO 18675 standard provides a test method to measure the shrinkage of partially sintered ceramic "milling blanks" for dental restorations after sintering. For this test, bars of milled ceramic are sintered, and the dimensions before and after sintering are used to calculate or verify the shrinkage. The standard includes a method for measuring non-isotropic shrinkage and warpage of the test bars.

Machinability

Lithium disilicate and zirconia are ceramic dental materials milled to create crowns and bridges. The ability to machine the ceramics to a precise shape depends on equipment, tooling, and milling parameters, which the material's manufacturer commonly specifies. For instance, the tool diameter, spindle speed, feed rate, "step over," and "step down" increments are needed for the various steps of roughing, semi-finishing inside and out, finishing inside and out, fine finishing, and fissure finishing. A "merlon" machining and fracture test in ISO 18675 shows the minimum machined thickness of a ceramic material (see Figure 6.4). Fractured merlons indicate that the machining process damaged the ceramic material. This test method combines the material, machine, tools, manufacturing strategy, and cutting parameters for partly sintered and fully dense blanks (preformed ceramics disc or ingots) for crowns and bridges. This test is practically designed for comparisons but is not a measurement of a material's inherent properties.

Water Solubility and Sorption

Dental restoratives usually need to be insoluble, but not universally. Two test methods are used based on weight, after soaking a material in water. Either the weight loss of the starting sample (often a disk) is measured or the dissolved remains in the soaking container are measured. The former is used for polymers, and the latter is used for testing endodontic sealers in the standards. The latter is also used for materials that may absorb and gain weight from water.

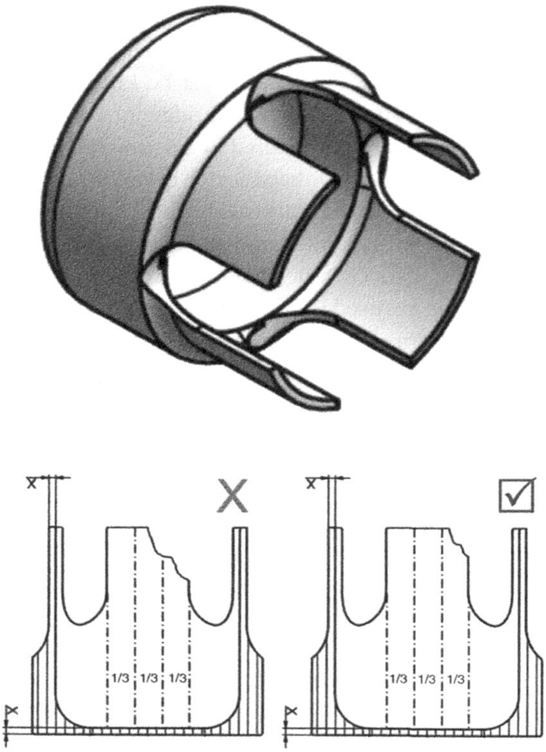

Figure 6.4 Geometry of standard merlon test specimens with an outer diameter of 1 cm (top), with unacceptable (X) and acceptable (✓) chipping of merlons after machining (bottom). ©ISO. This material is reproduced from ISO 18675:2022, with permission of the American National Standards Institute (ANSI) on behalf of the International Organization for Standardization. All rights reserved.

A polymeric restorative (Chapter 9) may only undergo minimal sorption and solubility (less than 40 μg/mm sorption and less than 7.5 μg/mm solubility after seven days in water) per ISO Standard 4049 or ADA 27 for polymeric restoratives. Leaching of residual monomers or hydrolytic degradation of the polymer matrix is detrimental; usually, the ceramic fillers in polymeric restoratives will be unaffected by water. Ceramic indirect restorations (Chapter 10) are expected to be insoluble.

Endodontic sealers (Chapter 8) should release less than 3% of their starting weight when configured as in ISO 6876 or ADA 57. Solubility of sealers can gradually cause loss of sealing ability and endodontic failure. However, water absorption is necessary for setting the tricalcium silicate-based ceramic cements in endodontics. Sparingly soluble ions are sometimes beneficial (e.g. fluoride, phosphate, calcium, or hydroxide ions) for surface mineralization or antimicrobial effects.

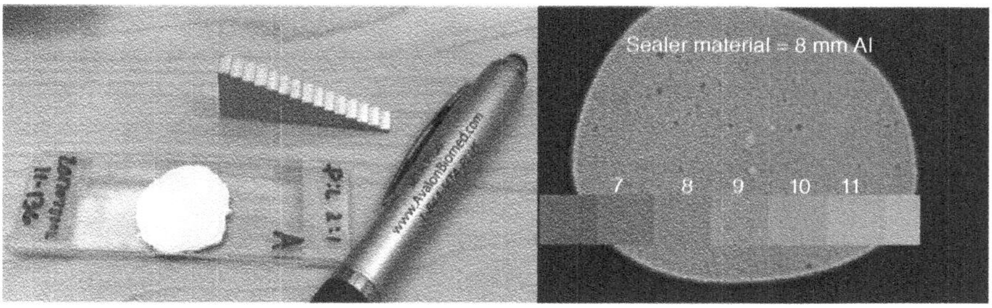

Figure 6.5 Radiopacity sample on the left with an Al step wedge and a pen to show scale, and digital image and analysis of radiopacity on the right.

Radiopacity

Insurance companies and dentists need X-rays to show where a restorative has been placed, including endodontic materials, and that requires radiopacity; radiopacity is also useful for the extraordinary circumstances when a dental material is aspirated or swallowed. Radiopacity is measured in samples 1 mm in thickness imaged concurrently with an aluminum (Al) step wedge using a dental X-ray machine with film or digitally. Aluminum is used as a comparative material because its radiopacity is similar to dentin and enamel. An example of the simple setup and an analyzed X-ray image are in Figure 6.5. The medical device radiopacity test methods are described in ISO 13116 and ASTM F640 standards. Values vary in the literature for radiopacity of dentin and enamel. Recent digital measurements for enamel and dentin are 2.1–4 and 1.3–2.5 mm of equivalent Al (50, 51). X-ray images are analyzed to compare the lightness of the material to the aluminum and determine what thickness of Al is equivalent to the 1-mm-thick sample. Lightness of the steps of aluminum can be graphed versus lightness; the radiopacity value can be easily interpolated by comparing the lightness of the aluminum thickness to the sample. Notably, radiopacity is linear only up to 5 mm of equivalent aluminum. Figure 6.5 includes an image of the step wedge superimposed in the Photoshop® analysis for radiopacity determination.

Fluidity

Fluidity is an indicator of viscosity and can be crucial in forming ceramics or in some aspects of dentistry, e.g., making replicas of teeth or filling a root canal system. Some ADA and ISO standards include tests of fluidity that are useful for comparing materials for the same use. For instance, a slump or fluidity test is used for dental plasters (ISO 6873/ADA 25) and flow/consistency tests under a load are used for elastomeric materials and root canal sealers. A fixed volume of material is tested in fluidity and flow/consistency tests, sometimes using a weighted sample; then, the diameter of the material is measured. Sometimes the requirements are a minimum (endodontic sealers) and/or a maximum diameter (impression materials). These dental tests (ISO 4823 and 6876, ADA 19 and 57) produce a figure of merit, rather than a viscosity.

Viscosity testing is quite complicated; so, the simplified testing methods are used in the ADA and ISO standards for comparisons of materials. Viscosity, with varying degrees of sophistication for torque analysis, is measured by manufacturers, using flow-cup, cone-plate, and rotational viscometers, but is not used in dental standards. Rotational rheometry is informative for developing any 3-D printing, tape-casting, and extrusion paste formulas as well as for traditional ceramic forming methods, including slip-casting as described in Chapter 7. Such testing helps manufacturers develop useful materials.

Setting Time

The hardening or setting time for a dental material is needed for practical clinical use. Setting times of dental materials are measured at room temperature or at body temperature, 37 °C, often using a Vicat needle or a Gillmore apparatus, as shown in Figure 6.6. These simple, hand-operated apparatuses use the penetration of an indenter in the surface, which is clinically similar to what a clinician would do to see if a material is set. Hand-held versions are not acceptable for accurate testing, the duration of the indenting should be brief, and the criterion should be "no further change" in the appearance of indentation over time. The Gillmore apparatus has two flat-tipped indenters and two weights for indenting.

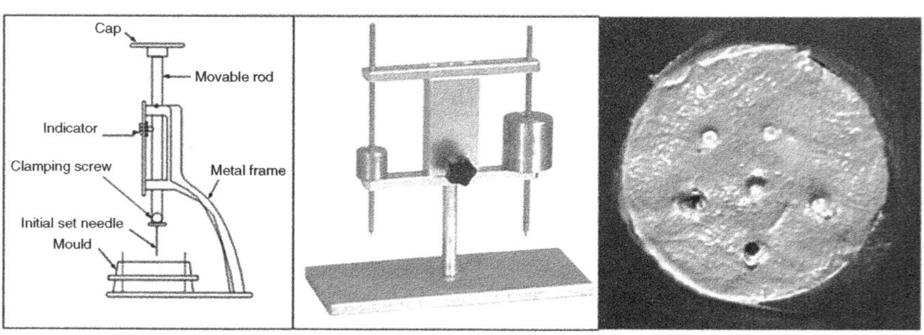

Figure 6.6 Manual setting time apparatuses: Vicat on the left, Gillmore in the center, and a series of Gillmore indentations as setting occurs is on the right. *Source:* Alpha Engineering Equipments. *Source:* (Middle Image) Alpha Engineering Equipments.

The lighter weight has the broader indenter, and the heavier weight has a smaller diameter indenter. The lighter and heavier "needles" are usually used to determine an "initial" and "final" setting time. The Gillmore test is used for concrete or mortar (ASTM C266 Test Method for Time of Setting of Hydraulic-Cement Paste by Gillmore Needles) and in dentistry (ISO 3107, 6876, 9917-1 and 9917-2); the Vicat apparatus is used in ISO 6873/ADA 25 for dental gypsum. These Gillmore and Vicat indentation methods can indicate when the next step in dentistry may be performed but do not truly indicate the chemical completion of a reaction or confirm the ability of the material to survive a load. Results can be variable and ambiguous, influenced by temperature variations, humidity, the lighting to observe the indentation, and especially the observer.

True setting determinations require more scientific measurements than the firmness of the surface, especially for polymeric materials, which are resilient. For instance, the setting times of ceramic-filled polymers for direct restorations are determined by temperature measurements as specified in ISO 4049/ADA 27 for polymer-based restorative materials.

Depth of curing (setting) is essential to determine for the light-curing monomers in direct restorative materials. One method is to light-cure material packed in a 6-mm diameter mold. The "cured" samples are removed from the mold, then the bottom is scraped to remove uncured monomer; the height of the remaining cylinder of material is considered the depth of curing. Curing of resin-based composite (monomer-ceramic) materials is highly influenced by the ceramic powder composition, including pigments, the index of refraction match to the polymeric matrix, the percentage of ceramic powder, the particle size distribution, and the components absorbance of the wavelength used for curing. Clinically, the diameter, proximity, and radiance of the curing light are critical – the closer and the larger the light's diameter and radiance leads to more curing. Uncured monomers are undesirable for direct restoratives.

Tribology – Wear Resistance

Over one's lifetime, teeth are eroded by frequent contact of the opposing teeth in speaking, chewing, and clenching and contact with foods and items we hold in our mouths, such as bones, nuts, pipes, fingernails, nails, or pins. Tooth wear is more commonly observed in older people on the anterior teeth's incisal edges. Tooth brushing is intended to remove debris from teeth but can contribute to minor mechanical wear from very vigorous brushing with a harsh toothbrush material or dentifrice. Besides mechanical erosion, chemical erosion occurs because we ingest acidic foods like vinegar and drink carbonated beverages, and oral bacteria form acids.

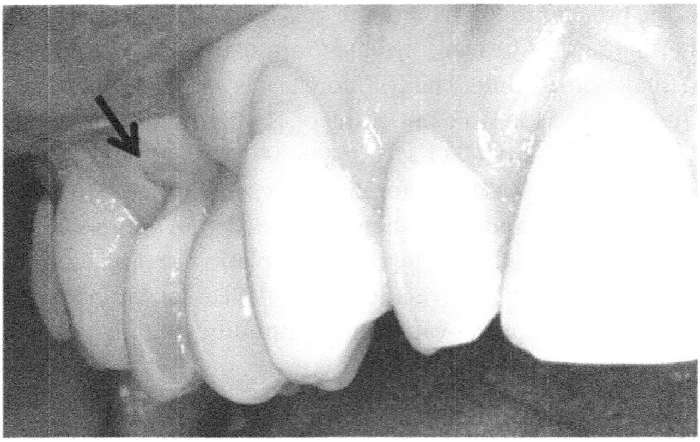

Figure 6.7 The arrow points to an abfraction lesion, and other cervical erosion lesions are present (52, 53).

Abfraction in the cervical region approximating the gums may also be seen in some older teeth, which is the gradual fracture and loss of enamel rods caused by chewing and concomitant tooth flexing from everyday stresses. See Figure 6.7 for an example of abfraction. Abfraction can be likened to beam bending of the tooth. This is a mechanical and cyclic fatigue phenomenon.

Many wear-testing devices have been developed to test restorative materials through simulated chewing and have been discussed in ISO technical report TR 14569-1 & 2. These tribology testers can be used to examine wear of restorative materials and wear of teeth by toothpastes or toothbrushes, simulated food, and opposing teeth. The sample preparation, antagonist, contact force and angle, time, and media for "chewing" vary, as do the wear measurements. Each testing device provides unique wear mechanisms and measurements, but they lead to diverse results among materials (54). Correlations with clinical results are unclear; however, the methods offer some discrimination of high- and low-wear materials (55, 56).

Thermal Expansion

The human body remains at a consistent 37 °C, but the temperature in the oral cavity varies with food and beverages – a temperature range of about 0–70 °C (57). Direct dental restorative materials ideally have a similar expansion to teeth for long-term performance, maintaining their adhesion and integrity. Bonding may be more important than thermal expansion match; however, the mismatch of the thermal expansion of silicate cements (Chapter 9) to teeth contributed to this restorative's shorter life span in the oral cavity.

Thermal expansion over a wider range of temperature (as high as 1500 °C) is also important for the design of indirect dental materials made by manufacturers and used by dental technicians, as described in Chapter 10. For instance, the thermal expansion coordination is critical for fusing multiple ceramics and metals – that is, for porcelain enamels and porcelains on alumina, lithium disilicate, and zirconia. Manufacturers test thermal expansion using thermomechanical dilatometry equipment (e.g. a push-rod dilatometer), which provides displacement and temperature information as a bar-shaped sample is heated. The bar is placed in an oven with a probe touching it, which transmits changes in length to a transducer that translates the motion into an electrical signal. The changes are recorded as the sample is heated at a constant rate, from which the thermal expansion is calculated per Kelvin (K), as described in ASTM Test Method E831. Most materials' thermal expansion is linear over a limited temperature range if no phase changes occur. Interferometry is a more precise method for this thermal measurement, but the equipment is more costly.

Thermocycling and Fatigue Testing

The oral temperature variation mentioned above has accounted for some materials' failures. Therefore, thermocycling protocols have been developed, especially for testing restorative materials and cements. Equipment has been developed that subjects the materials to thermal cycles between 5 and 55 °C, using a dwell time of 30 seconds at each temperature. After performing a protocol with a certain number of cycles, strength tests are performed to compare materials (58). No standard or consensus exists for thermocycling protocols; even the temperature extremes and the dwell times vary among testers (59, 60). This thermocycling test is unlike the severe thermal shock testing used for other applications of ceramics (61).

Fatigue of materials is the initiation and propagation of cracks in a material due to repeated (cyclic) loading and unloading, causing mechanical failure (breakage) at loads below the nominal fracture strength of the material (e.g., failure at a stress below that measured in a biaxial strength test). Fatigue testing is appropriate for testing dental materials because masticatory forces are applied over time. An example of a fatigue protocol that provides useful data for dentistry is applying a load of 80 N with a spherical stainless steel piston (diameter of 6 mm) at 2 Hz to samples submerged in distilled water at 37 °C. In one report, the samples were inspected after 10^4 and 10^6 cycles for the presence or absence of failure (62). Chipping and cracking occurred that differentiated among the ceramic indirect restoratives. Other fatigue protocols have been used (63, 64).

Measuring Color, Transparency, and Other Optical Properties

Colors have often been given names that are arbitrary and not internationally agreed upon, including the dental shade guides. The science of color designations and comparisons has been studied for many industries, such as the Pantone color system for opaque, printed colors, and the Munsell system for dentistry (65). However, the Commission Internationale de l'Eclairage (CIE) L * a * b* system is internationally accepted for dentistry and many other industries, where color matching is paramount. The CIE system describes colors by assigning values to the hue, chroma, and value, that is, the color of the rainbow/wavelength (0–360°), the intensity of that color (0–60), and the degree of whiteness (or blackness) (0–100). Hue, chroma, or lightness can be plotted in three dimensions as radial dimensions. Alternatively, Cartesian coordinates are used: L [lightness/whiteness], a* [red to green, −60 to +60], and b* [yellow to blue, −60 to +60]. See Figure 6.8 to visualize, in black and white, the spatial relationships of the two designations. CIE color differences (ΔE) are used to compare materials and effects; various thresholds, e.g., ΔE greater than 1 has been used for visual acceptance.

The CIE coordinates do not account for transparency, or the converse opacity, of a sample and measuring opacity is a subject of debate for translucent samples and color matching. Light that enters a partially transparent (translucent) material

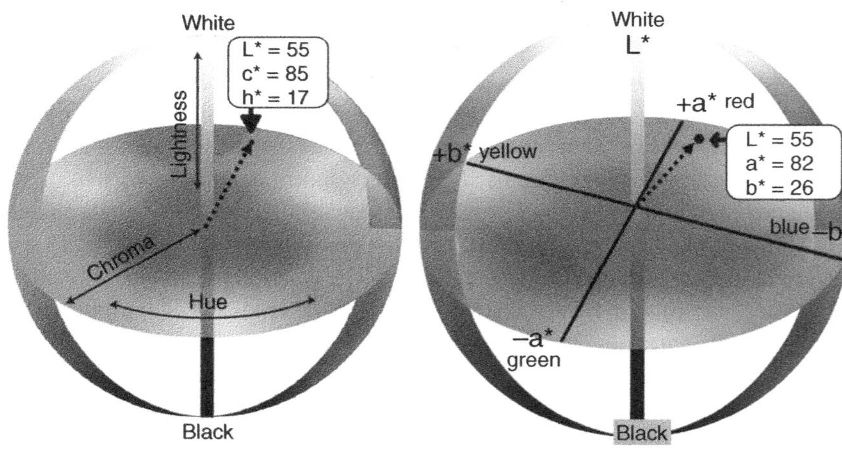

Figure 6.8 The color coordinates for the CIE color systems in radial notation (L*, h*, and c*) on the left and rectilinear notation (L*, a*, b*) on the right, with values for each set of with values for each set of color coordinates at the point of the dotted arrow.

encounters internal interfaces where light may be absorbed, reflected, or transmitted. No standard has been created to measure transparency; however, the "translucency parameter" may be used as a measure of opacity. The translucency parameter is defined as a material's color difference over a black versus over a white background (66). The contrast ratio is the ratio of the reflectance of a translucent material on a black backing to the reflectance on a white backing (67) determined with a spectrophotometer, which is also used to gauge opacity. Spectrophotometers are color-measuring equipment that are scientifically validated, but colorimeters are available for dentists for communication with dental laboratories.

Color stability is essential for restorative and endodontic materials (Chapters 8 to 10) and is determined by color measurements over time. Monomers may change color as they cure, especially over the first 24 hours after curing, or over longer times by exposure to light, hydrolytic degradation, or wear of the surface. Color changes are also affected by changes in gloss. Color-stability testing is covered in ISO 7491/ADA 80 standards.

Although color stability is usually inherent in ceramics, an exception is the use of bismuth oxide as a radiopaque component, used intracoronally. Bismuth oxide can change its oxidation state and color when exposed to alkaline materials or light, which has been a problem for some endodontic materials (Chapter 8) (68–70). Certain antibiotics also darken teeth from within when used for endodontic treatments.

Color measurement, color matching, color consistency (reproducibility), color stability, and determinations of discoloration are important to manufacturers, clinicians, and patients. Guidance on color measurement for dentistry is in ISO Technical Report 28642 and ADA 161, which describe three shade conformity issues for visual and instrumental methods for assessment. The color acuity of people making visual assessments is very important because color perception relies on the lighting and the viewer.

Opalescence and Fluorescence

The opalescence and fluorescence optical qualities of natural teeth are imitated by dental restorative materials. The "opal effect" occurs because of the scattering of light by internal particles, which is maximized when the internal particle's index of refraction is different from the matrix. Particles larger than 750 nm scatter all the visible light, making an object look white. When the internal particles are similar in size to the wavelengths of blue light (smaller than 400 nm, 0.4 μm), only blue and violet light are reflected or refracted. The result is that the color of an object with a fine, dispersed internal phase is different when viewed in transmitted light versus reflected light – opalescence. The key factors to maximize opalescence are: (1) a substance containing one or more internal phases, (2) the internal phases dispersed in the material are small in size, (3) the difference in the index of refraction between the matrix and the internal phases is large, and (4) the internal phase should have a high dispersion (larger index of refraction at shorter wavelengths) (71).

Opalescence has been created in dental composites by dispersing colloidal-sized (1 nm to 1 μm, 10^{-9} to 10^{-6} m) silica particles within the resin. The silica dispersion has two virtues: it adds viscosity to the resin and disperses light. Opalescence is created in dental glasses (e.g. for dental porcelains) by heat treatments that form very fine crystals or a phase-separated glass. Only some glass compositions can be heat-treated by the manufacturer to precipitate a finely dispersed crystal precipitate or phase-separated glasses – that is, two similar compositions of glass, where one forms droplets within the other matrix.

To create an opal, phase-separated glass, a homogeneous glass is heated causing the glass to precipitate microscopic droplets of a second glass within the matrix. The opacity of the resulting "opalized" glass is controlled by the difference in the refractive index between the phases, the volume percentage of each phase, and the size and distribution of the second phase, according to the principles described above. Manufacturing a consistent microstructure and opalescence in an "opal glass" is difficult because the temperature and time must be closely controlled throughout the processing. Rheinburger *et al.* patented a phase-separated glass for dentistry (US Pat. 5,432,130: 1995). Their glass forms droplets (immiscible glasses) in the matrix, 150–250 nm in diameter. The key components of the patented composition range were silica, boron oxide, phosphorus pentoxide, and ceria. An example of the microstructure, seen using transmission electron microscopy (TEM) of a phase-separated glass used in dentistry, was presented in Figure 5.5. This TEM picture shows the droplets, ranging in size from 50 to 500 nm, which create blue light scattering. Measuring opalescence is uncommon (66), and no special requirements exist in dentistry. Still, it can be observed visually by examining the material in reflected and transmitted light and observing a bluish and orangish cast, respectively.

Fluorescence is another optical property that can be quantified (66) by color measurements. The intensity and wavelength of the fluorescence can be observed when a material is exposed to UV wavelengths. Ideally, dental materials will mimic the combined visual effects of the pulp, dentin, and enamel in their color properties, including translucency, opalescence, and fluorescence.

Bioactivity

As noted in Chapter 5, bioactivity includes the in vivo precipitation of a surface layer of pseudo-apatite (HA). The formation of the hydroxyapatite layer precedes a cascade of healing reactions (72, 73) of the pulp or alveolar bone, which are not described here. This surface layer of HA obscures the underlying ceramic from the body's immune system to reduce the "foreign body" reaction by which the body identifies, attacks, and attempts to destroy (resorb) materials.

The ISO 23317 (In vitro evaluation for apatite-forming ability of implant materials) standard has a test method to determine if an apatite layer can be formed on materials. This in vitro test uses an acellular and protein-free simulated body fluid (SBF) with ion concentrations nearly equal to human blood plasma. Samples are soaked in the SBF solution with a volume equal to ten times the apparent surface area of disc-shaped samples for as long as four weeks at 37 °C. The formation of apatite layers on the samples, indicating bioactivity or biomineralization, can be detected by thin film X-ray diffraction spectrometry and scanning electron microscopy. The formation speeds of material may be compared, but the thicknesses of the apatite are not to be compared. Bioactivity has been very important for the in vivo success of pulpal and other endodontic treatment materials (Chapter 8).

Remineralization refers to the restoration of hydroxyapatite either in etched dentin or on enamel surfaces. If future dental materials can contribute to the remineralization of dentin or restore enamel, dentistry will be transformed.

Calcium hydroxide powder has been recognized as bioactive since the beginning of the 20th century for use as a bioactive pulp medicament (74) and a high pH, antimicrobial medicament (75). Calcium hydroxide particles do not set or form a hard layer and they gradually become bioinert by reacting to form calcium carbonate particles. Calcium hydroxide has been combined with some resins for a pulp medicament to create a "set" material (76).

The calcium silicate and calcium aluminate cements were recognized in the 1990s for their ability, like calcium hydroxide, to create a high pH (alkaline), antimicrobial environment and to form hydroxyapatite in contact with phosphate-buffered fluids (77) – bioactivity. The calcium silicate/aluminate cements biomineralize acellularly, beginning within 30 minutes of contact with SBF. See Figure 6.9 for an ex vivo example where a hydroxyapatite (HA) layer formed on a calcium silicate cement that had been placed in a tooth as a root-end filling; this root was soaked in phosphate-buffered saline, and then sagittally sectioned to illustrate bioactivity. The clinical and histological responses to the calcium silicate/aluminate cements are equal to or superior to calcium hydroxide (76, 78, 79), perhaps because the cements set and form a matrix with a reservoir of hydroxide and calcium ions, unlike materials containing calcium hydroxide particles. Bioactive calcium silicate and calcium aluminate cements have achieved prominence in pediatric dentistry and in endodontics for vital pulp and periapical tissue contact, which are discussed in Chapter 8.

"Bioactive glasses" and HA graft materials are also bioactive; they release ions into the tissue fluids, form a surface layer of HA, gradually dissolve, and are slowly resorbed (replaced) by bone tissue that advances between coarse graft particles, into the porosity of the granules.

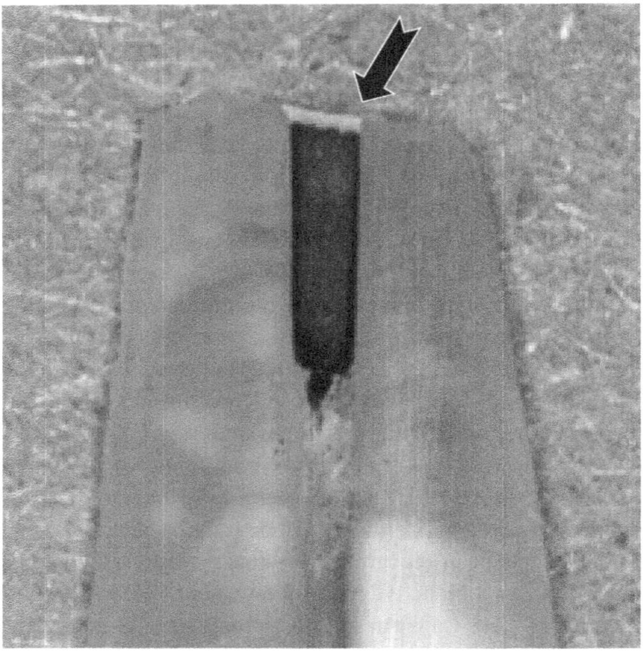

Figure 6.9 Optical image of a white bioactive layer (arrow) formed over a black, bioactive, calcium silicate cement root-end filling material. The tooth had been soaked in phosphate-buffered saline and then sectioned to reveal the precipitated mineralized layer.

Microscopy, Laser, and X-ray Analyses

Often, the best information about the performance of ceramics is obtained from studies of the microstructure via optical, scanning electron (SEM), transmission electron (TEM), or atomic-force (AFM) microscopy. The analyses of the phases, microstructures, and other spectra are complementary to the physical property test results. Ceramics are polished to a flat surface to see the grain boundaries in scanning and optical microscopy. Acid or thermal etching help the observer discern the size and distribution of the ceramic grains after sintering. Formerly, thin sections of ceramics were popular for optical microscopy with light and polarized light to identify phases.

Several techniques are used to analyze ceramics with various electron microscopes. Scanning electron microscopy (SEM) is important to examine powders, fracture surfaces, and interfaces using a rastered electron beam to create reflected electron images. The intensity of reflections into the detector increases with atomic number. Field Emission SEM (FESEM) uses an exceptional, narrow radius electron-emitting cathode for higher resolution images. Aberration-corrected SEM is used to compensate for imperfect "lenses" of the electron beam (80). Non-electrically conducting materials, such as ceramics, are coated with <100 Å (~10^{-8} m) of gold or carbon to enable clear images in any SEM.

An incident electron beam in an SEM will stimulate X-ray emission from a material; X-ray detectors augment scanning microscopy by identifying and showing the distribution of elements. This analysis technique is known as energy-dispersive X-ray spectroscopy (EDS, EDX, EDXS or XEDS), energy-dispersive X-ray analysis (EDXA or EDAX), or energy-dispersive X-ray microanalysis (EDXMA). A new detector for SEMs is available for simultaneous backscattered electron and X-ray detection, BEX. EDS detectors have significantly improved over the decades, enabling the detection of minor and trace elements; this has been achieved with digital electronics and improved detectors to achieve "higher counts" (signal) using less current and lower voltages. These advantages make EDX with an SEM more competitive with an electron microprobe microanalyzer (EPMA), which had been superior. The electron microprobe determines the chemical composition of small volumes (10–30 μm^3) using an electron beam and X-ray detection by wavelength. Elements from atomic number 3–94 can be measured as low as 100 ppm with an EPMA.

TEM requires an electron beam to be transmitted through a very thin sample, which reveals the grain structure and defects of very fine-grained (<1 µm) ceramics. TEM may include selected area diffraction (SAD) of X-rays emitted to identify crystal phases on a microscopic scale. TEM samples require careful preparation of thin samples, such as ion milling.

AFM or scanning probe microscopy (SPM) uses a small probe to obtain information about a material's topographic, magnetic, or chemical properties. The AFM probe has a very sharp tip, ~100 Å diameter, at the end of a small cantilever beam attached to a piezoelectric scanner assembly. Interatomic forces between the probe tip and the sample surface cause the cantilever to deflect, which is recorded by the change in the reflection of a laser beam aimed at the cantilever. A map of the surface is created from these data, having an area from 100 μm^2 to less than 100 nm^2; samples can be imaged in air or liquid. Larger samples can be analyzed, such as those used with an optical or scanning microscope. Surface roughness in the image area should not exceed about six microns.

Dentists use X-rays to visualize internal anatomical structures of various oral spatial areas, such as bitewing, periapical, and panoramic views, and manufacturers use dental X-ray equipment for measuring radiopacity. Additionally, dentists use the cone-beam computed technology (CBCT), developed since 1971, for procedures such as determining root fracture or selecting implant sites. CBCT X-ray equipment creates a series of X-ray images, which are converted with software to visualize the anatomy in three dimensions. Micro-CT equipment, X-ray microscopy (XRM) or μCT, is used by manufacturers and researchers for the microtomography or micro-computed tomography of samples smaller than a skull (<20 cm in diameter) with higher resolution than a CBCT image taken of the mouth. Micro-CT images have pixel sizes as small as 100 nm. The equipment and software assembles and can rotate 2D X-ray images as 3D models. Micro-CT non-destructively provides information about the micro-architecture of an item. Such equipment is useful to quantify the locations and sizes of gaps in dental materials in teeth. Gaps within root canal fillings and at the interface of tooth structures and a restorative material are always anathema.

Materials scientists use X-ray beams in other equipment for analyzing ceramics, particularly X-ray diffraction (XRD), to identify the elements or compounds (phases) present in crystalline materials. The XRD technique uses an incident X-ray beam of one wavelength; the X-ray beam is reflected at various angles by the crystals in a material; the detector records the characteristic pattern of intensities used for identification. This technique is predicated on the ceramics having the characteristic crystal forms of Figure 5.1. The chemical composition of compounds results in each material having a unique set of molecular crystal dimensions and angles for the axes. Software analysis is essential to discern multiple crystalline materials and may be semi-quantitative.

X-ray fluorescence (XRF) is another materials science analysis technique – entirely different from determining optical fluorescence discussed before; XRF is used to identify primary, minor, and trace elements present. An incident X-ray beam causes the ejection of some inner shell electrons, then an outer shell electron fills the vacancies created by the electron, and the fluorescent photons are detected by their energy or wavelength. The detection range of elements via XRF is beryllium to americium. XRF detectors are sensitive and may detect elements in concentration variations over six orders of magnitude. Micro-XRF uses a more focused beam to detect elements in structures as small as 20 μm and has been combined with an SEM for the study of minute samples in high and low vacuum. Portable XRF equipment has also been used for field work and the detection of trace elements (81).

Other electron microscopy techniques are less commonly used to identify ceramics in dentistry. Auger electron microscopy/spectroscopy (AEM) bombards a sample with X-rays or energetic electrons to cause the ejection of Auger core electrons, rather than the outer valence electrons involved in chemical bonding. The AEM spectra can be used to determine the identity of the emitting atoms and some information about their environment. The AES system examines a small sample volume (typically $10^{-30}\,\mu m^3$ or less), which is a benefit over EDX for pinpointing a phase. X-ray photoelectron spectroscopy (XPS) equipment uses an incident beam of X-rays to eject electrons from the near surface of a sample. The XPS spectra provide information on the elements present and how the elements are bonded, inferred from the energy and the number of electrons emitted. XPS equipment can detect all elements except hydrogen and helium. Multimodal imaging is a future for equipment, examples being Raman/SEM (82) and "Volume electron microscopy" (vEM) for 3D images of thicker samples (83).

Imaging techniques enable materials scientists to correlate observations of materials with performance testing, providing a basis for incremental improvement and innovations. The optical, electron, and X-ray images show the essence of the material structure to correlate with other properties. The X-ray analysis techniques identify the chemical contribution or distributions of elements or compounds.

Other Analyses

Micron and nano-sized ceramic powders have become the norm for dental materials. Particle size distributions are central to understand and control for ceramic powders performance in dentistry. Laser particle size analysis – laser diffraction analysis and laser diffraction spectroscopy – is commonly used by manufacturers for powder size analysis; it supplanted the step-wise sieve analysis used in the 20th century because sieves cannot be used to differentiate powder distributions finer than 400 mesh (38 µm), even with ultrasonic sieving. Laser diffraction analysis is based on the Fraunhofer diffraction principle that light scattered by a particle is proportional to the particle size, a method suitable for particle sizes from nanometers to millimeters. Such equipment requires a He–Ne laser or diode laser, a high-voltage power supply, and multiple detectors to analyze the diffracted light of a powder dispersed in a liquid; results yield the volume of each particle in the sample. Software is used to display the distribution of the particle sizes of a powder (see ISO 13320:2020 Particle size analysis laser diffraction methods) with the assumption the particles are spherical even though most particles are not.

Laser diffraction particle size analysis produces a calculated surface area. Other methods are more accurate for surface area measurements for powders and porous (e.g., partially sintered) materials based on physical adsorption using the Brunauer–Emmett and Teller (BET) theory for gas adsorption. A newer method is Small Angle X-ray Scattering (84).

Two thermal analysis techniques are useful for understanding the contents or behavior of materials: differential scanning calorimetry (DSC) and thermogravimetric analysis (TGA). Both techniques gradually heat a small sample; the change in the temperature of a sample is recorded for DSC and the weight change is recorded for TGA. DSC indicates endothermic or exothermic reactions such as phase changes. Thermogravimetry is used to measure moisture loss, evaporation, decomposition, or oxidation. Thermal properties of dental materials can affect their manufacture or performance.

Glass powders need index of refraction, softening point measurements, and thermal expansion for dentistry. The immersion and Becke line method is used to determine the index of refraction. This method places glass fragments into "immersion oils," standards with known index of refraction, for examination with a microscope. A bright line within the particle moves as the optical microscope's focus is slightly changed. The Becke line moves toward the higher refractive index materials when the distance (focus) is increased slightly. Repeated tests in different oils are used to match the glass to the standard oil to determine the index of refraction, so important for resin restoratives. The softening point of glass is used to determine the temperature below which the glass behaves as a rigid solid; it is a common quality control test to monitor variations in a glass composition. The softening point test requires a round glass fiber of the glass, 0.65 mm in diameter and 23.5 cm long to be heated in a furnace at the rate of 5 °C/min until the fiber elongates at 1 mm/min., which is called the softening temperature in ASTM C-338. Thermal expansion measurements can be used to confirm that a glass composition of each new batch remains the same as prior batches, as a quality control or product development measure. Softening point and thermal expansion testing have been used for dental porcelain enamels.

Ion release may be necessary to understand a material's performance, such as its dissolution in a liquid. A pH meter will show if acidic or alkaline (basic) ions are released. Wet chemical analyses identify the metal ions in eluted liquids although newer techniques have supplanted wet chemistry. Atomic absorption spectroscopy (AAS) and atomic emission spectroscopy (AES) equipment quantitatively determine elements using light absorption by metallic ions dissolved in a liquid (such as an acid), nebulizing, and heating with a flame to excite the atoms and cause characteristic photon emission. Other techniques use inductively coupled plasma with mass spectrometry (ICP-MS) or with optical emission spectroscopy (ICP-OES) to detect elements faster and at lower concentrations than AAS or AES. ICP-MS uses an argon (Ar) plasma to convert a sample into ions that are measured using a scanning quadrupole mass filter MS and a detector. The ICP is at atmospheric pressure; the MS and detector operate in a vacuum chamber. ICP-OES uses an optical spectrometer to measure the light emitted from elements as they pass through the plasma. An ICP-MS provides much lower detection limits than ICP-OES.

Compounds can be "deciphered" using infrared absorbance, such as Fourier-transform infrared spectroscopy (FTIR). FTIR measures how much light is absorbed over a range of wavelengths. Fourier-transform spectroscopy shines a multi-wavelength beam and measures how much of IR light is assimilated by the sample at various wavelengths. The light passes into a Michelson interferometer – a specific configuration of mirrors, one of which is moved by a motor. Wavelengths of light are modulated by the thin sample, creating a spectrum. A computer analysis of the data is used to infer the absorption at each wavelength. Another technique, UV–vis spectroscopy, shines a monochromatic light beam at a sample to measure how much UV and visible light is absorbed over a range of wavelengths. Compounds are also determined and measured by liquid or gas chromatography with a coupled mass spectrometer (LC/MS and GC/MS). Gas chromatography, also known as vapor-phase chromatography (VPC) or gas–liquid partition chromatography (GLPC), requires vaporization of compounds without causing their decomposition. As with GC, liquid chromatography relies on passing the material, dispersed and diluted in a liquid, through a column of absorbent media, and the residence time is characteristic of the substances.

Raman spectroscopy records the vibrational modes of molecules bombarded with lasers or X-rays. An incident laser beam is reflected from a material, and the modified energy is correlated to known molecular vibrations, revealing the composition, similar to IR analysis. A spectrum is recorded from which molecules are discerned. Raman spectroscopy analyzes a tiny volume ($<1\,\mu m$ in diameter, $<10\,\mu m$ in depth). Water does not interfere with Raman spectral analysis, making it suitable for the microscopic examination of hydrated ceramics. A Raman system has an optical microscope, a laser, a monochromator or polychromator, and a detector (such as a charge-coupled device (CCD) or photomultiplier tube (PMT)). Many variations are used for Raman spectroscopy, including FTIR-Raman and UV lasers.

Less common is nuclear magnetic resonance (NMR) analysis, which requires more expensive equipment than the other costly analytical equipment mentioned. An NMR spectrometer uses a spinning sample holder inside a very strong magnet, a radio-frequency emitter, an antenna surrounding the sample, and electronic controls. This technique records the re-orientation of atomic nuclei with non-zero nuclear spins in an external magnetic field. Less than 1 g of sample is non-destructively analyzed. The NMR active nuclei, such as ^{1}H or ^{13}C, in a magnet will absorb the radio frequencies at a frequency characteristic of the isotope, and the atomic constituents can be identified. The resonant frequency, energy of the radiation absorbed, and the intensity of the signal are proportional to the strength of the magnetic field.

This overview of analytical equipment serves to introduce the reader to the types of tools that materials scientists use to understand the composition and correlate with other properties observed. Many techniques are used in combination to understand and develop dental ceramics.

Summary of Testing Dental Ceramics

This chapter presented an informal overview of some testing methods used for ceramics to assess the performance of dental and other industrial ceramics. It is not a thorough or all-inclusive list of every dental material test; many inventive methods and equipment have been used to evaluate special effects or properties needed for performance and comparisons of dental ceramics. Notably, some tests for dental materials are simplistic and suitable for dental researchers or graduate students to perform efficiently and compare materials; other tests require expensive equipment, software, and the ability to interpret the spectra from an instrument. How suitable these tests are for indications of clinical performance is always subject to debate in the literature. An excellent example of materials science fabrication and characterization of dental materials is in reference (85).

This potpourri of analysis techniques facilitates identification of components, their percentages, and understanding of the performance of dental materials. The testing of ceramics is an indirect but essential process for dental research and manufacturing. Most of the testing equipment mentioned in this chapter rely on electronic controls; ceramics in electronics are inescapably important to the testing and the items being tested.

Ceramics in Chapter 6

The following ceramics and other inorganic materials were mentioned in this chapter:

- alumina
  - glass-bonded alumina
  - sapphire
- bioactive glass
  - silica, calcia, phosphorus pentoxide
  - silica, magnesia, boron oxide
- calcium aluminate cement
- calcium hydroxide
- calcium silicate cement
- diamond
- gypsum
- hydroxyapatite
- porcelain, with leucite
- silica, quartz
- silicon carbide
- zirconia

References

1 Darvell, B.W. (2023). Mechanical test relevance – a personal perspective on some methods and requirements. *Front Dent Med* 3: 1–14.

2 Zhang, Y.R., Du, W., Zhou, X.D., and Yu, H.Y. (2014). Review of research on the mechanical properties of the human tooth. *Int J Oral Sci* 6 (2): 61–69.

3 Chun, K., Choi, H., and Lee, J. (2014). Comparison of mechanical property and role between enamel and dentin in the human teeth. *J Dent Biomech* 5: 1–7.

4 Bechtle, S., Ozcoban, H., Lilleodden, E.T. et al. (2012). Hierarchical flexural strength of enamel: transition from brittle to damage-tolerant behaviour. *J R Soc Interface* 9: 1265–1274.

5 Banks, R.G. (1990). Conservative posterior ceramic restorations: a literature review. *J Prosth Dent* 63 (6): 619–626.

6 Fei, X., Li, Y., Zhang, Q. et al. (2024). Novel pit and fissure sealant with nano-CaF(2) and antibacterial monomer: fluoride recharge, microleakage, sealing ability and cytotoxicity. *Dent Mater J* 43 (3): 1–13.

7 Stifler, C.A., Jakes, J.E., North, J.D. et al. (2021). Crystal misorientation correlates with hardness in tooth enamels. *Acta Biomater* 120: 124–134.

8 Ismail, H.S., Morrow, B.R., Ali, A.I. et al. (2024). Effect of different storage media on elemental analysis and microhardness of cervical cavity margins restored with a bioactive material. *Restor Dent Endod* 49 (1): 1–16.

9 Arola, D.D., Gao, S., Zhang, H., and Masri, R. (2017). The tooth: its structure and properties. *Dent Clin N Am* 61 (4): 651–668.

10 Cui, B., Li, J., Wang, H. et al. (2017). Mechanical properties of polymer-infiltrated-ceramic (sodium aluminum silicate) composites for dental restoration. *J Dent* 62: 91–97.

11 Iwamoto, N. and Ruse, N.D. (2003). Fracture toughness of human dentin. *J Biomed Mater Res A* 66 (3): 507–512.

12 Chen, Y., Maghami, E., Bai, X. et al. (2023). Which dentine analogue material can replace human dentine for crown fatigue test? *Dent Mater*: official publication of the Academy of Dental Materials 39 (1): 86–100.

13 Sheets, J., Wee, A., Simetich, B., and Beatty, M. (2020). Effect of water dilution on full-arch gypsum implant master casts. *Prosthesis* 2 (4): 266–276.

14 Kim, J.H., Im, Y.W., Oh, S. et al. (2019). Characterization of an anti-foaming and fast-setting gypsum for dental stone. *Dent Mater*: official publication of the Academy of Dental Materials 35 (12): 1728–1739.

15 O'Brien, W.J. (2008). *Dental materials and their selection*, 4the, 425. Hanover Park, IL: Quintessence Pub. Co.

16 Ali, M., Okamoto, M., Watanabe, M. et al. (2022). Biological properties of lithium-containing surface pre-reacted glass fillers as direct pulp-capping cements. *Dent Mater*: official publication of the Academy of Dental Materials 38 (2): 294–308.

17 Krishnan, M., Tiwari, B., Seema, S. et al. (2014). Transparent magnesium aluminate spinel: a prospective biomaterial for esthetic orthodontic brackets. *J Mater Sci Mater Med* 25 (11): 2591–2599.
18 Krell, A. and Bales, A. (2011). Grain size-dependent hardness of transparent magnesium aluminate spinel. *Int J Appl Ceram Technol* 8 (5): 1108–1114.
19 Adcock, J.M., Sidow, S.J., Looney, S.W. et al. (2011). Histologic evaluation of canal and isthmus debridement efficacies of two different irrigant delivery techniques in a closed system. *J Endodont* 37 (4): 544–548.
20 Starling, L.B. (1985). Transfer molded "All Ceramic Crowns": the cerestore system. In: *Proceedings of conference on recent developments in dental ceramics*, Ceramic engineering and science proceedings (ed. W. Smothers), 41–56. The American Ceramic Society.
21 Denry, I.L. and Rosenstiel, S.F. (1993). Flexural strength and fracture toughness of dicor glass-ceramic after embedment modification. *J Dent Res* 72 (3): 572–576.
22 Zhang, Y. and Kelly, J.R. (2017). Dental ceramics for restoration and metal veneering. *Dent Clin N Am* 61 (4): 797–819.
23 Scherrera, S.S., Kelly, J.R., Quinn, G.D., and Xu, K. (1999). Fracture toughness (KIc) of a dental porcelain determined by fractographic analysis. *Dent Mater*: official publication of the Academy of Dental Materials 15: 342–348.
24 Darvell, B.W. (2009). *Materials science for dentistry*. Oxford Boca Raton: Woodhead Pub.; CRC Press.
25 Vallerini, B.F., Pinelli, L.A.P., Silva, L.D. et al. (2025). Assessment of the chemical solubility of experimental and commercial lithium silicate glass-ceramics. *Dent Mater*: official publication of the Academy of Dental Materials 41 (3): e8–e17.
26 Gali, S. and K R. (2019). Zirconia toughened mica glass ceramics for dental restorations: wear, thermal, optical and cytocompatibility properties. *Dent Mater*: official publication of the Academy of Dental Materials 35 (12): 1706–1717.
27 Kim, H.K. (2020). Optical and mechanical properties of highly translucent dental zirconia. *Materials (Basel)* 13 (15): 3395.
28 Naliani, S., Sutanto, D., Evelyna, A., and Hizkia, M.A. (2021). Compressive strength and Weibull distribution of lithium disilicate dental ceramics. *Makassar Dent J* 10 (3): 201–203.
29 Nandini, S. (2010). Indirect resin composites. *J Conserv Dent* 13 (4): 184–194.
30 Cho, K., Rajan, G., Farrar, P. et al. (2022). Dental resin composites: a review on materials to product realizations. *Compos Part B* 230: 1–22.
31 Bala, O., Arisu, H.D., Yikilgan, I. et al. (2012). Evaluation of surface roughness and hardness of different glass ionomer cements. *Eur J Dent* 6 (1): 79–86.
32 Lohbauer, U. (2009). Dental glass ionomer cements as permanent filling materials? – properties, limitations and future trends. *Materials* 3 (1): 76–96.
33 Osiewicz, M.A., Werner, A., Roeters, F.J.M., and Kleverlaan, C.J. (2022). Wear of bulk-fill resin composites. *Dent Mater*: official publication of the Academy of Dental Materials 38 (3): 549–553.

34 Daabash, R., Alshabib, A., Alqahtani, M.Q. et al. (2022). Ion releasing direct restorative materials: key mechanical properties and wear. *Dent Mater*: official publication of the Academy of Dental Materials 38 (12): 1866–1877.

35 Gauthier, M.M. (ed.) (1995). Crystallography and engineering properties of ceramics. In: *Engineered materials handbook desk edition*, 691–1188. ASM International.

36 Bayne, S.C. (2013). Beginnings of the dental composite revolution. *J Am Dent Assoc* 144 (8): 880–884.

37 Bowen, R.L. (1963). Properties of a silica-reinforced polymer for dental restorations. *J Amer Dent Assoc* 66 (1): 57–64.

38 Morrell, R. (1998). *Biaxial flexural strength testing of ceramic materials*. Centre for Materials Measurement and Technology National Physical Laboratory.

39 Miura, D., Ishida, Y., Miyasaka, T. et al. (2020). Reliability of different bending test Methods for dental press ceramics. *Materials (Basel)* 13 (22): 1–10.

40 Xiao, H., Wang, X., and Long, C. (2021). Theoretical model for determining elastic modulus of ceramic materials by nanoindentation. *Materialia* 17: 1–8.

41 Liao, Y., Gruber, M., Lukic, H. et al. (2020). Fracture toughness of zirconia with a nanometer size notch fabricated using focused ion beam milling. *J Biomed Mater Res B Appl Biomater* 108 (8): 3323–3330.

42 Quinn, G.D., Salem, J., Bar-on, I. et al. (1992). Fracture toughness of advanced ceramics at room temperature. *J Res Natl Inst Stand Technol* 97 (5): 579–607.

43 Wang, A., Hu, P., Zhang, X. et al. (2017). Accurate measurement of fracture toughness in structural ceramics. *J Eur Ceram Soc* 37 (13): 4207–4212.

44 dos Santos, D.M., Monteiro, R.V., Athayde, F.R.F., and De Souza, G.M. (2023). In vitro and practical guide for the analysis of bond strength to ceramics. *Cer Intl* 49 (11): 17099–17108.

45 Perdigao, J., Araujo, E., Ramos, R.Q. et al. (2021). Adhesive dentistry: current concepts and clinical considerations. *J Esthet Restor Dent*: official publication of the American Academy of Esthetic Dentistry [et al] 33 (1): 51–68.

46 Bourgi, R., Kharouf, N., Cuevas-Suárez, C.E. et al. (2024). A literature review of adhesive systems in dentistry: key components and their clinical applications. *Appl Sci* 14 (18): 1–51.

47 Khan, S.A., Tushar, Nezam, S. et al. (2020). Comparison and evaluation of linear dimensional accuracy of three elastomeric impression materials at different time intervals using vision inspection system: an in vitro study. *J Int Soc Prev Comm Dent* 10 (6): 736–742.

48 Kar, S., Tripathi, A., Singh, J., and Ramkumar, J. (2022). Comparison of dimensional accuracy of elastomeric impression materials using 3D laser scanner. *Med J Armed Forces India* 78 (Suppl 1): S55–S60.

49 Kumari, N. and Nandeeshwar, D.B. (2015). The dimensional accuracy of polyvinyl siloxane impression materials using two different impression techniques: An in vitro study. *J Indian Prosth Soc* 15 (3): 211–217.

50 Salzedas, L.M.P., Louzada, M.J.Q., and Filho, A.B.O. (2006). Radiopacity of restorative materials using digital images. *J Appl Oral Sci* 14 (2): 147–152.

51 An, S.Y., Lee, D.H., and Lee, K.B. (2015). Radiopacity for contemporary luting cements using digital radiography under various exposure conditions. *J Prosthodont*: official journal of the American College of Prosthodontists 24 (8): 642–646.

52 Nascimento, M.M., Dilbone, D.A., Pereira, P.N. et al. (2016). Abfraction lesions: etiology, diagnosis, and treatment options. *Clin Cosmet Investig Dent* 8: 79–87.

53 Marus, R. (2011(June)). Esthetic and predictable treatment of abfraction lesions. *Inside Dentistry* 7 (6): 1–3.

54 Heintze, S.D., Barkmeier, W.W., Latta, M.A., and Rousson, V. (2011). Round robin test: wear of nine dental restorative materials in six different wear simulators – supplement to the round robin test of 2005. *Dent Mater*: official publication of the Academy of Dental Materials 27 (2): e1–e9.

55 Koletsi, D., Iliadi, A., Eliades, T., and Eliades, G. (2019). In vitro simulation and in vivo assessment of tooth wear: a meta-analysis of in vitro and clinical research. *Materials (Basel)* 12 (21): 1–15.

56 Wang, R., Zhu, Y., Chen, C. et al. (2022). Tooth wear and tribological investigations in dentistry. *Appl Bionics Biomech* 2022: 2861197.

57 Barclay, C.W., Spence, D., and Laird, W.R.E. (2005). Intra-oral temperatures during function. *J Oral Rehabil* 32 (12): 886–894.

58 Alrahlah, A. (2018). Diametral tensile strength, flexural strength, and surface microhardness of bioactive bulk fill restorative. *J Contemp Dent Prac* 19 (1): 13–19.

59 Morresi, A.L., D'Amario, M., Capogreco, M. et al. (2014). Thermal cycling for restorative materials: does a standardized protocol exist in laboratory testing? A literature review. *J Mech Behav Biomed Mater* 29: 295–308.

60 Gale, M.S. and Darvell, B.W. (1999). Thermal cycling procedures for laboratory testing of dental restorations. *J Dent* 27: 89–99.

61 Meng, Q., Zhang, K., He, R., and Qu, Z. (2024). A review of thermal shock behavior of ceramics: fundamental theory, experimental methods, and outlooks. *Int J Appl Ceram Technol* 21 (6): 3789–3811.

62 Alessandretti, R., Borba, M., and Della Bona, A. (2020). Cyclic contact fatigue resistance of ceramics for monolithic and multilayer dental restorations. *Dent Mater*: official publication of the Academy of Dental Materials 36 (4): 535–541.

63 Drummond, J.L. (2008). Degradation, fatigue, and failure of resin dental composite materials. *J Dent Res* 87 (8): 710–719.

64 Drummond, J.L., Lin, L., Al-Turki, L.A., and Hurley, R.K. (2009). Fatigue behaviour of dental composite materials. *J Dent* 37 (5): 321–330.

65 O'Brien, W., Oh, W.-S., and Piché, P. (2012). Color parameters of the chromascop shade guide. *Dent J* 1 (1): 3–11.

66 Yu, B., Ahn, J.S., Lim, J.I., and Lee, Y.K. (2009). Influence of TiO_2 nanoparticles on the optical properties of resin composites. *Dent Mater*: official publication of the Academy of Dental Materials 25 (9): 1142–1147.

67 Johnston, W.M. (2014). Review of translucency determinations and applications to dental materials. *J Esthet Restor Dent*: official publication of the American Academy of Esthetic Dentistry [et al] 26 (4): 217–223.

68 Camilleri, J. (2014). Color stability of white mineral trioxide aggregate in contact with hypochlorite solution. *J Endodont* 40 (3): 436–440.

69 Valles, M., Mercade, M., Duran-Sindreu, F. et al. (2013). Influence of light and oxygen on the color stability of five calcium silicate-based materials. *J Endodont* 39 (4): 525–528.

70 Krug, R., Ortmann, C., Reich, S. et al. (2022). Tooth discoloration induced by apical plugs with hydraulic calcium silicate-based cements in teeth with open apices-a 2-year in vitro study. *Clin Oral Investig* 26 (1): 375–383.

71 Primus, C.M., Chu, C.C., Shelby, J.E. et al. (2002). Opalescence of dental porcelain enamels. *Quintessence Int* 33 (6): 439–449.

72 Guo, S. and Dipietro, L.A. (2010). Factors affecting wound healing. *J Dent Res* 89 (3): 219–229.

73 Choudhury, H., Pandey, M., Lim, Y.Q. et al. (2020). Silver nanoparticles: advanced and promising technology in diabetic wound therapy. *Mater Sci Eng C Mater Biol Appl* 112 (110925): 1–16.

74 Arandi, N.Z. (2017). Calcium hydroxide liners: a literature review. *Clin Cosmet Investig Dent* 9: 67–72.

75 Gluskin, A.H., Lai, G., Peters, C.I., and Peters, O.A. (2020). The double-edged sword of calcium hydroxide in endodontics: precautions and preventive strategies for extrusion injuries into neurovascular anatomy. *J Am Dent Assoc* 151 (5): 317–326.

76 Leye Benoist, F., Gaye Ndiaye, F., Kane, A.W. et al. (2012). Evaluation of mineral trioxide aggregate (MTA) versus calcium hydroxide cement (Dycal®) in the formation of a dentine bridge: a randomised controlled trial. *Int Dent J* 62 (1): 33–39.

77 Sarkar, N.K., Caicedo, R., Ritwik, P. et al. (2005). Physicochemical basis of the biologic properties of mineral trioxide aggregate. *J Endodont* 31 (2): 97–100.

78 Accorinte Mde, L., Holland, R., Reis, A. et al. (2008). Evaluation of mineral trioxide aggregate and calcium hydroxide cement as pulp-capping agents in human teeth. *J Endodont* 34 (1): 1–6.

79 Hilton, T.J., Ferracane, J.L., and Mancl, L. (2013). Northwest practice-based research collaborative in evidence-based D. Comparison of CaOH with MTA for direct pulp capping: a PBRN randomized clinical trial. *J Dent Res* 92 (7 Suppl): 16S–22S.

80 Joy, D.C. (2008). The aberration-corrected SEM. In: *Biological low-voltage scanning electron microscopy*, 107–127. Springer.

81 Sharps, M.C., Martinez, M.M., Brandl, M. et al. (2021). A dual beam SEM-based EDS and micro-XRF method for the analysis of large-scale Mesoamerican obsidian tablets. *J Archaeol Sci Rep* 35: 102781.

82 Cardell, C. and Guerra, I. (2016). An overview of emerging hyphenated SEM-EDX and Raman spectroscopy systems: applications in life, environmental and materials sciences. *Trends Anal Chem* 77: 156–166.

83 Peddie, C.J., Genoud, C., Kreshuk, A. et al. (2022). Volume electron microscopy. *Nat Rev Methods Primers* 2 (1): 1–53.

84 Schlumberger, C., Scherdel, C., Kriesten, M. et al. (2022). Reliable surface area determination of powders and meso/macroporous materials: small-angle X-ray scattering and gas physisorption. *Microporous Mesoporous Mater* 329: 1–8.

85 Fischer, N.G., de Souza Araujo, I.J., Daghrery, A. et al. (2025). Guidance on biomaterials for periodontal tissue regeneration: fabrication methods, materials and biological considerations. *Dent Mater*: official publication of the Academy of Dental Materials 41 (3): 283–305.

7

Forming Ceramics

Ceramic items in our everyday lives originate from forming and firing powders to form a solid item. The properties of the final ceramic start with the formula and powders used for processing via the forming and firing steps described here. Glass items are melted, and then cast, blown, molded, drawn, or quenched to form an object or a powder. Polycrystalline ceramics are formed and sintered from 500 to 3000 °C. Shrinkage is an ever-present consideration that has been the bane – and bailiwick – of ceramic engineers and dental technicians. The forming and firing techniques used for dental powders have imitated industrial processes: hot and cold pressing, slip casting, "ceramming" of glasses, 3D printing of ceramic powders, and Copy or Computer-Aided Design & Milling (CAD-CAM). Although costly, CAD-CAM equipment is being used by about 70% of US practices and dental laboratories. The 3D printing techniques are commonly used for polymeric devices, such as models (Chapter 14) and nightguards.

Most ceramics originate with processing minerals found in nature that are processed into powder. Other ceramic powders are precipitated from chemically purified compounds. For instance, the sol–gel chemical process starts with dissolving a colloidal solution (sol) of chemicals as a precursor for creating a gel, followed by chemical precipitation (1, 2). Typical precursors are metal alkoxides, an alkaline solution of alcohol with the metal ions connected to the alcohol. The precipitated gel is dried and fired to a higher temperature to create a powder, which is usually processed by milling, grinding, and sieving. The sol-gel process is used to produce ceramic nanoparticles.

Fumed silica nanoparticles are ubiquitous in dentistry, especially toothpastes, and also for cosmetics and food; fumed silica is a thickener and stabilizer for pastes. The fume is made by injecting microscopic droplets of silicon tetrachloride into a flame (pyrogenic process), resulting in amorphous silica nanoparticles (~100 to 300 nm) that often form larger branched "chains," (3) as shown in

Ceramics in Dentistry: Materials, Manufacturing, and Clinical Applications,
First Edition. Carolyn M. Primus.

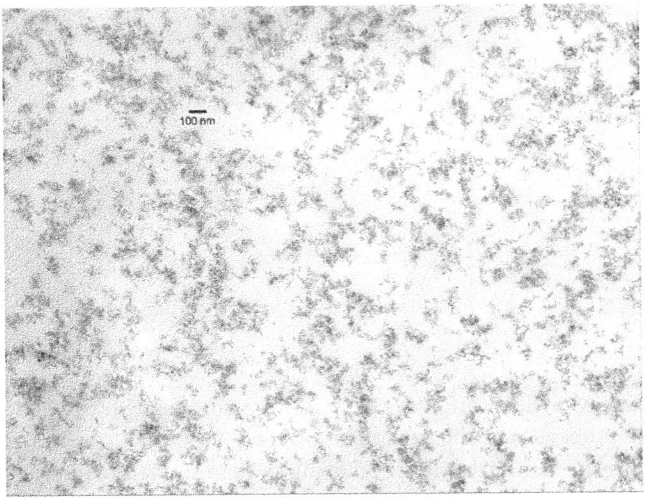

Figure 7.1 Transmission electron micrograph image of fumed silica nanoparticles dispersed in a dental adhesive. Note the fractal nature (never-ending pattern across the scale) of the silica filler. *Source:* Courtesy of Solventum Company.

Figure 7.1. Silica sols (solutions) of such particles also have broad uses in dentistry, as well as other medical devices and cosmetics.

Other ceramic powders are made by grinding minerals or purified ceramics into the desired particle size range. Purity of the powder depends on the source and the prior processing of the material. Crushing of minerals or chunks of glass is used for the primary powder processing, followed by grinding, wet or dry, in ball, rod mills, and fluid energy (air impact) mills. Dry milling includes "balls" of various shapes and sizes that tumble with the powder in a rotating or vibrating container to impart energy and create finer (smaller) particles. Wet milling uses balls or beads in equipment that tumbles, vibrates, agitates (stirred or attrition) or uses planetary motion; the latter combining centrifugal and Coriolis motions. The batches vary from 1 to 700 L in industrial mills and can create micron-sized particles.

Powders are often processed to extract a certain size fraction, be it coarse, fine, or a blend with dry, ultrasonic, vibratory, or air sieves (classifiers) to create the size fractions of powders suitable for the next step of processing. Fine powders of ceramics ($<10\,\mu m$) are often desired for smooth mixtures and easier forming but are complicated by the agglomeration of particles. Some powders are granulated by pressure filtering or spray drying of a thin slurry of the powders to facilitate the next consolidation step.

Forming Polycrystalline Ceramics

Glass and crystalline ceramic powders are blended, formed, and fired to manufacture solid ceramic items. The powders may be blended via dry or "wet" methods with water, organic liquids, or polymers. The blending is comparatively simple for the lower viscosity liquid-powder mixtures; viscous mixtures require more energy and sophisticated equipment. The processing parameters for powder mixing and blending are many: the composition of the dry and liquid ingredients, the starting particle size, the equipment's method of combining, and the time. Some ceramic powders are blended and then fired to create different compounds, which may also be ground into a new powder; Portland cement (calcium silicate cement) powder is the most common example of firing to create the desired phases. The forming of a ceramic item is dependent on the particle size distribution of the powders, their composition, and the assortment of additives used to form the powders into an object. The strongest ceramics are formed into solid objects using methods to minimize pores, machining flaws (surface cracks), and include little glass content. More translucent polycrystalline ceramics are usually formed with a glass powder.

Ceramic powders, pastes, or suspensions of powders are fashioned into shapes via techniques such as dry-pressing, injection molding (IM), extrusion, slip casting, cold isostatic pressing, or tape-casting. See Figure 7.2 for diagrams of these methods. The goal is to compact ceramic powders into a shape suitable for heat treating, preferably having a shape that is as close to the final shape desired (near net shape), which means less machining will be required after firing. Uniaxial dry-pressing is a technique to compress powders, using a single- or double-action mold; it requires very little binder additive. However, density gradients in the compacted powder can sometimes be detected after sintering; for more uniformity, cold isostatic pressing of powders is used. For hydrostatic (isostatic) pressing, the powders are packed into a polymer bag, which may have a rudimentary shape. The bag is uniformly compressed using about 250 MPa hydrostatic pressure from an oil, sometimes warm, that surrounds the bag, to form a compacted powder of density of 40–60% having fewer density gradients than uniaxial compaction. Slip casting requires ceramic powders to be suspended in a relatively low-viscosity, aqueous liquid. The powder suspension is poured into a mold; the water is gradually absorbed by the porous mold, gradually forming a thick layer of ceramic powder on the walls of the mold. The excess slip suspension is poured out of the mold, and the green shape of the molded ceramic is carefully separated from the mold. For IM, a ceramic powder is mixed with organic additives to form a dough that is forced with pressure into a mold; heat and pressure may be used to ensure the dough completely fills the mold's cavity. Extrusion is like IM, but a continuous object, such as a rod or tube, is formed. Tape-casting is another forming method that makes a thin, flexible ribbon of ceramic from a suspension

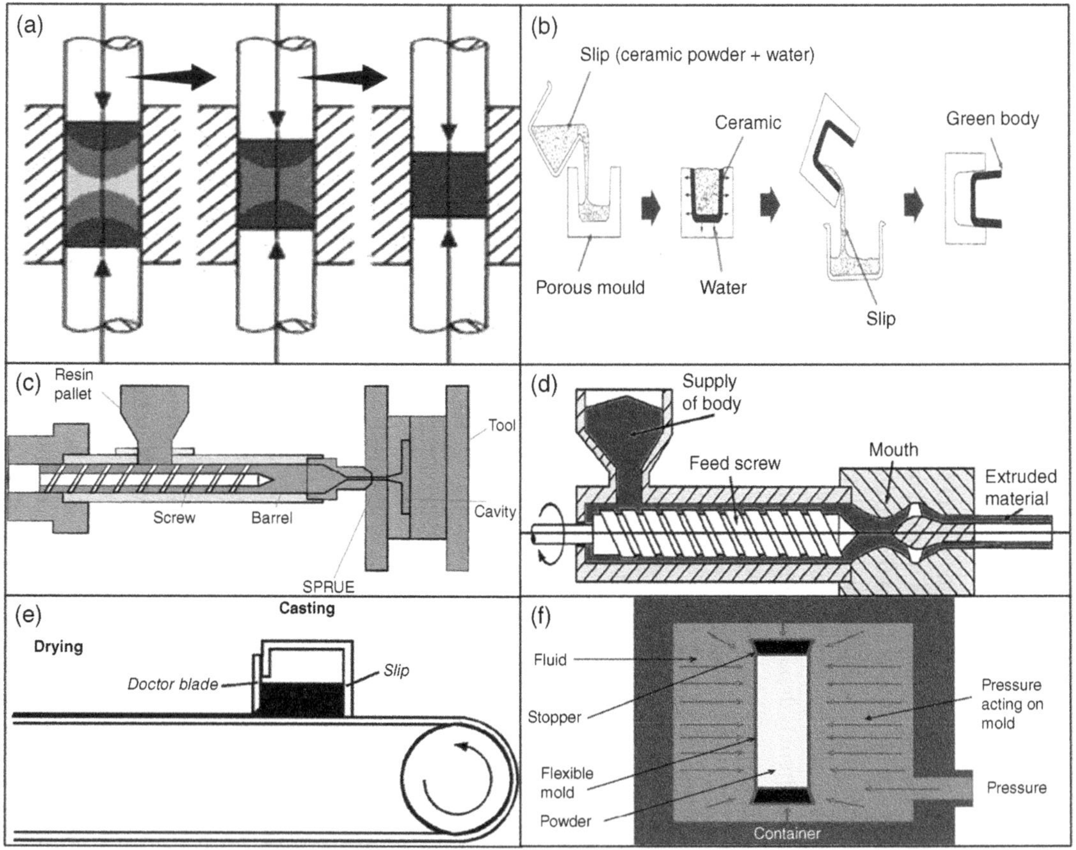

Figure 7.2 Schematics of the methods of forming ceramic powders: (a) dry-pressing or uniaxial hot-pressing, (b) slip casting, (c) injection molding, (d) extrusion, (e) tape-casting, and (f) isostatic (hydraulic) cold- or hot-pressing.

compressed on a flat surface; this method is essential for making the flat electronic substrates so important in modern devices. After any forming processes, the ceramic items are considered to be "green" and usually require drying, debinding (removal of organics), and sintering (firing), which are described later.

Three-dimensional printing of ceramic powders is accomplished via several methods, including selective laser sintering, inkjet printing, stereolithography (digital light processing), and nanoparticle ink-jetting. The 3D forming techniques for ceramics require organic liquids combined with ceramic powders in a thick slurry (or ink) to form the shapes using manufacturing. The 3D techniques are very beneficial for complex or custom objects and rapid prototyping. Unlike IM, molds are not needed for 3D printing; however, software and equipment are necessary to create a computerized design (CAD) for dispensing and stabilizing the ceramic suspension to the design. The composition, rheology, and 3D printing parameters of the ceramic-organic pastes are crucial to creating shapes and avoiding defects at the boundaries between printing "passes" or layers. To date, dental laboratories are more likely than dentists to use 3D printing which is currently used for constructing models and nightguards. These 3D printing items do not require ceramic fillers; no subsequent heat treatment is needed.

Unique methods of forming ceramics are evolving, especially for fibrous or porous ceramics. Examples are solutions electrospinning of membranes, electrowriting (use of electric field to guide polymer printing), and "fused deposition" – extrusion and "printing" of molten thermoplastics, for instance, for periodontal tissue engineering (4).

Any forming technique must be carefully performed because defects made during forming will usually remain after the firing process. For instance, pores in a slip-cast item will not be eliminated during sintering, and density gradients in cold-pressed powders will be present after firing. After forming, the "green" ceramics may be suitable for machining, trimming, or cutting, but are fragile compared to those after sintering.

Sintering

Firing was serendipitously developed in human history as a method to transform dried, molded clay into bricks, porcelain toilets or sinks, and tableware. Firing is a multistep process that materials engineers call sintering, which consolidates (densifies) green ceramic objects without melting the entire object. The goal of forming and sintering ceramic powders is to create strong, fully dense, (pore-free) ceramics suitable for their application.

The first phase of firing is the removal of water and organics used in forming the molded/formed green ceramics. The formula of a ceramic powder batch is crucial for forming and firing. The water or organic additives are dissipated by evaporation, sublimation, or decomposition by raising the temperature. This "burn-out" phase, also denoted as drying and debinding, is often executed with slow and stepwise heating to about 600 °C, which is a temperature at which most organic materials are evaporated or decomposed. Carbonate and nitrate salts (e.g. K_2SO_4 Na_2CO_3) are sometimes included in a powder formula that also decompose at temperatures from 300 to 1200 °C, releasing gases but leaving behind the metal oxide (i.e. potassia, soda; K_2O, Na_2O). Gases, including carbon dioxide or nitrous oxides from the salts or organics, are released during burn-out, the gaseous product of decomposition. The burn-out phase to eliminate binders is fraught with hazards such as rapid gas release that can create large pores and distort the green shape, which are irreversibly deleterious events. Some salts melt at lower temperatures than they decompose, which is another complication for burn-out that potentially causes distortion. After eliminating the organic binders, an even more porous, fragile ceramic shape remains. Firing of the fragile ceramic is continued in an oven (kiln, furnace) for strengthening via sintering.

Sintering occurs at a higher temperature when the ceramic powder particles bond, pores are eliminated, and a strong solid ceramic object is created. Sintering causes compacted particles to coalesce via a thermodynamically driven phenomenon – the reduction of surface energy. The surface-to-air contact area is replaced with the lower energy particle-to-particle contact. The particle contacts create grain boundaries that accommodate the misorientation of the crystals (Figure 5.1). Sintering can be performed with powders of ceramics, metals, and polymers. Even ice sinters: ice cubes in water and alcohol will stick together as they melt; ice crystals will coalesce in the freezer (5). Snowflakes sinter to form ice crystals at temperatures near −15 °C, a phenomenon studied for glaciers. Sintering starts to occur roughly above one-half the melting temperature of a compound in absolute temperature (Kelvin). For instance, alumina has a melting point of 2345 K (2072 °C), and sintering is measurable above 1273 K (1000 °C) (6). Exceptions to this rule exist for clever new sintering methods discussed below. Heat gives the molecules more energy to diffuse, rearrange, and reduce the surface area by forming the lower-energy interparticle contacts.

The science of sintering was developed in the latter half of the 20th century by ceramic engineers. They identified these sintering mechanisms: surface transport (surface diffusion or evaporation-condensation) and solid state diffusion (bulk transport), including grain boundary diffusion, volume diffusion, plastic or viscous flow, and dislocation migration (more common in metals) (7, 8). Sintering mechanisms cause three phenomena: reduction of pores with concomitant adhesion of particles, change of particle shape to form connected "grains," and growth of the powder particles (grain growth). The dominant mechanism depends on the composition, the powder size distribution, and the firing schedule. Sintering has

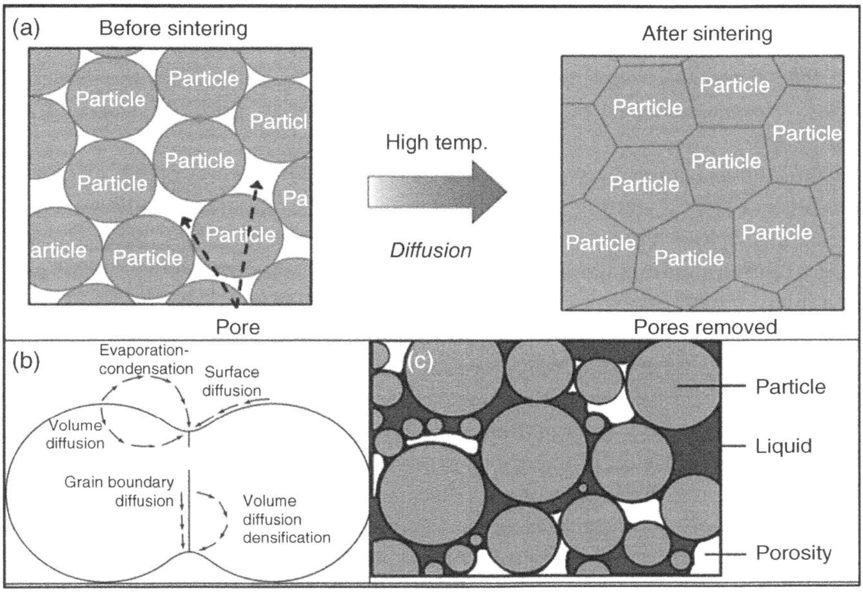

Figure 7.3 Models of sintering showing: (a) ideal spherical particles forming fully dense grains after sintering, (b) motion of molecules during mechanisms of sintering, and (c). liquid-phase sintering where a partially dense material has been formed after sintering (some pores remain) – this is akin to viscous flow of a glass phase between crystalline particles. [The dislocation migration mechanism is not depicted.]

been modeled as the contact between two idealized spherical particles, as shown in Figure 7.3. As sintering occurs, the particle-to-particle contacts flatten and form "necks" which bond the powder particles. The necks grow, reducing the pores in size and number during sintering. Ceramic powder particles are mostly irregular and angular shapes, rarely spherical as depicted; however, the concept of coalescing and flattened contacts ("necking") is useful. As densification progresses, surface diffusion slows, and grain boundary diffusion becomes dominant. In addition to the sintering mechanisms, reactions may occur to form new ceramic phases, particularly when mineral and a glass powders are combined.

The surface diffusion and evaporation-condensation sintering mechanisms do not cause shrinkage but do strengthen a powder compact by reducing the surface area and expanding the interparticle contacts (neck growth) between the particles; these mechanisms usually dominate at lower temperatures than the bulk transport mechanisms. The bulk diffusion sintering mechanisms cause shrinkage of the powder compact, as much as twenty linear percent, because these mechanisms eliminate pores and allow grains (crystals) to grow. Smaller grains may be engulfed by larger grains, eliminating some grain boundaries, which is another thermodynamic driving force. Sometimes, shrinkage may appear non-uniform because shrinkage occurs more easily in denser areas and toward the center of mass; complex shapes of the "green" ceramic may undergo non-uniform shrinkage.

Liquid-phase sintering occurs under conditions where solid powder particles are present with a wetting (low contact angle), lower melting (liquid) phase. A prime example is the sintering of tungsten carbide with cobalt, used to make many tools, including dental instruments (Chapter 17). Cobalt powder can melt in a mixture with tungsten carbide powder, and the liquid cobalt wets the carbide grains, penetrating between them and inducing particle rearrangement with its lower viscosity. With some solubility of the tungsten carbide in the cobalt, densification occurs faster, eliminating pores and increasing strength and rigidity afterward. Porcelains sinter via liquid-phase sintering, where the glass acts as a wetting liquid on any higher melting crystals present. The crystalline particles may react with or dissolve in the viscous glass at elevated temperature. Wetting and capillary action contribute to liquid-phase sintering densification.

Usually, sintering is performed without pressure; however, pressure may be applied to accelerate sintering, using uniaxial (from one direction) or isostatic (hydraulically from all directions) force, analogous to the powder forming methods shown in Figure 7.2a and f. New methods for sintering other than radiant heating have been tested (9), such as cold, flash, ultrafast high temperature, microwave, spark plasma, combustion, and photonic sintering methods. These methods may reduce fuel consumption, sintering time, and cost. For instance, "cold" sintering is done below 300 °C and requires a low viscosity (fluid) paste of oxides – and perhaps polymers – that is compressed with up to 600 MPa; densification occurs at temperatures that may be less than 50% of the conventional sintering temperature. A final heat process may be needed after cold sintering.

Ultrafast sintering uses two carbon felt pads, surrounding a thin, green ceramic (< 5 mm thick); full density can be achieved within seconds via unprecedented heating and cooling rates (typically 10^{-3} °C/min), as high as ~3000 °C. Heating is achieved by radiation and conduction in vacuum or an inert atmosphere by heating the graphite pads with electrical current. Flash sintering requires the powder compact to be in an oven between metallic connections that impart a high electrical field (volts/cm), which causes faster densification at a lower temperature than conventional sintering (10). A burst of light occurs when the ceramic begins to conduct electricity at an elevated temperature. This method is similar to flash-spark-plasma and microwave sintering methods. Microwave sintering, which was first tried in the 1960s, occurs when the microwaves of decimeter to millimeter (10^{-1} to 10^{-3} m) wavelength are absorbed by a powder compact, heat the ceramic's surface, and the heat dissipates within. This method was first used for cemented carbides containing cobalt metal and tungsten carbide. Combustion sintering/synthesis, also known as self-propagating higher-temperature synthesis, requires a compacted column of reactant powders to be heated until an exothermic reaction occurs. The combustion/reaction front moves rapidly through the mixture, creating temperatures of up to 3000 °C, to densify ceramic powders with nano-sized grains. Photonic sintering relies on millisecond-long, white light pulses from a xenon flash lamp, creating heating rates up to 108 °C/min. These fascinating heating methods are not currently known to be used for dental ceramics but may be used in the future.

The microstructure of a ceramic item after firing is dependent on the composition, the forming process, the "burn-out," and the sintering. The heating rate, maximum temperature, holding time(s), and atmosphere (air, vacuum, oxygen, hydrogen, or inert gas), influence the final ceramic microstructure. The microstructure controls the properties of strength, toughness, hardness, corrosion resistance, and wear resistance. The density, surface area, and grain size are studied for the effects of ceramic forming and firing methods. Finer powders, higher temperatures, and longer times often improve powder compact densification and properties.

Machining

Machining of a ceramic object may be required to achieve the precise shape needed, even for 3D printed ceramics. Machining can be done in the green state, after partial sintering, or in the final, fired state after sintering. Strong, fully dense ceramics are most difficult to machine; the ceramic may fracture or may wear out the machining tools. Partially sintered materials have been denoted as biscuit, bisque, pre-sintered, or partially sintered; they are an "in-process" material, which needs to have a final firing; some surface diffusion or bulk sintering is performed by the manufacturers to give strength to the material. For instance, partially sintered zirconia dental materials are strong enough to be handled and suitable for computer-aided milling into the shape of a dental crown or bridge in a dental laboratory. After milling, the final sintering process to "full density" is performed. This has replaced an earlier product of dense, magnesia-stabilized zirconia; it was difficult to machine and has been abandoned.

Lithium disilicate and zirconia have been a triumph of CAD-CAM for dentistry. Lithium disilicate crowns are machined in the partially cerammed state, described later, followed by a final ceramming step. Partially sintered zirconia is CAD-CAM processed, and then the final firing to full density is performed. Machining in the partially cerammed or sintered state is successful because of the manufacturers' excellent reproducibility of shrinkage. For some anatomical details, dentists and dental technicians may use small, rotary instruments to make the final, precise machining adjustments after the final heat treatment.

Cement Manufacture

Calcium silicate and calcium aluminate cements are ubiquitous in our built environment as floors, driveways, patios, roads, bridges, sewer systems, industrial furnaces, building blocks, and every skyscraper. These calcium-based cements do not occur naturally; they are made by firing minerals at high temperatures (~1500 °C) and quenching the reacted powders. The raw materials for calcium silicate cements usually include calcium carbonate, silica, and alumina powders from varied sources of minerals. Sometimes waste materials are included to keep costs low for the construction commodity grades, but not for dental materials. The raw materials' powders are blended, formed into pellets a few centimeters in diameter, and loaded into a kiln/furnace. Inclined rotary kilns having an automatic feed system for the raw material pellets are commonly used for continuous industrial cement firing; the pellets slowly tumble from the higher, cooler end to the hot, lower end of the kiln. The first phase of firing is the decomposition of calcium carbonate, releasing carbon dioxide. It is interesting to note that the carbon dioxide release from cement manufacture has become an environmental concern because concrete – which contains about 10–30% cement powder by volume – is the second most used substance in our world, next to water! The pellets continue to be heated and reach a peak temperature of about 1500 °C where the calcia, silica, and alumina oxides quickly react, forming the calcium silicate and calcium aluminate cement compounds described in Chapter 5. For calcium silicate cements, minor amounts of iron oxide compounds may be present in the raw minerals to lower the firing temperature required to form the tri/dicalcium silicate phases, by the ferrite's liquid-phase sintering contribution. The fired pellets are expelled as "clinker" at the lower, hot end of the inclined rotary kiln, for rapid quenching with air. Quick cooling ensures that the most water-reactive phases of calcium silicate are maintained, avoiding the formation of the gamma-dicalcium silicate; this phase is not as reactive with water as the other allotropes. The clinker nodules of cooled cement are transferred for grinding and sieving into a cement powder with a mean particle size ideally smaller than 50 μm. Non-continuous, rotary, or stationary kilns are also used for making smaller amounts (batches) of specialized cements, such as those used in dentistry. After grinding the clinker, calcium silicate cement powder is usually blended with calcium sulfate to control (slow) the hydration (setting time) of the cement, which also depends on the tricalcium aluminate content.

Calcium silicate and calcium aluminate cements appear to be just two compounds, but six cement phases are commonly present in these two materials, as

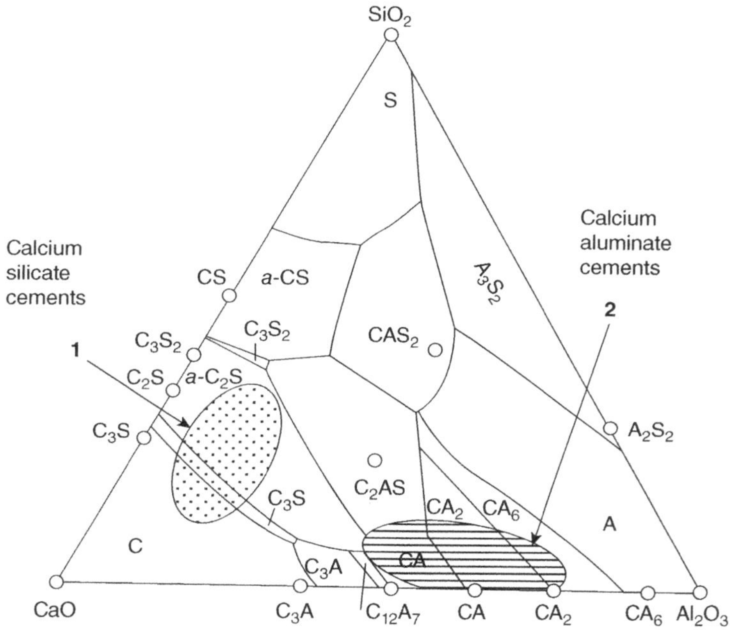

Figure 7.4 Ternary phase diagram for calcia (CaO, C), silica (SiO_2, S), and alumina (Al_2O_3, A), showing the range of compositions for the calcium silicate (area 1) and calcium aluminate (area 2) cements. The various compounds are abbreviated.

noted in Chapter 5. Materials scientists refer to phase diagrams, which show the equilibrium melting and solidification temperature of metals and ceramics, sometimes under high pressure. These depictions of the equilibrium phases are used to understand what compounds (phases) can be manufactured for a particular composition after firing to a particular temperature. The compositional ranges for the calcium silicate and the calcium aluminate cements (water-reactive compositions) are outlined in the ternary (three-component) phase diagram shown in Figure 7.4. Only a small range of compositions is suitable for manufacturing the silicate and aluminate calcium cements. The compositional ranges are non-overlapping; therefore, the two calcium cements (silicate and aluminate) must be fabricated separately.

The proportions of the phases vary within each compositional range. A phase diagram also shows how much of one material can be dissolved in another at equilibrium. For instance, a small amount of alumina can be dissolved in the calcium silicate phases, and some silica may be dissolved in the calcium aluminate phases.

The phase diagram also shows that the calcium silicate cement powders are primarily composed of crystals of two water-reactive compounds (phases): tricalcium silicate and dicalcium silicate, which are denoted as $3CaO.SiO_2$, Ca_3SiO_5, alite (haturite), and $2CaO.SiO_2$, Ca_2SiO_4, belite (larnite). Tricalcium aluminate ($3CaO.Al_2O_3$) is usually present in calcium silicate cement because of alumina mixed with most silicate raw materials. Depending on the iron oxide content of the raw materials, tetracalcium aluminoferrite ($4CaO.Al_2O_3.Fe_2O_3$, ferrite) may also be present, which lowers the firing temperature needed to make calcium silicate cement. Lower firing temperature is more economical in manufacturing, but this black iron-containing phase darkens the cement. White calcium silicate cements have a low iron content (<1%). Each brand of cement around the world is unique in the proportions of the major and minor phases, additives, and impurities.

Two, non-cement (non-water-reactive) calcium silicate phases also exist – wollastonite and rankinite (calcium silicate, $CaO.SiO_2$, $CaSiO_3$, and tricalcium disilicate, $3CaO.2SiO_2$, $Ca_3Si_2O_7$) (11); these are avoided in cement making. The lime-alumina boundary of the phase diagram in Figure 7.4 shows the six calcium aluminate compounds that exist: tricalcium aluminate, dodecacalcium hepta-aluminate, monocalcium aluminate, calcium dialuminate, and monocalcium hexa-aluminate ($3CaO.Al_2O_3$, $12CaO.7Al_2O_3$, $CaO.Al_2O_3$, $CaO.2Al_2O_3$, and $CaO.6Al_2O_3$). The reactivity (speed of setting with water) of calcium aluminates increases with the calcium oxide content, making tricalcium aluminate the most reactive among all these compounds. Industrial calcium aluminate cement usually contains calcium monoaluminate ($CaO.Al_2O_3$) and monocalcium dialuminate ($CaO.2Al_2O_3$) with only minor amounts of other phases. Calcium aluminate cements are manufactured similarly to the calcium silicate cements, combining limestone (calcium carbonate) and alumina in a rotary kiln. Some calcium aluminate cement powders are have excess alumina powder; alumina is handy in calcium aluminate cements as insulation of kilns at high temperature. Calcium aluminate cements for dental products are not known to contain alumina, which is inert.

The calcium silicate and calcium aluminate cements phases react with water, forming a hard mass composed of the remnants of the original cement particles, coated by a hydrated layer and surrounded by a matrix of the cement hydrates and alkaline, hydroxide reaction products. The calcium silicate and calcium aluminate cements are important in treating the pulp and roots, in contact with bone. See Chapter 8.

Forming Single-Crystal Ceramics

A few dental and industrial applications require large (macroscopic) single crystals, formed by crystallizing a molten ceramic. Silica, alumina, and zirconia are commercially important as single crystals. Silica single crystals are well-known semi-precious gemstones. Alumina single crystals, such as sapphires, are naturally occurring and have also been made with the flame-fusion technique of

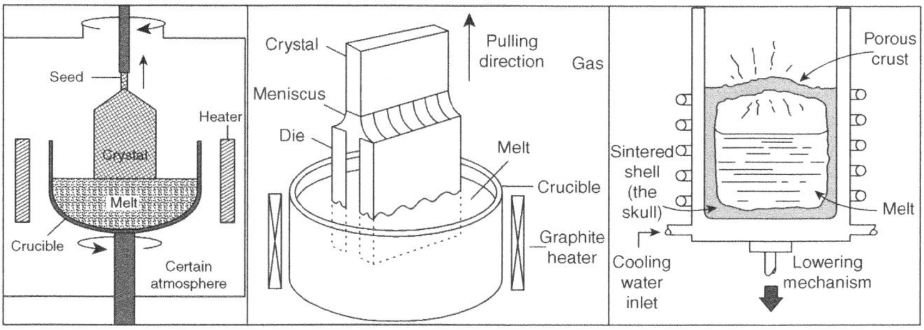

Figure 7.5 The Czochralski (left), the edge-defined, and film-fed growth (center), for drawing sapphire orthodontic brackets out of molten alumina. Skull melting method for zirconia is on the right.

Verneuil using an oxy-hydrogen torch. Sapphire crystals have been made for dental uses via the Czochralski method, or the edge-defined, film-fed growth (US Pat. No. 4,639,218) methods (Figure 7.5). With either method, a seed crystal of sapphire is inserted into molten alumina (at >2072 °C), and long crystals are drawn, which when cooled are cut into orthodontic brackets.

Zircon ($ZrSiO_4$) gemstones are naturally occurring, but the cubic zirconia ($cZrO_2$) crystals are "lab-made" and a common substitute for diamonds in jewelry. The high melting point of zirconia (2715 °C) makes it difficult to find a container for melting zirconia and making single crystals; the "skull melting" process is used. Radio frequency (RF) induction (12) at 800 kHz –2MHz and power up to 600 kW is used to heat graphite or zirconium (metal) rods. Embedded in a batch of zirconia powder. The graphite or Zr metal heat the zirconia powder until it starts to melt in the center of the powder batch. The outer part of the zirconia powder is cooled with copper coils and circulating water, creating a temperature gradient or a "skull" (shell) around the molten zirconia; the shell that does not melt or contaminate the zirconia. The graphite oxidizes and vaporizes, and the zirconium metal oxidizes and remains in the molten mass. The temperature is controlled for forming large crystals by gradually lowering the heating elements or reducing the power to lower the temperature causing crystals to grow in the molten zirconia.

Glass Making

Glasses are made via unique melting processes that differ from creating polycrystalline ceramics. Conventionally, a mixture of ceramic powders is blended and heated to temperatures up to 1600 °C for melting a glass. The components in the blended powders usually contain silica, fluxes (to lower the glass forming temperature), and stabilizers (to add water resistance to the glass). Oxides and less expensive but carbonates or nitrates are sometimes included. Salts release gases when heated, but their residual metal oxide becomes part of the glass, similar to the burn-out phase before sintering. The mixture of molten oxides is held at a high enough temperature to allow the decomposition gases to dissipate, making a homogeneous liquid without bubbles – a process called glass “fining.” When fluoride is needed in a glass formula, compounds such as calcium fluoride (CaF_2), aluminum fluoride (AlF_3), magnesium fluoride (MgF_2), or cryolite (Na_3AlF_6) are included in the batch formula. The fluoride compounds are used because fluorine (F_2) is a gas. Prolonged, high temperature heat causes vaporization of fluoride from glass as hydrogen fluoride (HF) gas, which is a potent acid and a hazard. Evaporation reduces the fluoride. Decomposition and vapor losses must be considered in batch calculations. Glass batch formulas are usually based on experimental trials where the resulting glass is analyzed and tested to see how much of each oxide is retained after melting. Batch formulas are trade secrets of manufacturers.

Manufacturing of glass may be continuous or batch processes but the high-volume continuous processes used for window glass or glass fibers are uneconomical for dental glasses. Dental glasses are melted in platinum, silica, or refractory (alumina–zirconia–silica) crucibles. Cascading silica or refractory crucibles within kilns have also been used as a method to homogenize a small batch. The container for melting is important because the molten glass may erode it which changes the glass composition and can create defects, such as small inclusions of the crucible in the glass. After melting and fining, the hot liquid is cooled quickly to create glass and avoid devitrification (precipitation of crystals).

Glass powders (frits) are made by quenching a stream of molten glass in water or between water-cooled steel rolls. For instance, elevated, glass melting kilns are used to melt a batch of glass, probably no more than a few hundred kilograms in a crucible or vat. A plug in the bottom is removed to drain the glass into a vat of water. The glass is removed from the water and milled to form a powder. Milling a glass into powder may introduce contamination from abrasion of the milling media or the lining of the mill; contamination will usually add opacity or color and may change some properties of the frit. To avoid potential problems, manufacturers use hard grinding media and avoid metal or soft polymer liners of grinding mills.

Dental glass ingots have been cast in a mold or made from glass powders (cold pressing powders followed by sintering).

Glass-Ceramming

Uncontrolled crystallization, or devitrification, has plagued many glass formulas when unwanted crystals form during the cooling of a cast-glass object, often causing cracking. Glass-ceramics are cast-glass objects that are specially heat-treated to selectively form beneficial crystals within the glass for higher strength, stiffness, or hardness; better chemical durability; lower thermal expansion; or certain optical properties. This "ceramming" heat treatment is usually a two-stage process, as depicted in Figure 7.6. First, the cast-glass object is heated to a temperature slightly above the annealing point of the glass (13), where the viscosity of the glass is roughly 10^{13} Poise; at this temperature, crystals can nucleate but grow slowly. The nucleation temperature is chosen to enable many crystal nuclei – sometimes nanometers in size – to form on glass imperfections, nucleating agents in the glass, stochastically in the bulk, or at the surface. Nucleating agents are the most reliable for creating a uniform, reproducible glass-ceramic microstructures (13). Phosphorus pentoxide dissolved in a glass is common to use to start nucleation or phase separation of the glass. Fluoride, vanadia, chromia, or molybdenum oxide can also cause nucleation, as can some sulfides or metal colloids.

After a selected duration for nucleation, the temperature of the glass is slowly raised to a higher temperature where the nucleated crystals grow faster forming small uniform crystals that impart the desired properties of the glass-ceramic. The crystal growth rate rises with temperature and then falls to zero as the liquid temperature for the glass is approached so the "growth" temperature is carefully chosen; see Figure 7.6. The heat treatment changes how much and what crystals are precipitated (e.g. lithium metasilicate or lithium disilicate) and the crystal's form (e.g. spherulites or plate-like). The size and shape of the object also influence the microstructure because competing crystallization occurs on the surface and within an object. The ceramming heat treatment influences the residual glass in its percent and composition, contributing to the glass-ceramic's properties. Crystals are usually more dense than the original glass; therefore, shrinkage occurs during the ceramming process. In some instances, the higher density of the crystals can lead to deleterious pore formation. However, this change in dimensions is usually less than the firing shrinkage for sintering powder compacts. Overall, the ceramming process must be carefully determined to ensure control and reproducibility in fabricating an item, such as a dental crown or bridge; extensive experimentation is required with microstructural and chemical analyses.

Coatings and Thin Films

Thick ceramic coatings (a few millimeters) can be made by thermal-spraying. Powders are melted and sprayed onto a surface where they are quenched and solidify. The powders are heated with a plasma or a flame; the molten powder particles are entrained in the gas stream and form in "pancake"-like microstructures. Plasma arc discharge jets have a temperature quenched on the surface > 15,000 K, which makes it possible to spray the most refractory oxides as well as metals. Variations of the thermal spray processes exist, including detonation thermal-spraying and

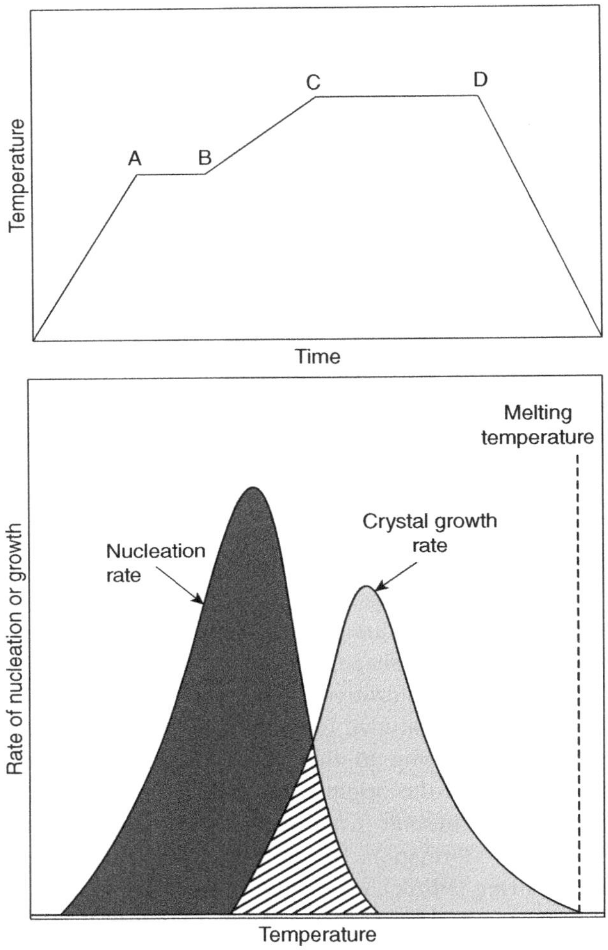

Figure 7.6 Top – Schematic heat treatment for glass-ceramming where the A–B region is the nucleation time/temperature and C–D is the crystal growth time/temperature. *Source:* Adapted from [13]. Bottom – A schematic depicting the rates of nucleation and crystal growth to illustrate why two temperatures are chosen for the ceramming process. The relative nucleation and growth rates may vary in their magnitude depending on the glass composition. *Source:* Adapted from [14].

vacuum plasma spraying (15). Hydroxyapatite coatings made by such methods are applied to the threads of some dental implants (Chapter 16).

Thin films of ceramics are used to improve the performance of some cutting tools or electronics, and even orthodontic brackets. The prominent methods for creating thin coatings are sputtering and chemical vapor deposition. Sputtering is performed by bombardment of a metal with a plasma that ejects microscopic particles. A substrate to be coated is placed in a vacuum chamber containing a low pressure of inert gas, usually argon; a negative charge is applied to a source material, creating the plasma that ejects atoms from the source and impacts the substrate. These thin films may be invisible on the substrate. Sputtering is the thin film deposition manufacturing process at the core of today's semiconductors, disk drives, CDs, and optical devices industries. Reactive sputtering is a variation that forms compounds on the substrate when the plasma includes oxygen or nitrogen molecules. Sputtering is also needed for scanning electron microscope preparation of samples, such as applying a conductive metal to the ceramic.

Chemical vapor deposition (CVD) is a family of processes that deposit a film of a material from a vapor via a chemical reaction occurring on, or in the vicinity of, a heated substrate surface. The films' results depend on the gas composition and the gas–solid chemical reactions. As the precursor gases pass over the surface of the heated substrate, chemical reactions form a solid phase on the substrate. Several CVD processes are used to deposit coatings atmospheric pressure, metal-organic, low-pressure, laser, photochemical, chemical vapor infiltration, chemical beam epitaxy, plasma-assisted, and plasma-enhanced. The substrate's temperature, the gas pressure, and gas composition influence the occurrence of reactions and coating results. The CVD process can produce coatings of uniform thickness and properties, with a low porosity on complex shapes (16). Nitrides are a common CVD coating (e.g. CrN or TiN) to improve wear resistance.

Summary of Forming Methods for Dental Ceramics

The techniques to make ceramic powders, form ceramics, and make ceramic coatings described in this chapter have been appropriated from industry to make the ceramic powders, pastes, and solid objects used in dentistry. Many ceramic powders are needed in dental products, particularly those in paste form. Raw materials, powders, or single crystals are created using methods from sol–gel precipitation, melting, grinding, and firing. The ceramic powders and pastes enable the dentist or dental laboratory technician to customize treatments for a patient that fill and replace missing anatomy or create the precise fit of a device such as a crown or bridge. Ceramic powders are crucial for the endodontic sealers and gutta-percha points in Chapter 8, direct restorations in Chapter 9, indirect restorations in Chapter 10, cements in Chapter 11, hygiene materials in Chapter 13, impression or duplicating materials in Chapter 14, and abrasives in Chapter 17. Some ceramic powders are self-setting cements with water, but diverse ceramic powders are incorporated into polymers for restoratives, cements, and adhesive cements that are essential for clinical dentistry.

Many ceramic powders are consolidated into solid ceramic items via the usual ceramic methods of dry-pressing, injection molding (IM), and extrusion. The 3D printing method is less common but rising in popularity. Ceramic objects are made by sintering the consolidated powders, creating the desired properties in a fully dense ceramic solid. Glass-ceramics have been uniquely adapted for dental restoratives, and they require a controlled heat treatment different from sintering. Coating techniques have imparted new features for medical devices and dental instruments, such as hydroxyapatite on titanium implants and nitride coatings for instrument durability.

Manufacturers develop formulas and processes to make, test, verify, and validate materials for products they introduce to the market. The manufacture of products is behind the scenes to the dentist or technician; however, sophisticated powder-making, forming, and firing methods are crucial for creating successful dental treatment materials. This chapter was written to give the dental and medical device professionals insights into the complexity of making ceramics for their niche purposes.

Ceramics in Chapter 7

The following ceramics or inorganic materials were mentioned in this chapter:

- alumina
- calcia
- calcium aluminate cement
  - monocalcium alumina
  - monocalcium dialuminate
  - calcium alumino ferrite
  - tricalcium aluminate
  - dodecacalcium hepta-aluminate
  - monocalcium hexa-aluminate
- calcium carbonate
- calcium silicate cement
  - wollastonite, calcium silicate
  - alite, haturite, tricalcium silicate
  - belite, larnite, dicalcium silicate
  - rankinite
- calcium sulfate

- chromium nitride
- clay
- hydroxyapatite
- iron oxide
- lithium disilicate
- phosphorus pentoxide
- porcelain
- potassia
- silica
  - fluoride glass with calcium, aluminum, or magnesium fluoride or cryolite
- soda
- titanium nitride
- zircon
- zirconia

References

1 Levy, D. and Zayat, M. (2015). *The sol-gel handbook*, 1508. Wiley-VCH Verlag GmbH & Co.

2 Schubert, U. (2015). Chemistry and fundamentals of the sol–gel process. In: *The sol-gel handbook*, 1–28. Wiley-VCH Verlag GmbH & Co.

3 Boldridge, D. (2010). Morphological characterization of fumed silica aggregates. *Aerosol Sci Technol* 44 (3): 182–186.

4 Fischer, N.G., de Souza Araujo, I.J., Daghrery, A. et al. (2025). Guidance on biomaterials for periodontal tissue regeneration: Fabrication methods, materials and biological considerations. *Dent Mater* 41 (3): 283–305.

5 Blackford, J.R. (2007). Sintering and microstructure of ice: a review. *J Phys D Appl Phys* 40 (21): R355–R385.

6 German, R.M., Suri, P., and Park, S.J. (2009). Review: liquid phase sintering. *J Mater Sci* 44 (1): 1–39.

7 Fulrath RM, Pask JA. Ceramic microstructures: their analysis, significance, and production: proceedings of the third international materials symposium "Ceramic Microstructures--Their Analysis, Significance, and Production,". Huntington, N.Y.: R. E. Krieger Pub. Co.; 1966. 1008 p.

8 German, R.M. (2016). Sintering trajectories: description on how density, surface area, and grain size change. *J Mater* 68 (3): 878–884.

9 Guillon, O., Rheinheimer, W., and Bram, M. (2023). A perspective on emerging and future sintering technologies of ceramic materials. *Adv Energy Mater* 25 (18): 1–11.

10 Cologna, M., Rashkova, B., and Raj, R. (2010). Flash sintering of nanograin zirconia in <5 s at 850°C. *J Am Ceram Soc* 93 (11): 3556–3559.

11 Yunus, S.N.H., Fhan, K.S., Johar, B. et al. (2021). Phase analysis of bio-based derived tricalcium disilicate from 2CaO: 1SiO2 By X-ray diffraction. *J Phys Conf Ser* 1–7.

12 Xu, J., Lei, X., Jiang, X. et al. (2009). Industrial growth of yttria-stabilized cubic zirconia crystals by skull melting process. *J Rare Earths* 27 (6): 971–974.

13 Grossman, D.G. (1988). The science of castable glass ceramics. In: *Proceedings of the fourth international symposium on ceramics perspectives in dental ceramics. Perspectives in dental ceramics* (ed. J.D. Preston), 117–133. Quintessence.

14 Wen, S., Wang, Y., Lan, B. et al. (2019). Pressureless crystallization of glass for transparent nanoceramics. *Adv Sci* 6 (17): 1–9.

15 Martin, E. and Daniel, K. (2012). Thermal spraying of oxide ceramic and ceramic metallic coatings. In: *Ceramic coatings* (ed. S. Feng). Rijeka: IntechOpen p. Ch. 6.

16 Pierson, H.O. (1999). Fundamentals of chemical vapor deposition. In: *Handbook of chemical vapor deposition (CVD)*, Seconde (ed. H.O. Pierson), 36–67. Norwich, NY: William Andrew Publishing.

8

Saving Teeth Through Endodontics

Teeth are a remarkable combination of hard and soft tissues. Hard tissue is on the outside (enamel), with underlying semi-soft tissue (dentin) and a core of soft pulp tissue, all anchored in the alveolar bone via cementum tissue and its surrounding periodontal ligament fibers. The pulp tissue connects the tooth's neural and vascular systems to our circulatory and nervous systems through the foramina at the apices, tips of the roots. Endodontics is a specialized branch of dentistry that focuses on the pulpal system within the tooth to keep it alive and healthy, or failing that, keeping the tooth in place and avoiding its extraction.

Teeth are constantly challenged by bacteria, mastication, bruxing, thermal insults, occlusal contact forces, chemicals, and occasional trauma. The pulp's nerves transmit these thermal changes, motion, and pain sensations. Traumatic injury to teeth can rupture the blood vessels at the apical foramen (opening) where the pulpal tissues enter the alveolar bone; such an injury may necessitate endodontic treatment, as described in this chapter. With age and life challenges, instances arise where pulp protection is needed, lest the pulp and dentin become sensitive or infected.

Common endodontic procedures are treating vital pulp, removing and sealing the pulpal space (root canal therapy), and surgery to treat disease just beyond the root tips (apices). Some of these procedures are performed by general dentists; others are performed by pediatric dentists, oral surgeons, and endodontists. Endodontic treatments are described below, highlighting the contributions of ceramics to vital pulp, orthograde root canal, and surgical interventions. For an in-depth understanding of endodontic procedures, other references (1–3) should be consulted.

Ceramics in Dentistry: Materials, Manufacturing, and Clinical Applications,
First Edition. Carolyn M. Primus.

Incipient Caries and Tooth Sensitivity

Bacteria attack tooth enamel and dentin from the outside, and dentists are trained to detect decay and treat caries. Ideally, bacteria are stopped from damaging the enamel before the decay reaches the dentin where it causes sensitivity, pain, and pulpal disease. Prevention and maintentance are discussed in Chapter 13.

Several inorganic silver compounds have been used in dentistry since the 1800s to combat enamel decay, although Chinese use of silver precedes this time by 1200 years (4). Silver's antibacterial property has been exploited by using solutions of nitrate (25%), fluoride (40%), and in ammonium nitrate known as Howe's ammoniacal silver nitrate solution (5); silver and tin fluoride have sometimes been administered together. Adding ammonia to a silver nitrate solution makes it alkaline rather than acidic, the latter being capable of deleterious etching of enamel. Each of these silver compounds has been applied to caries on enamel to "sterilize" the lesion and stop the caries from progressing deeper into enamel. The mechanisms of silver's interactions with hydroxyapatite and bacteria are complex (6), but can be described as silver precipitation from salt solutions, which hardens the decayed (demineralized) dentin or enamel, and blocks the dentinal tubules. The drawback has been that silver compounds stain the teeth, leaving harmless black spots. These silver compounds are not suitable for pulp contact, indirect pulp capping, or treating reversible pulpitis because inflammation and necrosis of the pulp has been reported for silver compounds on pulp tissue (7). Silver treatments fell out of use when the effects of fluoride were recognized; however, silver diamine fluoride (SDF) solution, combining silver and fluoride, is currently popular for pediatric and geriatric patients to minimize tooth anatomy removal; see Chapter 13. Notably, SDF does blacken carious tissue, its main drawback.

Dentin hypersensitivity is common and originates from the nerves in the dental pulp. Normally, the dentinal tubules are below the gumls embedded in alveolar bone, but gum recession may expose the orifices of these tubules to mechanical, thermal, chemical, or osmotic provocations (8). Transient sensitivity is considered reversible pulpitis (pulpal inflammation) ascribed to the exposure of coronal or radicular (root) dentinal tubules in the oral cavity. Exposure of the tubule orifices to liquid in the oral cavity causes motion of the tubules' fluid back and forth. This tiny motion stimulates the pulpal nerves, signaling pain, via complex mechanisms (9). The treatment of tooth sensitivity has been to occlude (cover the entrance of) these tubules on the exterior of the tooth to stop the fluid from moving and irritating the pulpal nerves. SDF, hydroxyapatite, fluoride compounds, calcium magnesium phosphate ($CaMgPO_4$), and potassium nitrate (KNO_3) solutions or pastes are used in medicaments and toothpastes to combat tooth sensitivity. Organic (resin) varnishes temporarily reduce sensitivity; some contain tricalcium phosphate, $Ca_3(PO_4)_2$, to help occlude the tubule openings. Anti-sensitivity materials are self-applied in home care or professionally applied topically (Chapter 13).

Notes to Clarify Calcium Silicate/Aluminate Cements in Endodontics

All the following descriptions of endodontic treatments include the use of calcium silicate/aluminate cements. These cements may be the most innovative use of ceramics in dentistry because these common ceramics have been found to support healing and osteogenesis in addition to having good dimensional stability to seal root canals. Calcium silicate/aluminate ceramics have vastly improved vital pulp therapy, root canal sealing, perforation treatment, root-end surgery, apexification, and revascularization procedures.

The use of these calcium cements in the modern era (>1990) began with an invention (US Pats. 5,415,547 and 5,769,638) by an endodontist and his patient, who was an expert in cement and concrete. The inventors denoted the cement as Mineral Trioxide Aggregate, MTA (10), which was later commercialized as ProRoot® MTA; their invention contained 80% calcium silicate cement and 20% bismuth oxide and was mixed with water to set. The calcium silicate cement imbued the mixture with three essential benefits for endodontics: the ability to harden/set with water, bioactivity (formation of hydroxyapatite on the surface), and antibacterial properties (calcium hydroxide is a reaction product formed as the cement sets).

The first such calcium silicate cement endodontic products were powders that were mixed with water into a thick consistency for plugging perforations or root-end filling. The products were derided for their impurity and similarity to industrial Portland cement, tendency for difficult handling, washout (be displaced), slow setting, discoloration, problems with mixing, and high cost (11). The original, experimental MTA invention was maligned as having arsenic (12) because the original invention used a construction-grade calcium silicate cement. Dental manufacturers are careful to avoid contamination such as that prohibited for glass ionomer cements in ISO 9917-1, which limits acid soluble lead (<100 ppm) and arsenic (<2 ppm).

The cement portion of the experimental MTA was relatively coarse, dark gray cement; it contained tri- and dicalcium silicate with lesser amounts of tricalcium aluminate, tetracalcium aluminoferrite, and calcium sulfate; the latter slowed the setting time to about two hours, longer than desired. Over time, new products were developed with finer powders (13), different phase proportions, color stable, lower cost, and and new liquids that provided better handling, washout resistance (14), and setting times as brief as 15 minutes (15, 16). For instance, two dental products have been advertised as "fast-setting, mineral trioxide aggregate-derived pozzolan cements" (17–19); although the components are not disclosed, the products may include fine amorphous silica and calcium hydroxide. However, the pozzolanic hydration reaction may cause shrinkage (20), an undesirable effect for these dental cements. No clinical or physical benefits have been published for such dental cements, although faster setting has been claimed (17) through releasing beneficial calcium and hydroxide ions, which is common for all the calcium cements described.

The dark gray color of the original ProRoot MTA was a hazard for being seen through thin tissue. A white version of ProRoot MTA was developed to overcome this issue (US Pat. 7,892,342 B2), which had no tetracalcium aluminoferrite phase (or iron oxide of any type). All the current calcium silicate/aluminate cement products are white and do not contain the ferrite cement phase, unlike the original ProRoot MTA. Another discoloration hazard appeared over time with these endodontic cements, particularly in primary teeth (21). Teeth would gradually darken, which was an esthetic but not a clinical problem. The problem was traced to the use of bismuth oxide. Bismuth oxide is a useful radiopaque material but is prone to discoloration by exposure to light or sodium hypochlorite (see Figure 8.1). The sensitivity of bismuth to light and oxidation causes the valence state to change (Bi^{+3} to Bi^{+5}), which changes the color. Zirconia has been a popular alternative to bismuth oxide as a radiopaque powder in calcium silicate/aluminate cements. Both monoclinic and tetragonal powders of zirconia have been used in these cement products, but they are not as radiopaque as tantalum oxide or calcium tungstate, which are also used. Few of the calcium cement products contain bismuth oxide.

Calcium silicate cements are used below the gum line to avoid their gradual dissolution by the acidic environment of the oral cavity. Some products now include monocalcium aluminate cement (22, 23) for its higher acid resistance and faster setting, especially when combined with calcium silicate cement (US Pat. 12,171,898).

Mixing of powders and liquids is not a favorite task of dental assistants or dentists because of concerns about getting the proportions of components correct. In response to this feedback, unit-dose products have been commercialized. Also, newer calcium silicate/aluminate cement products are available as single pastes of the cement dispersed in an organic liquid. The organic liquid creates the paste but doesn't allow setting of the cement. The premixed cement pastes are more convenient for dentists but set more slowly compared to powders mixed with a water-based liquid; these pastes must absorb water from the body to set. The cement paste products are made as thick pastes having a putty-like consistency,

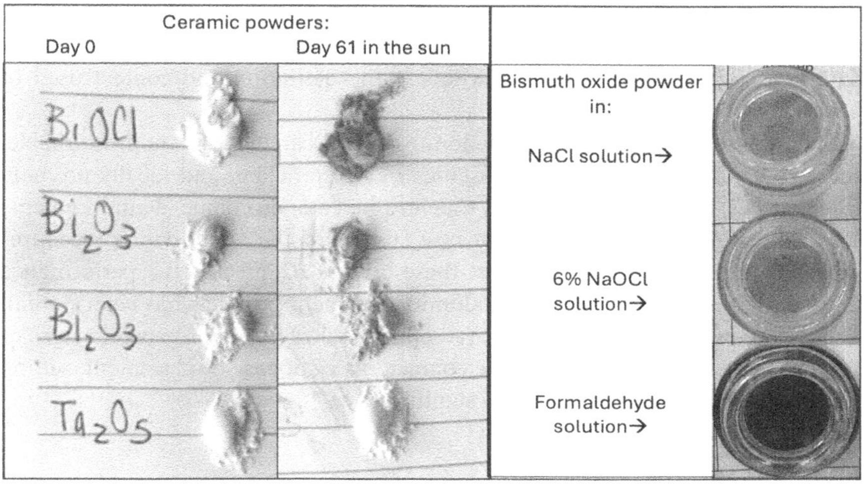

Figure 8.1 Examples of bismuth compound discoloration (vs. Ta_2O_5) when exposed to sunlight (left). Note the lack of discoloration for the materials with tantalum oxide. Both NaOCl solutions and formaldehyde also discolor bismuth oxide (right).

akin to Play-Doh (24, 25); these pastes are suitable for vital pulp therapy, perforations, or root resorption, as described below. Other cement pastes are offered in a thinner paste form which are used for root canal sealing, also described below; for these procedures, thin, syrupy mixtures are needed to penetrate the intricacies of the root canal system.

Dozens of calcium silicate/aluminate cement products are available worldwide in various formats – powder-water, powder-gel, or premixed pastes – as individual doses or in multi-dose containers. These newer cement products offer improved handling, washout resistance, and lower prices, making them much more suitable for endodontic, general, and pediatric dentistry (24). However, many dental authors have erroneously stated that all "MTA" products contain bismuth oxide, are coarse, and set slowly, which is passé for modern calcium cement products. Dentists need to read the literature skeptically and use the Safety Data Sheets. The key advances from industrial cement materials are higher purity, finer powders (13), radiopacity, and new liquids for faster setting.

Confusing names are used for these "MTA-type materials"; the original moniker for this type of cement cannot be shaken (26). Other terms such as "tricalcium silicate" and "tri/dicalcium silicate-based" are suitable, but "bioceramics" is annoying to materials scientists who know that bioceramics include so many more materials than this one type of material (27); in fact, bioceramics is the subject of this text! Cement is another confusing term having multiple meanings;

calcium silicate/aluminate cements use the hydraulic (water-reactive) definition. Cement also refers to the process of adhering one item to another, such as a crown to a tooth, or the material itself, which is the definition and context used in Chapter 11.

Materials for endodontics must be non-toxic, non-carcinogenic, non-resorbable, radiopaque, antimicrobial, bacteriostatic, and bactericidal, and ideally promote osteogenesis and cementogenesis. Calcium silicate/aluminate dental cements have been shown to be the current best choice for the endodontic procedures described below because they meet these criteria. Clinically, the performance among prominent calcium silicate/aluminate cement products has been similar, despite the differences in additives, radiopaque powders, and the percentages of cement (~40–90%), even though the characteristics of ease of placement, setting time, radiopacity, and cost (24) vary significantly.

Vital Pulp Therapy

Pathogenic oral microbes dissolve enamel and dentin tissues via the caries process, gradually approaching the pulp. Trauma may also open an access through the hard tissue to the pulp, allowing bacterial infection (28). When an infection invades the dentinal tubules, a dentist may seek to arrest the decay by removing the infected part of the enamel and dentin with a drill or excavator instrument, then place a direct restorative material to cover the underlying tooth and replace the tooth shape (Chapter 9). Before the restoration, a vital pulp therapy material may be placed. The least invasive procedure is the placement of a "base" (material) in a deep cavity preparation (Figure 8.2); these are thermally insulating and block bacteria from advancing nearer to the pulp. The first base material was a sheet of gutta-percha containing about 75% zinc oxide; zinc phosphate cement and zinc oxide-eugenol medicaments have also been used as base materials. Heat transfer is complex and depends on the material's heat capacity, thickness, and density, but ceramic materials usually provide insulation of the pulp from hot liquids, even under an amalgam or metal crown. Nowadays, glass ionomers, calcium hydroxide medicaments, and calcium silicate/aluminate cements are more commonly used as base materials for thermal insulation rather than zinc oxide-containing materials. Table 8.1 shows that zinc phosphate and zinc oxide-eugenol cements are more insulating (lower thermal conductivity) than metals or ice, but less insulating than calcium silicate cement, or non-dental insulators made of corkboard or glass.

A cavity liner is a barrier material against microbes that is needed when the cavity preparation is even thinner remaining dentin over the pulp, as in Figure 8.2; this is denoted as indirect pulp therapy. Some of the same materials are used as a

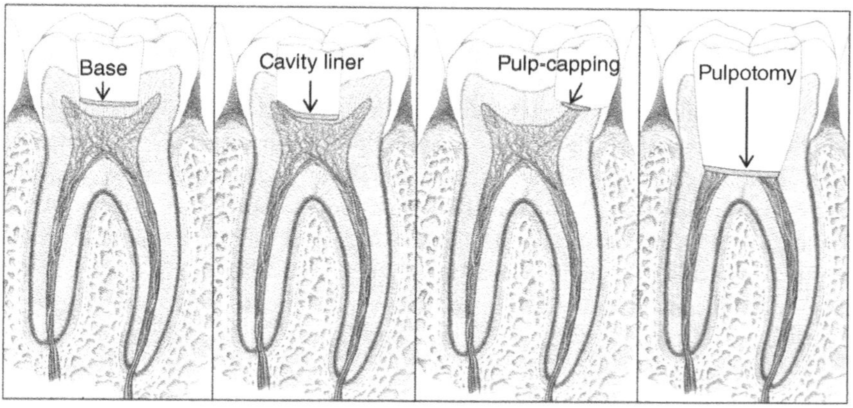

Figure 8.2 Diagrams of interventions for endodontic vital pulp therapy. The solid, light gray areas indicate where the cement is placed on/near the pulp (arrows). Live pulpal tissue is shown in and emanating from the roots. *Source:* Illustrations by N. Deutsch.

Table 8.1 Thermal conductivity of selected materials.

Material	Approximate thermal conductivity (29) (mcal/cm·s·K)
Dentin	1–2.3
Enamel	1.6–2.2
Resin-based composite resin	0.3
Tricalcium silicate cement	0.7
Glass	2.0–2.5
Zinc phosphate cement	2.5–3.1
Zinc oxide-eugenol	4.0
Amalgam	5.4
Stainless steel	38
Gold	740

base or a cavity liner; however, calcium silicate/aluminate cements are becoming more common than others in indirect pulp therapy. The advantage of calcium silicate/aluminate cements is their ability to form a hard layer that blocks bacteria (communication) through the tubules that lead to the pulp. Calcium silicate cements precipitate a thin layer of hydroxyapatite at the tubules orifices to protect the pulp from the ingress of bacteria from the cavity. Ideally, a cavity liner will stimulate the pulp to secrete protective reparative dentin near the liner material as shown in the histological optical photo in Figure 8.3.

If microbes reach the pulp, or the dentist breaches the pulp during a restorative treatment, a "pulp capping" material is needed to seal the opening to the pulp chamber as depicted in Figure 8.2. If the pulp exposure is small and properly sealed, the pulp can create new dentin to reseal the pulp chamber via the phenomenon of dentinal bridging, which is the formation of reparative dentin under the capping material, similar to that in Figure 8.3. A wide variety of materials have been used for this vital pulp treatment (30), especially calcium hydroxide, zinc oxide-eugenol cement, zinc oxide-polycarboxylate cement, tricalcium phosphate particles, hydroxyapatite particles, tetracalcium phosphate cement, and calcium silicate/aluminate cements.

Calcium hydroxide medicaments were introduced in 1920 for pulp treatments. They are known to support pulp healing and dentinal bridging (reparative dentin) via the bioactive action of calcium and hydroxide ions released from this slightly soluble material. Calcium hydroxide is applied to pulp tissue when mixed with water, non-setting organic liquids, or resins (28), the most well-known being Dycal® resin. The pulp's histological response to $Ca(OH)_2$ is the formation of porous reparative dentin (31, 32); reparative dentin is good but porosity is undesirable. Zinc oxide-eugenol cements (ZOE, described in Chapter 5) near the pulp can reduce inflammation; however, in direct pulpal contact, ZOE cements produce chronic inflammation and necrosis. Polycarboxylate cement is "innocuous" on the pulp (33), despite its initial acidic pH of 1.5 that quickly rises to 4 during setting, but it is neither antibacterial nor does it induce dentinal bridging. Tricalcium phosphate particles reduce pulp inflammation but cause unpredictable dentin bridging, as does tetracalcium phosphate. Carbon dioxide lasers and

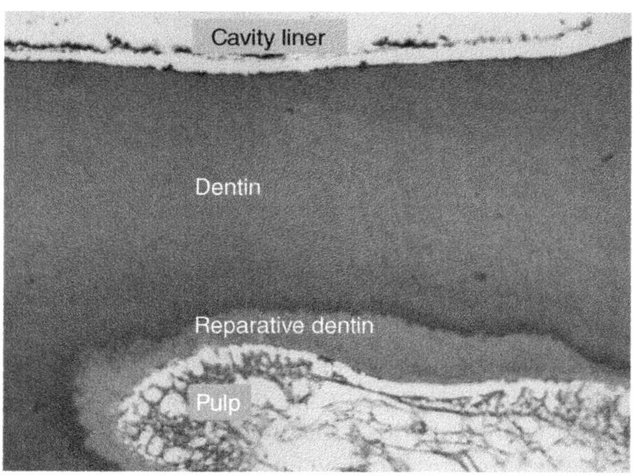

Figure 8.3 Histology of a canine (dog) tooth 60 days after a cavity liner was placed showing the healing by formation of reparative dentin somewhat distant from the cavity preparation that had been lined (filled) with a calcium silicate cement.

neodymium-doped yttrium-aluminum-garnet lasers have been used on pulp tissue exposures to coagulate the pulp and stimulate reparative dentin (34) but are not the best practice. Glass ionomer cements and Resin Modified Glass Ionomer Cements (RMGIC) described in Chapter 9 are excellent bacterial and thermal barriers that have good biocompatibility when used in close approximation to the pulp. However, their acidity makes them unsuitable for direct contact with the pulp as they cause chronic inflammation.

The current best practice for pulp-capping is to use bioactive calcium silicate/aluminate cement products. These calcium cements are known for their ability to support the healing of pulpal and periapical tissues as seen in the reviews of the dental uses of calcium silicate and calcium aluminate cements (26, 35–40). Such calcium cement products are available in many formats (25). These are bioactive cements that set in the teeth, creating a hard barrier that bacteria cannot penetrate. These cements are used as thick pastes for vital pulp therapy. They are not designed to have pores for osseous ingrowth or resorption, unlike bioactive glasses or calcium phosphate cements and are not resorbable. Some products require the mixing of a powder and a liquid; others are available as pre-mixed pastes that set on contact with body fluids.

If the pulp exposure is large or untreated, microbes invade the coronal pulp tissue. Such infections require a partial or complete pulpotomy procedure, which is the removal of the infected coronal portion of the pulp. The goal of this treatment is to remove unhealthy pulpal tissue and leave healthy pulp tissue in the remaining root canal system as depicted in Figure 8.2. This procedure is common in primary teeth but is now being used more for permanent teeth (41, 42). After removing the unhealthy tissue in the pulp chamber, a material must be placed on the pulpal wound to seal this tissue and prevent further ingress of bacteria. Until the 2000s, formocresol – a mixture consisting of formalin, cresol, and glycerin – was regularly placed on the pulp remnants in the pulpotomy (pulp tissue removal) procedure. Formocresol contains formaldehyde and has a fixative effect on the upper layer of pulp cells; although successful (43, 44), formocresol has been criticized for its odor and carcinogenic component. Ferric sulfate ($Fe_2(SO_4)_3$) solution (15.5%) is a strong astringent and has been an alternative to formocresol, which is also not bioactive; ferric sulfate is a water-soluble ceramic salt. Both have been supplanted by calcium silicate/aluminate cement products that are more biocompatible and better for stimulating reparative dentin for healing.

The high (alkaline) pH, and release of calcium ions from bioactive cements onto the pulp tissue is beneficial. The high pH can degrade bacterial cells' DNA and cellular proteins to help kill the bacteria. The associated release of calcium ions supports healing by causing the bioactive reaction described previously; that is, hydroxyapatite is precipitated on the cement's surface where body fluids are present, between the cement and the pulp. After the hydroxyapatite layer forms, the pulp tissue begins a cascade of reactions to stimulate reparative dentin. New dentin forms between the hydroxyapatite and the pulp tissue. Furthermore, calcium silicate cements do not shrink during setting, creating a seal to protect the remaining pulp.

Some of the vital pulp therapy products have been combinations of resins and ceramics: calcium hydroxide, calcium-based cements, and radiopaque powders. These products include chemical and photo-initiators for curing (hardening/polymerizing) the resins with blue light, as described in Chapter 9. Either alone or combined with resins, calcium hydroxide and silicate cements are well-recognized for use on pulp tissue to support healing of the pulp after a direct or indirect "insult" (36, 45, 46). However, combining ceramic powders with resins reduces the effectiveness of bioactivity (47, 48) because the materials contain less bioactive powder and the resins encase the cement particles to prevent as large a bioactive effect. One dual-curing resin-cement product has been indicated for pulpotomies; the other resin/cement products are indicated for pulp-capping or cavity lining. Light-curing deep in the tooth at the bottom of the pulp chamber is difficult to accomplish and can leave undesirable uncured monomers on the pulp. These resin products are unsuitable for endodontic procedures, other than pulp-capping or pulpotomies, as described next.

Root Canal Therapy

Untreated tooth caries (decay) that progresses more deeply into the pulp and root canals of teeth causes an irreversible pulpitis or pulpal necrosis. The worst infections spread throughout the root canal system, beyond the root apex (tip), and start to dissolve the alveolar bone. This disease of apical periodontitis causes pain and loosens teeth. Such infections progress via the formation of recalcitrant biofilms – multi-species bacterial colonies – within the roots and dentinal tubules. Biofilms have high resistance to antimicrobial agents, so antimicrobial drugs delivered systemically are ineffective in the root canal system. Therefore, dentists have developed specific endodontic treatment techniques known as root canal treatment/therapy/procedures to eliminate such infections. Root canal therapy removes the entire pulp tissue system, leaving the dentin and enamel, and is referred to as a pulpectomy – see Figure 8.4. The tooth is "devitalized."

Root canal treatment starts with drilling a small, conservative access, through the enamel and coronal dentin. When the pulp is reached, it is removed with a tapered instrument. Next, the root canals are "instrumented" to minimally enlarge the canals and remove residual pulp tissue. Stainless steel and nickel-titanium (NiTi) alloys are used, some with titanium nitride coating; diamond-like carbon coatings are in the future. A myriad of instruments with different diameters,

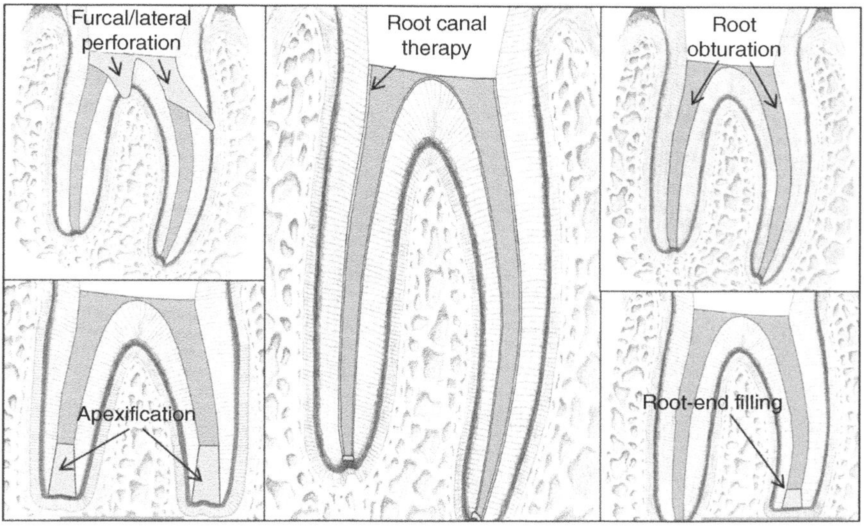

Figure 8.4 Diagram of interventions for root canal and surgical procedures. The solid, light gray areas indicate where the calcium cement is placed (arrows) to seal the root canal from the alveolar bone. The medium gray areas indicate the placement of gutta-percha. Illustrations by Naomi Deutsch.

tapers, and shapes are needed because thorough removal of pulp tissue is not easy. Instruments are also used to shape the canal system, removing some dentin and residual bacteria. During and after instrumentation, the root canals are flooded with liquids (irrigants, described below) to help remove tissue and kill the microbes and remove the biofilm that caused the infection. These liquids are used to contact all the root canal passageways, which often have a complicated pulpal anatomy, as depicted in Figure 8.5. Residual microorganisms hinder the long-term success of root canal treatment; their removal from the anatomical complexities is crucial. After cleaning and shaping, calcium hydroxide pastes may be placed in the instrumented root canals as a temporary, antimicrobial medicament for one or two weeks. After the pulpectomy, instrumentation, and irrigation, the final step of root canal therapy is obturation.

Lasers based on ceramics – neodymium/erbium doped with yttrium aluminum garnet (Nd/Er:YAG), or yttrium garnet doped with erbium-chromium, yttrium–scandium–gallium–garnet (YSGG) – are being used to assist with pulp tissue removal by ablation. Lasers also "activate" irrigants by inducing motion to help with the debridement of tissues after shaping and to kill microorganisms. The laser's wavelength varies from 1 to 3 μm and the power is about 10 W.

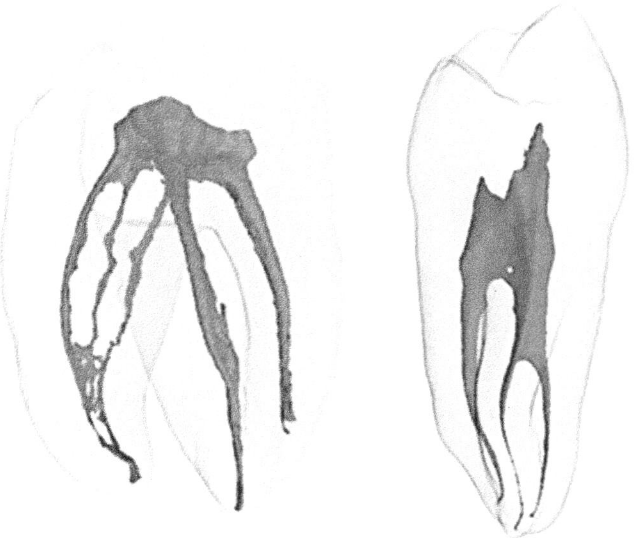

Figure 8.5 Diagrams of the anatomical complexities of the root canal (dark gray), which vary among the teeth and individuals. Multiple passageways are present. *Source:* With permission of Ahmed et al. (49)/John Wiley & Sons.

Endodontic Obturating Materials

After the pulp is removed and the root canals are "prepared", the root canal system of a tooth must be obturated (filled) with a material; without obturation a direct passageway would exist for the passage of oral bacterial into the alveolar bone. In the 1800s, obturation materials began being developed, including zinc phosphate cement, a material that was also used as a filling material and as a cement (Chapter 11) to hold restorations in place. The acidity of zinc phosphate was known to be a hazard for filling root canals because of the potential for dissolution of the dentin; careful proportioning of the phosphoric acid solution and the zinc oxide powder is always imperative for this cement.

Contemporary root canal therapy is completed by obturation of the root canal system using two materials: gutta-percha and a root canal sealer. Dental gutta-percha is a rubbery solid that is used just to take up space in the root canal. Gutta-percha was made using a naturally occurring sap from Palaquium gutta trees, but synthetic trans-polyisoprene is now used to avoid allergies from the natural resin that contains components other than polyisoprene. The rubber powder is blended with ceramic powders such as ZnO, TiO_2 and radiopaque powders such as $BaSO_4$. The rubber content is only about 15% by weight. Pigments and plasticizers are also part of the formula that make these cones pink. The gutta-percha formulas in the early 20th century included chloroform and paraformaldehyde, but these are no longer used (50). Chloroform softens the gutta-percha but is unsuitable in the periapical tissue; furthermore, it evaporates from the gutta-percha and the rubber shrinks, leaving a bacterial pathway. An alternative obturation material was proposed in the 1990s, which contained polycaprolactone polymer combined with bioactive glass, bismuth oxychloride, and barium sulfate. At first it was hailed as the "monoblock" sealing system – paired with its dual-cure, self-etch, methacrylate resin-based Epiphany root canal sealer – but its long-term performance was poor, and it was discontinued (51, 52). Exploration is ongoing of materials to completely fill the root canal system with only one material.

Gutta-percha formulas are molded by manufacturers into various sizes of long (~16 mm), tapered (2–6%), conical forms to insert into the root canals. These firm but somewhat flexible gutta-percha cones are shown in Figure 8.6. The larger end of the tapered cones is color-coded, conforming to the scheme in ISO 6877/ADA 78 to conveniently indicate their diameter. Gutta-percha is a thermoplastic and is sometimes warmed (below 65 °C, its nominal melting point) to enhance its

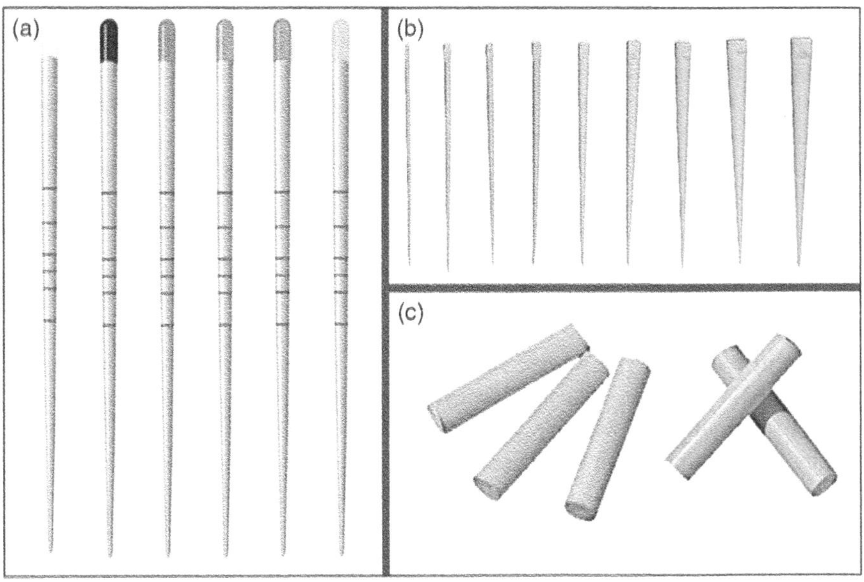

Figure 8.6 Photos of gutta-percha materials for nonsurgical endodontics, not at the same scale. (a) Standard 2% tapered points with color-coded tips and depth markings, (b) points of various tapers, (c) enlarged view of gutta-percha pellets for softening in the coronal (most distant from the apex) region of the canal, over the points.

conformance to the irregularities of the root canal system; heat is also used to cut off the larger end of points, which do not remain in the root canal. Another innovative technique has been to mold gutta-percha onto a core material, such as titanium or radiopaque polymers (e.g., polydimethylsiloxane or polysulfone); this is known as carrier-based obturation. A special warming device is used to soften the coating before the insertion of the obturator into the canal. Also, pellets of gutta-percha (depicted in Figure 8.6) can be warmed, injected, and compacted (using coronal pressure) using equipment akin to a hot glue gun for injection. Even with heat, gutta-percha cannot fill all of the root canal anatomy having complex isthmus, anastomoses, and accessory or lateral canals. A syrupy, root canal sealer must be used with the gutta-percha to fill the interstices where the gutta-percha cannot penetrate. Several placement and compaction methods are used for completing the obturation with gutta-percha points and sealer (53, 54).

Root Canal Sealers

Root canal sealers have been used since the mid-1800s to fill root canals after pulpectomy. By the 20th century, both gutta-percha and sealer pastes were used in tandem. Howe's silver solution was used by some early endodontists to coat the canals and occlude the tubules from within the tooth as part of root canal therapy. Root canal sealers evolved from merely resinous, non-setting substances that adapted to the root canal walls into formulated pastes containing ceramic powders that set. The early powder-liquid formulas (50) included formaldehyde or chloroform solutions to provide an anesthetizing effect and to soften the gutta-percha. The liquids were mixed with powders such as zinc oxide, zinc sulfate, kaolin clay, anhydrous alum (usually potassium alum, $KAl[SO]_2$), and other components to gradually harden in the root system. Careful insertion was required to avoid "overextension" into the periapical area, where formaldehyde would harm the bone tissue. Performance of the chloroform sealers was inferior to later formulas (55).

The extirpation of the pulp creates a wound at the apex. Root canal sealers should provide closure at the apex and allow healing of this wound in the alveolar bone. In the early 20th century, Dr. Bernhard Gottlieb had his own formulas for healing this wound using dentin powder to induce sealing near the apex, presaging tissue engineering (50). Others copied him and used bone or ivory powders, but widespread use did not occur.

Many formulas of root canal sealers are currently available (56), which are distinguished by their chemical matrix: zinc oxide-eugenol, salicylate, fatty acid, glass ionomer, silicone, epoxy resin, self-curing methacrylate resins, and calcium silicate/aluminate cements. All root canal sealers contain a ceramic radiopaque powder; endodontists want to see that the root canal was filled on an x-ray image.

The usual, higher atomic number ceramic powders have been incorporated into the matrices of root canal sealers, such as barium sulfate, bismuth oxide or carbonate, calcium tungstate, and tantalite (tantalum oxide). Zinc oxide, fumed silica, zirconia, titania, and clays are less radiopaque, although these powders are often included in root canal sealers to add white color, enhance paste stability, some radiopacity, and increase the viscosity of the organic matrices. Silver particles have been part of some ZnO-eugenol sealers to add radiopacity and antibacterial action. Most of the sealer products contain two components that the dentist must mix into a treacly, medium-viscosity paste that self-hardens via a chemical reaction in the root canal. Light-curing is nearly impossible in a root canal, so light-cured polymers are not used, unlike the direct restoratives of Chapter 9.

By 1925, zinc oxide-eugenol (ZOE) sealers were prominently in use, which were less viscous versions of ZOE formulas for cements or pulp medicaments. ZOE sealer variations were known as Wach's, Rickert's, and Grossman's sealers, each containing zinc oxide for mixing with their unique eugenol-containing liquids, and some remain in use. The auxiliary ceramic powders included bismuth subnitrate (bismuth oxynitrate, $Bi_5O(OH)_9(NO_3)_4$), calcium phosphate (undisclosed which particular phosphate), bismuth subcarbonate (bismuth oxycarbonate, $Bi_2O_2[CO_3]$), magnesia (MgO), sodium borate (probably borax, $Na_2B_4H_{20}O_{17}$), and barium sulfate ($BaSO_4$). Silver and calcium hydroxide powders were/are popular additions in some root canal sealers.

Epoxy resin sealers were invented in the mid-20th century and have been widely used because of their adhesion and intimate coating of root canal dentin, good handling, high radiopacity (~10 mm equivalent Al), low solubility, and low shrinkage. The original epoxy-bisphenol product was a powder-liquid mixture including silver, bismuth oxide, and titania. Unfortunately, the first products released some formaldehyde during setting. Later products were developed as two-paste products that do not release formaldehyde during setting.

Calcium hydroxide powder has been added to zinc oxide-eugenol, polydimethylsiloxane, disalicylate, epoxy resin, methacrylate, and calcium silicate cement root sealers; the hope was that the calcium and hydroxide ions would provide beneficial antibacterial effects within the root canal system. Calcium hydroxide powder does not set; therefore the powder was added to formulas that did set. The antibacterial effects and characteristics have not been dramatically better than those of sealers without $Ca(OH)_2$ (57).

The first calcium silicate/aluminate cement endodontic products were used for root-end filling and perforations, procedures described later. But these products had unsuitable handling for root canal sealing because they were cement powder mixed with water and did not create a lubricating paste to help insert the gutta-percha. Furthermore, the flow and film thickness required in ISO 6876 for root canal sealers couldn't be achieved. Refinements in new products, such as finer powders and other liquids, containing salts, organic liquids, or resins, have made calcium silicate/aluminate cement-based products popular as root canal sealers (35). Many brands of calcium silicate/aluminate cement root canal sealers are available worldwide.

Calcium silicate/aluminate cement sealers have a high pH, form hydroxyapatite on their surface within the root canal, and are compatible with wet tissue; both contribute to sealing the canal. Some of these ceramic cement sealer products are powder-liquid systems where the liquid is water-based; the powder and liquid are mixed into the smooth, syrupy consistency desired to coat gutta-percha and root canal walls. Setting begins when the powder and liquid are mixed. Newer calcium silicate/aluminate sealers are manufactured as a single paste, which contains the ceramic cement powder suspended in a water-miscible organic liquid and do not require mixing. The unique feature of these pastes is that setting occurs by reacting with the water in the body. In vivo, the organic liquid is gradually displaced (dissolved in tissue fluid), and the cement powder absorbs water from the tissue fluids so that the cement hardens and becomes impervious. This single paste idea is appealing for dentists because no mixing is needed, and the proportions of each component are properly allocated. No-mix pastes are akin to the light-curable restoratives in Chapter 9. A few root canal sealer products combine calcium silicate/aluminate cements with resin in two-paste products; the pastes are mixed, and the resins chemically set, encapsulating the cements. As with vital pulp therapy, the presence of resins leads to the presence of less bioactive cement.

Another paste sealer concept combines bioactive glass and radiopaque ceramic powders – bismuth oxide (Bi_2O_3), lanthanum oxide (La_2O_3), and samarium oxide (Sm_2O_3) – in a glycerin solution for, perhaps, enhanced antimicrobial ability (58). Calcium phosphate powders are also used in some sealers to enhance biocompatibility.

The properties of root canal sealers are important; they are pastes of medium viscosity, similar in consistency to ketchup or syrup depending on the brand. These materials are classified as Type 1 materials, per ISO 6876:2025 for endodontic sealing materials Revision 4. The sealer requirements, codified in ISO 6876 and ADA 57, and other desirable properties for these sealers are listed in Table 8.2a and b. Root canal sealers must set and must exhibit certain attributes of flow, radiopacity, insolubility, and dimensional stability and have the ability to achieve a thin film to fill the root canal anatomy; an illustration of the usual sealer consistency is in Figure 8.7. Intimate contact is needed among the sealer, gutta-percha, and dentin to achieve the desired goal of an impervious barrier to the ingress of bacteria from the mouth through the tooth; these characteristics are indirectly measured by flow and film thickness. The sealer pastes are either manually coated on the gutta-percha points, or a small amount is injected into the canals before the gutta-percha cones are inserted. Radiopacity is needed to ensure that the material

Table 8.2a ISO 6876:2012 and ADA 57:2021 requirements.

Test (unit)	Requirements for root canal sealers, Type 1	Features for surgical materials, Type 2
1. Extraneous matter	No observable extraneous matter No segregation of paste	
2. Flow (mm)	>17	Not applicable
3. Working time (hr:min)	If setting <30 min., flow >17 mm, 15 s before stated working time	State working time
4. Setting time (hr:min)	• If <0:30 min: <110% stated initial set • If 0:30–72:00 hours: within stated range, initial set; no requirement for effective (final) set	State setting time
5. Film thickness (μm)	<50	Not applicable
6. Solubility and disintegration (%)	• <3.0 • No evidence of disintegration	
7. Radiopacity (Thickness of equivalent Al, mm)	≥3	
8. Linear dimensional stability (%)*	±1	

* ADA 57:2021 only.

Table 8.2b Additional desirable characteristics of endodontic sealers and surgical materials.

Feature	Desirable characteristics of sealers	Desirable characteristics of surgical materials
9. Retreatable	Can remove "completely" if a retreatment is required	Not applicable
10. Bioactivity	Forms HA on surface	
11. Antimicrobial	Able to kill planktonic bacteria and biofilms	
12. Dentinal tubule penetration	Penetrate dentinal tubules to kill bacteria and contribute to sealing	
13. Seal the root canal	Be adherent to gutta-percha and dentin walls, not shrink, fully coat surfaces and anatomy	Be adherent to dentin walls, not shrink, fully coat surfaces and anatomy

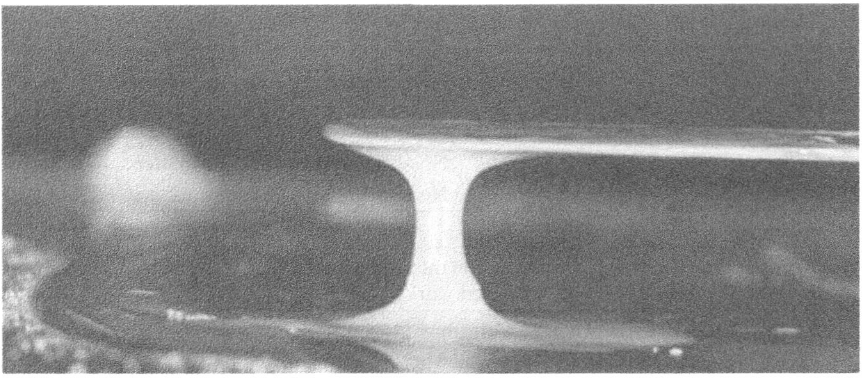

Figure 8.7 A root canal sealer is shown that has elasticity between a glass mixing plate and the spatula, illustrating the desired consistency.

is properly distributed in the roots and not beyond; endodontic radiographs are taken through the alveolar bone, so higher radiopacity is needed than for the coronally placed materials. Solubility in water and the expansion or contraction of sealers during or after setting are deleterious and, when excessive, will reduce the long-term success of the root canal therapy. The working and setting times for the sealers should be stated in products' directions for use to assist with clinical treatment planning and technique. Quick curing is required for the light-cured restorative materials of Chapter 9 but endodontic sealers have longer working and setting/curing times – usually more than 15 minutes allowing the dentist to thoroughly fill the root canal anatomy, which may have multiple canals. Setting time for the sealers may be as lengthy as 24 hours, long after the patient leaves the operatory. Other desirable characteristics for root canals are the ability to remove (most of) the materials (sealer and gutta-percha) if retreatment (described later) is required and having bioactivity or antimicrobial properties that can help inactivate microbes in infected tubules and enhance sealing ability.

No endodontic sealing test has been universally accepted. Various methods have been used to compare materials based on microleakage methods with bacteria, bacterial metabolites, dyes, radioactive isotopes, electrochemical and liquid pressure. The techniques have had variable results and problems with reproducibility; sealing tests are no longer published by prominent endodontic journals. Unfortunately, no combination of materials and obturation techniques has proved to form an impermeable seal (59). Micro-CT images have shown that no root canal sealer creates a 100% contact, nor 100% density; pores remain in the canals as passageways for bacteria from the oral cavity into the alveolar bone (60). Imperfect obturation may be the fault of the sealers' wetting ability but may also be affected by the clinician's skill and the limitations of obturation techniques. Vacuum-assist equipment may reduce porosity after obturation (61) in the future.

Perforations and Resorption

Unfortunately, dentist-induced problems occur (iatrogenic effects) during root canal therapy, which is often the perforation of the root canal wall by an endodontic instrument. The dentist may have encountered problems following the root canal to the apex because of the curvature, calcification (narrowing) of the canals, instrument choice, or inexperience. See Figure 8.4 for diagrams of furcal and lateral perforations. Perforation creates a passageway from the root canal to the periodontal ligament and the alveolar bone, a likely avenue for infection. A pathway between the inside and outside of a tooth's root can also be caused by a specific pathosis, known as root resorption (Figure 8.4). Such channels for bacteria from within the tooth to the bone are not conducive to healing; therefore, perforations and root resorptions must be obturated. The best prognosis for perforations requires several conditions: quickly treated (within hours), be smaller than 0.2 mm in diameter, be more coronal than apical, be within the alveolar not the crestal or apical bone and preferably without periodontal disease. Perforation requires a material that seals the dentin wall. Resorption also requires sealing the dentin, usually with a material applied from within the root canal. These treatments are done simultaneously with the root canal therapy described above.

The materials used for such perforations are considered as Type 2 root canal sealers in ISO 6876:2025 Revision 4; such sealing materials have a viscosity like peanut butter, much higher than the Type 1 root canal sealers. The Type 2 requirements a insolubility and radiopacity, as noted in Table 8.2. Ideally, Type 2 materials set faster than Type 1 root canal sealers; however, for slower setting materials, washout resistance is important. Calcium hydroxide-containing materials, zinc oxide-eugenol, and amalgam have been used historically for filling perforations, but with limited success (62). In comparison, calcium silicate/aluminate cements have been successfully used to manage such unfortunate occurrences (10, 63–65); these Type 2 cement products are the same as those used for pulpotomy therapy.

Retreatment

Root canal therapy is a very reliable method to maintain a tooth within the alveolar bone (66, 67), avoiding extraction. Although successful, cases do arise where the root canal treatment must be revised, a procedure called retreatment. The initial treatment of the tooth may be deficient due to some unforeseen characteristics such as an unidentified canal, tooth fracture, insufficient obturation to the apex of all the roots, or ongoing apical infection that did not heal. For retreatment, a dentist removes the prior obturation materials as much as possible and identifies the cause of ongoing pain or lack of healing. Chloroform is used, on a temporary basis, to soften the gutta-percha and enhance its removal. Rotary instruments are also used to remove the first treatment's obturation materials – sealer and gutta-percha. Then, the root canal system is rinsed (irrigated) and refilled (obturated) as in the first treatment, with the goal that the infection is sufficiently removed for the surrounding bone to heal. Notably, some of the ceramic particles present in the root canal sealers from the first treatment are likely to have been pushed deep into the dentinal tubules; such embedded particles will remain after the endodontist repeats the shaping, cleaning, and obturation steps. Luckily, such remnant ceramic particles are biocompatible anodynes!

Concern has arisen about retreatment of teeth that have been obturated using a calcium cement sealer because such materials are viewed as having the strength of concrete. In practicality, calcium cement sealers form a rather thin layer, and their strength is diluted by the presence of inert radiopaque components and the amount of liquid used in the paste; tests show equal removal of these cements compared to epoxy sealers (68–70).

In rare cases to save a tooth, the entire canal system may be obturated with a calcium silicate/aluminate cement without gutta-percha – Type 1 and Type 2 materials may be used in combination for this. The set cement can strengthen a tooth and be antimicrobial. Such a situation may be needed with a fractured tooth, or when the risk of osteonecrosis could occur if extracted (71). After complete obturation with calcium silicate/aluminate cement, another retreatment is inadvisable; ultrasonic instruments would be needed at a minimum.

Post-operative pain can be problematic for root canal treatment, which has been attributed more to technique than to the materials used (72). However, ongoing pain or swelling and non-healing periapical lesions may require surgery as described below.

Endodontic Surgery and Other Endodontic Treatments

In some cases, orthograde root canal therapy doesn't resolve an abscess at a root tip, and root-end surgery may be appropriate to save the tooth from extraction (73). Surgery requires the amputation of a few millimeters of an infected root tip following the steps of accessing the root tip through the buccal tissue and bone, curettage, and root-end resection (amputation). Next, the canal with that severed root must have a small cavity (crater) created, often with ultrasonic instruments. Then, Type 2 root canal sealing material must be placed as a thick paste in the crater made in the remaining root tip. This is called retrograde filling to seal the interior of the root from communicating with the surrounding bone and stem the ingress of the infection from the coronal portion of the tooth to the alveolar bone. The soft tissue is sutured over the site and the bone will gradually fill in the area and heal.

The materials used for root-end filling have changed dramatically since the 1800s when the procedure was first performed (74). Silver nitrate ($AgNO_3$) was used for disinfection and zinc (oxide)-phosphate cement was used to seal the root-end. Zinc oxide-eugenol products and amalgam have also been used to seal the end of surgically amputated roots, as mentioned for perforation treatment. These materials have been supplanted by calcium silicate/aluminate cements having superior results (75, 76). See Figure 8.4 for a diagram of a healed resected root tip where the bone has regenerated around the amputated root tip.

Apexification is a procedure related to root-end filling used for immature teeth, that is, roots that are shaped like a blunderbuss. The apexification procedure is performed to encourage immature teeth to lengthen and close their apices, after an infection has been detected throughout and around such roots, such as from trauma. For this treatment (Figure 8.3), the pulp is removed, and a Type 2 calcium cement paste is placed in the root tips, with sealer and gutta-percha above the cement.

Endodontics extends beyond the procedures discussed above to include treatment for conditions including dens invaginatus and evaginatus, internal or cervical root resorption, osteonecrosis, and horizontal or vertical root fracture. Calcium-based hydraulic ceramic cements are often used to treat these conditions. An uncommon treatment is replantation or transplantation, which are valiant efforts to save a tooth by first extracting it, treating the tooth, and then quickly replacing the tooth in a socket. The treatment goal is avoidance of root resorption and to reunite the periodontal ligament on the tooth to the bone. The current accepted procedure includes partially or totally filling (Figure 8.4, obturation) the root canal system with a calcium silicate/aluminate cement (77) before replantation or transplantation.

Regenerative Endodontic Therapy

The roots of permanent teeth are not fully developed in adolescents; the apical opening is wider than in fully developed teeth, which have a narrow apex. Trauma or caries can lead to the pulp becoming necrotic in these developing teeth. Revascularization is a current regenerative treatment procedure for necrotic immature teeth to encourage the body to complete root development and an alternative to apexification described above.

The regenerative procedure requires drilling to expose the pulp for its extirpation, followed by root canal disinfection and "conditioning" with sodium hypochlorite (NaOCl) then ethylenediaminetetraacetic acid (EDTA, amino-polycarboxylic acid, $C_{10}H_{16}N_2O_8$). Asepsis is achieved by filling the pulp and root canal space with antibiotics for a few days. Disinfection is followed by removal of the antibiotics and the stimulation of apical bleeding (with a pointed instrument) to recruit undifferentiated, apical, mesenchymal stem cells to enter the roots. Within the root system, a blood clot forms and serves as a tissue engineering scaffold (78, 79). Then, a collagenous matrix is placed over the blood clot, topped by a bioactive cement, and covered with a restorative material to prevent leakage and reinfection. The calcium silicate/aluminate cements are placed in the upper end of the canal (coronal), not at the root apex as is done for apexification. This new therapy is used to form new vital tissue in the tooth, which may function like pulp tissue. Usually single-rooted anterior teeth are treated with the goal of completing the formation of the root apex over the ensuing years of adolescence.

Root Canal Irrigants

In the 20th century, root canal irrigation became an important step with the primary goal to kill microbial inhabitants inside infected teeth (80). The anatomically intricate root canal system cannot be adequately accessed by any current instruments or equipment, so liquid medicaments are necessary to assist in achieving the desired goal. Irrigants are used during and after the reshaping of the root canal walls with metal instruments. Ideally, the irrigants are antimicrobial, lubricating, capable of dissolving organic or inorganic tissue, non-irritating, stable, non-staining, and suitable for use in the presence of blood, serum, and tissue protein with a low surface tension. Also, they should not have negative effects on live cells, particularly in the periapical region, nor interfere with the sealer or gutta-percha used afterward, be easy to use/remove, and have a low cost per use. Substantivity is also a benefit. Several liquids partially meet these goals as noted below.

The first such liquid used for endodontic irrigation of the root canal system was a solution of hydrogen peroxide (3–5% H_2O_2), an inorganic substance. Sodium hypochlorite (NaOCl), also inorganic, has supplanted hydrogen peroxide, with its superior antimicrobial action. Milton's solution (1 or 2% chlorine in 16.5% sodium chloride, also inorganic) has been used but has fallen out of favor because of its salt content, which in conjunction with the hypochlorite, is highly corrosive to endodontic instruments. Usually sodium hypochlorite solution (NaOCl, 1–8%) is used before, during, and after the root canal is shaped with instruments to kill bacteria and achieve some dissolution of collagen. Ethylenediaminetetraacetic acid solution (17% $C_{10}H_{16}N_2O_8$) is also commonly used to loosen the dentin swarf (smear layer) created by the metal endodontic instruments during shaping of the root canal anatomy. The current common practice is to use EDTA and NaOCl solutions in succession.

Other organic disinfectants have been tested or are in use including peracetic acid (2% CH_3CO_3H, weaker than acetic acid), chlorhexidine gluconate (2% $C_{22}H_{30}Cl_2N_{10}$) (81), etidronic acid (18% etidronate, HEBP, $C_2H_8O_7P_2$), and maleic acid (7% $C_4H_4O_4$) solutions. Combination liquids have been used, such as chlorhexidine with EDTA and triclosan (TCS, $C_{12}H_7Cl_3O_2$), doxycycline hyclate/citric acid (4%/3.25%), and EDTA with cetrimide, in addition to herbal irrigants and other combinations with doxycycline. The effectiveness of the irrigants is dependent on the active ingredient, its concentration, use of heat, time in the canal, and the methods of dispensing/removing in the canal (82). Interactions of successive irrigants must be considered (83) to avoid precipitation reactions of potentially toxic salts. Ceramic powders are not usually a component of irrigants, but nanosized diamonds suspended in solution removed of hard tissue debris created by the cleaning and shaping of root canals (84).

Impact of Ceramics on Endodontic Procedures

Modern endodontic treatments have been transformed by materials and procedures. Improved materials include better metallic instruments, the use of more antimicrobial and calcium chelating irrigants, improved solutions and agitation techniques for irrigating, ceramic-containing sealers, and ceramic-powder-filled gutta-percha. Better procedures include emphasis on bacteria and biofilm eradication concomitant with rubber dams, development of apexification and revascularization protocols, and the use of retreatment and improved apical surgical techniques. Ceramic powders are included in every endodontic sealer and surgical material, providing radiopacity, bioactivity, or antimicrobial benefits.

Hydraulic calcium silicate/aluminate cements have revolutionized endodontic treatments in the last three decades. Reference (85) has extensive examples of using these cements for root canal, surgical, perforation, and vital pulp therapy procedures. See Figure 8.8 for two histology photos illustrating the beneficial healing of teeth supported by these ceramic cements; the periodontal ligament and cementum have healed over an amputated root where a calcium silicate cement was placed in the root-end, and organized dentin was formed in response to a pulpotomy treated with calcium silicate cement. These prosaic ceramic cements have unique benefits of bioactivity and the reliable sealing with dimensional stability that have made the current standard of care. In fact, these ceramic cements have started a trend toward more vital pulp therapy and less primary root canal therapy to maintain vital primary and permanent teeth (86).

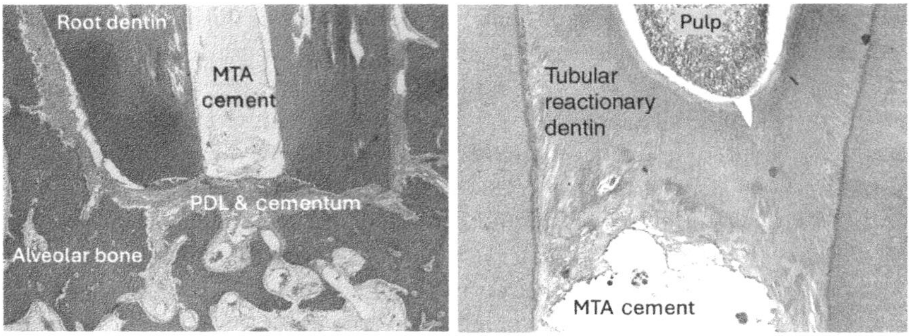

Figure 8.8 (Left) Histology in a canine subject showing a root tip healed after surgical amputation and root-end filling with a calcium silicate cement (MTA); note that high-quality, dense bone has formed over the root tip with a normal periodontal ligament (PDL). (Right) Histology of the pulp after a pulpotomy; note the high-quality, tubular dentin that has formed to separate the pulp from the calcium silicate cement (MTA) placed on the pulp tissue.

The next chapter is about direct restorative treatments other than amalgam. The consensus is that the resin composites trumped use of amalgam, despite composites' lesser longevity and greater tendency for secondary decay (87), which can cause a need for the endodontic treatment described in this chapter.

Ceramics in Chapter 8

The following ceramics and other inorganic materials were mentioned in this chapter:

- barium sulfate
- bismuth oxide
- bismuth oxychloride
- calcium aluminate cement
- calcium carbonate
- calcium hydroxide
- calcium magnesium phosphate
- calcium silicate cement: alite, belite
- calcium sulfate
- calcium tungstate
- ceria
- clay
- ferric sulfate

- hydrogen peroxide
- hydroxyapatite
- lanthana
- magnesia
- monopotassium phosphate
- potassium iodide
- potassium nitrate
- pozzolanic cement
- samaria
- silica
- fumed
  - for ionomer cement
    - bioactive glass
- silver fluoride
- silver iodide
- silver nitrate
- sodium hypochlorite
- tantalum oxide, tantalite
- tetracalcium phosphate
- tin fluoride
- titania
- titanium nitride
- tricalcium phosphate
- yttrium aluminum garnet and variations
- zeolite
- zinc oxide
- zinc phosphate, hopeite

References

1 Gutmann, J.L. and Harrison, J.W. (1994). *Surgical endodontics*, 468. St. Louis: Ishiyaku EuroAmerica.

2 Gutmann, J.L. (1997). *Problem solving in endodontics: prevention, identification, and management*, 496. Maryland Heights, MO: Mosby.

3 Dumsha, T.C. and Gutmann, J.L. (2008). *Clinician's endodontic handbook*, 240. Lexi-Comp Incorporated.

4 Gao, S.S., Zhao, I.S., Duffin, S. et al. (2018). Revitalising silver nitrate for caries management. *Int. J. Environ. Res. Public Health* 15 (1): 80.

5 Peng, J.J., Botelho, M.G., and Matinlinna, J.P. (2012). Silver compounds used in dentistry for caries management: a review. *J. Dent.* 40 (7): 531–541.

6 Zhao, I.S., Gao, S.S., Hiraishi, N. et al. (2018). Mechanisms of silver diamine fluoride on arresting caries: a literature review. *Int. Dent. J.* 68 (2): 67–76.
7 Zaeneldin, A., Chu, C.H., and Yu, O.Y. (2023). Dental pulp response to silver-containing solutions: a scoping review. *Dent J (Basel).* 11 (5): 1–12.
8 Sun, Y., Sanders, A.M., Pashley, D.H. et al. (2025). Beyond hydrodynamics: the role of ion channels in dentine hypersensitivity. *J. Dent.* 157: 105745.
9 Aminoshariae, A. and Kulild, J.C. (2021). Current concepts of dentinal hypersensitivity. *J Endodont* 47 (11): 1696–1702.
10 Lee, S.-J., Monsef, M., and Torabinejad, M. (1993). Sealing ability of a mineral trioxide aggregate for repair of lateral root perforations. *J Endodont* 19 (11): 541–544.
11 Junqueira, M.A., Cunha, N.N.O., Caixeta, F.F. et al. (2018). Clinical, radiographic and histological evaluation of primary teeth pulpotomy using MTA and ferric sulfate. *Braz. Dent. J.* 29 (2): 159–165.
12 Primus, C.M. (2006). Comments on "arsenic release provided by MTA and Portland cement" by Duarte MA, et al. *Oral Surg. Oral Med. Oral Pathol. Oral Radiol. Endod.* 101 (4): 416–417. author reply 7–8.
13 Komabayashi, T. and Spangberg, L.S. (2008). Comparative analysis of the particle size and shape of commercially available mineral trioxide aggregates and Portland cement: a study with a flow particle image analyzer. *J Endodont* 34 (1): 94–98.
14 Formosa, L.M., Mallia, B., and Camilleri, J. (2013). A quantitative method for determining the antiwashout characteristics of cement-based dental materials including mineral trioxide aggregate. *Int. Endod. J.* 46 (2): 179–186.
15 Quintana, R.M., Jardine, A.P., Grechi, T.R. et al. (2019). Bone tissue reaction, setting time, solubility, and pH of root repair materials. *Clin. Oral Investig.* 23 (3): 1359–1366.
16 Ha, W.N., Nicholson, T.M., Kahler, B., and Walsh, L.J. (2017). Rheological characterization as an alternative method to indentation for determining the setting time of restorative and endodontic cements. *Materials (Basel).* 10 (12): 1451.
17 Choi, Y., Park, S.J., Lee, S.H. et al. (2013). Biological effects and washout resistance of a newly developed fast-setting pozzolan cement. *J Endodont* 39 (4): 467–472.
18 Jang, J.H., Kang, M., Ahn, S. et al. (2013). Tooth discoloration after the use of new pozzolan cement (Endocem) and mineral trioxide aggregate and the effects of internal bleaching. *J Endodont* 39 (12): 1598–1602.
19 Park, S.J., Heo, S.M., Hong, S.O. et al. (2014). Odontogenic effect of a fast-setting pozzolan-based pulp capping material. *J Endodont* 40 (8): 1124–1131.
20 Bentz, D.P. (2008). A review of early-age properties of cement-based materials. *Cem. Concr. Res.* 38 (2): 196–204.
21 Hutcheson, C., Seale, N.S., McWhorter, A. et al. (2012). Multi-surface composite vs stainless steel crown restorations after mineral trioxide aggregate pulpotomy: a randomized controlled trial. *Pediatr. Dent.* 34 (7): 460–467.

22 de Oliveira, I.R., TL, A., Parreira, R.M. et al. (2015). Characterization of calcium aluminate cement phases when in contact with simulated body fluid. *Mater. Res.* 18 (2): 382–389.

23 Walsh, R.M., Woodmansey, K.F., He, J. et al. (2018). Histology of NeoMTA Plus and Quick-Set2 in contact with pulp and periradicular tissues in a canine model. *J Endodont* 44 (9): 1389–1395.

24 Abukabbos, H., Tomar, S., and Guelmann, M. (2018). Cost estimates for bioactive cement pulpotomies and crowns in primary molars. *Pediatr. Dent.* 40 (1): 51–55.

25 Primus, C. (2023). Bioactive ceramics for pediatric dentistry. In: *Contemporary endodontics for children and adolescents*, 1ste (ed. A.B. Fuks, M. Moskovitz, and N. Tickotsky), 149–186. Springer.

26 Primus, C.M., Tay, F.R., and Niu, L.N. (2019). Bioactive tri/dicalcium silicate cements for treatment of pulpal and periapical tissues. *Acta Biomater.* 96: 35–54.

27 Raghavendra, S.S., Jadhav, G.R., Gathani, K.M., and Kotadia, P. (2017). Bioceramics in endodontics – a review. *J Istanb Univ Fac Dent.* 51 (3 Suppl 1): S128–S137.

28 Komabayashi, T., Zhu, Q., Eberhart, R., and Imai, Y. (2016). Current status of direct pulp-capping materials for permanent teeth. *Dent. Mater. J.* 35 (1): 1–12.

29 Shen, C., Rawls, H.R., and Esquivel-Upshaw, J.F. (2021). *Phillips' science of dental materials*, 13the, 448. Philadelphia: Elsevier, Inc.

30 Qureshi, A., Soujanya, E., Nandakumar et al. (2014). Recent advances in pulp capping materials: an overview. *J. Clin. Diagn. Res.* 8 (1): 316–321.

31 Fuks, A.B. (2002). Current concepts in vital primary pulp therapy. *Eur. J. Paediatr. Dent.* 3 (3): 115–120.

32 Hilton, T.J., Ferracane, J.L., and Mancl, L. (2013). Northwest practice-based research collaborative in evidence-based D. Comparison of CaOH with MTA for direct pulp capping: a PBRN randomized clinical trial. *J. Dent. Res.* 92 (7 Suppl): 16S–22S.

33 el Kafrawy, A.H., Dickey, D.M., Mitchell, D.F., and Phillips, R.W. (1974). Pulp reaction to a polycarboxylate cement in monkeys. *J. Dent. Res.* 53 (1): 15–19.

34 Cengiz, E. and Yilmaz, H.G. (2016). Efficacy of erbium, chromium-doped:yttrium, scandium, gallium, and garnet laser irradiation combined with resin-based tricalcium silicate and calcium hydroxide on direct pulp capping: a randomized clinical trial. *J Endodont* 42 (3): 351–355.

35 Aminoshariae, A., Primus, C., and Kulild, J.C. (2022). Tricalcium silicate cement sealers: do the potential benefits of bioactivity justify the drawbacks? *J. Am. Dent. Assoc.* 153 (8): 750–760.

36 Torabinejad, M., Parirokh, M., and Dummer, P.M.H. (2018). Mineral trioxide aggregate and other bioactive endodontic cements: an updated overview – part II: other clinical applications and complications. *Int. Endod. J.* 51 (3): 284–317.

37 Parirokh, M. and Torabinejad, M. (2010). Mineral trioxide aggregate: a comprehensive literature review – Part I: chemical, physical, and antibacterial properties. *J Endodont* 36 (1): 16–27.

38 Darvell, B.W. and Wu, R.C. (2011). "MTA"-an hydraulic silicate cement: review update and setting reaction. *Dent. Mater.*: official publication of the Academy of Dental Materials 27 (5): 407–422.

39 Primus, C., Gutmann, J.L., Tay, F.R., and Fuks, A.B. (2021). Calcium silicate and calcium aluminate cements for dentistry reviewed. *J. Am. Ceram. Soc.* 105 (3): 1841–1863.

40 Eid, A.A., Gosier, J.L., Primus, C.M. et al. (2014). In vitro biocompatibility and oxidative stress profiles of different hydraulic calcium silicate cements. *J Endodont* 40 (2): 255–260.

41 Ahmed, M.I., El Hilaly Mohamed Eid, G., and Youssef, H.A. (2021). Clinical and radiographic assessments of potassium nitrate in polycarboxylate versus mineral trioxide aggregate as pulpotomy biomaterials in immature mandibular first permanent molars: a randomized clinical trial. *J Endodont* 47 (11): 1672–1682.

42 Silva, E., Pinto, K.P., Belladonna, F.G. et al. (2023). Success rate of permanent teeth pulpotomy using bioactive materials: a systematic review and meta-analysis of randomized clinical trials. *Int. Endod. J.* 56 (9): 1024–1041.

43 Lin, Y.T. and Lin, Y.J. (2020). Success rates of mineral trioxide aggregate, ferric sulfate, and sodium hypochlorite pulpotomies: a prospective 24-month study. *J. Formos. Med. Assoc.* 119 (6): 1080–1085.

44 Strange, D.M., Seale, N.S., Nunn, M.E., and Strange, M. (2001). Outcome of formocresol/ZOE sub-base pulpotomies utilizing alternative radiographic success criteria. *Ped Dent.* 23 (3): 331–336.

45 Davaie, S., Hooshmand, T., and Ansarifard, S. (2021). Different types of bioceramics as dental pulp capping materials: a systematic review. *Ceram. Int.* 47 (15): 20781–20792.

46 Prati, C. and Gandolfi, M.G. (2015). Calcium silicate bioactive cements: biological perspectives and clinical applications. *Dent. Mater.*: official publication of the Academy of Dental Materials 31 (4): 351–370.

47 Peskersoy, C., Lukarcanin, J., and Turkun, M. (2021). Efficacy of different calcium silicate materials as pulp-capping agents: randomized clinical trial. *J Dent Sci.* 16 (2): 723–731.

48 Gong, V. and Franca, R. (2017). Nanoscale chemical surface characterization of four different types of dental pulp-capping materials. *J. Dent.* 58: 11–18.

49 Ahmed, H.M.A., Versiani, M.A., De Deus, G., and Dummer, P.M.H. (2017). A new system for classifying root and root canal morphology. *Int. Endod. J.* 50 (8): 761–770.

50 Abrishami, A.M.V. and Gutmann, J.L. (2022). Historical perspectives on the evolution of root canal sealer/cements. *J. Hist. Dent.* 70 (2): 107–118.

51 Stiegemeier, D., Baumgartner, J.C., and Ferracane, J. (2010). Comparison of push-out bond strengths of resilon with three different sealers. *J Endodont* 36 (2): 318–321.

52 Barborka, B.J., Woodmansey, K.F., Glickman, G.N. et al. (2017). Long-term clinical outcome of teeth obturated with resilon. *J Endodont* 43 (4): 556–560.

53 Almasri, A., Abduljalil, M., and Aksoy, U. (2024). Efficacy of different irrigation activation techniques on dentinal tubule penetration of the novel AH-plus bioceramic sealer. *Appl. Sci.* 14 (2): 701.

54 Yang, R., Tian, J., Huang, X. et al. (2021). A comparative study of dentinal tubule penetration and the retreatability of EndoSequence BC Sealer HiFlow, iRoot SP, and AH Plus with different obturation techniques. *Clin. Oral Investig.* 25 (6): 4163–4173.

55 Orstavik, D., Kerekes, K., and Eriksen, H.M. (1987). Clinical performance of three endodontic sealers. *Endod Dent Traumatol.* 3 (4): 178–186.

56 Komabayashi, T., Colmenar, D., Cvach, N. et al. (2020). Comprehensive review of current endodontic sealers. *Dent. Mater. J.* 39 (5): 703–720.

57 Desai, S. and Chandler, N. (2009). Calcium hydroxide-based root canal sealers: a review. *J Endodont* 35 (4): 475–480.

58 Saud, A.N., Koç, E., Özdemir, O. et al. (2025). Evaluation of antibacterial and biocompatibility of radiopaque bioactive glass-based endodontic cements. *Ceram. Int.* 51 (10): 12645–12653.

59 AliGhamdi, A. and Wennberg, A. (1994). Testing of sealing ability of endodontic filling materials. *Endod Dent Traumatol.* 10 (6): 249–255.

60 Kim, J., Vo, K., Dhaliwal, G.S. et al. (2024). Micro-CT determination of the porosity of two tricalcium silicate sealers applied using three obturation techniques. *J. Oral Sci.* 66 (3): 163–168.

61 Li, J., Bergeron, B.E., Chao, J. et al. (2020). Micro-computed tomography evaluation of root canal filling quality with apical negative pressure. *J. Dent.* 100: 103431.

62 Hashem, A.A. and Wanees Amin, S.A. (2012). The effect of acidity on dislodgment resistance of mineral trioxide aggregate and bioaggregate in furcation perforations: an in vitro comparative study. *J Endodont* 38 (2): 245–249.

63 Hashem, A.A. and Hassanien, E.E. (2008). ProRoot MTA, MTA-Angelus and IRM used to repair large furcation perforations: sealability study. *J Endodont* 34 (1): 59–61.

64 Ford, T.R., Torabinejad, M., McKendry, D.J. et al. (1995). Use of mineral trioxide aggregate for repair of furcal perforations. *Oral Surg. Oral Med. Oral Pathol. Oral Radiol. Endod.* 79 (6): 756–763.

65 Main, C., Mirzayan, N., Shabahang, S., and Torabinejad, M. (2004). Repair of root perforations using mineral trioxide aggregate: a long-term study. *J Endodont* 30 (2): 80–83.

66 Imura, N., Pinheiro, E.T., Gomes, B.P. et al. (2007). The outcome of endodontic treatment: a retrospective study of 2000 cases performed by a specialist. *J Endodont* 33 (11): 1278–1282.

67 Balto, K. (2011). Tooth survival after root canal treatment. *Evid Based Dent.* 12 (1): 10–11.

68 Shim, E., Son, J.W., Kwon, J. et al. (2025). Retrieval of AH plus bioceramic and ceraseal versus AH plus in endodontic retreatment. *J. Clin. Med.* 14 (6): 1–17.

69 Sapana, S., Arya, A., Nandanwar, A. et al. (2024). Comparison of retreatability of AH plus sealer and bioceramic sealer with solvent, retreatment files and diode laser: a CBCT and SEM analysis. *J Pharm Bioallied Sci.* 16 (Suppl 4): S3528–S3530.

70 Kim, K., Kim, D.V., Kim, S.Y., and Yang, S. (2019). A micro-computed tomographic study of remaining filling materials of two bioceramic sealers and epoxy resin sealer after retreatment. *Restor Dent Endod.* 44 (2): 1–9.

71 Vescovi, P., Campisi, G., Fusco, V. et al. (2011). Surgery-triggered and non surgery-triggered bisphosphonate-related osteonecrosis of the jaws (BRONJ): a retrospective analysis of 567 cases in an Italian multicenter study. *Oral Oncol.* 47 (3): 191–194.

72 Zamparini, F., Lenzi, J., Duncan, H.F. et al. (2024). The efficacy of premixed bioceramic sealers versus standard sealers on root canal treatment outcome, extrusion rate and post-obturation pain: a systematic review and meta-analysis. *Int. Endod. J.* 57 (8): 1021–1042.

73 Stueland, H., Orstavik, D., and Handal, T. (2023). Treatment outcome of surgical and non-surgical endodontic retreatment of teeth with apical periodontitis. *Int. Endod. J.* 56 (6): 686–696.

74 Gutmann, J.L. and Gutmann, M.S. (2010). Historical perspectives on the evolution of surgical procedures in endodontics. *J. Hist. Dent.* 58 (1): 1–42.

75 von Arx, T. (2016). Mineral trioxide aggregate (MTA) a success story in apical surgery. *Swiss Dent J.* 126 (6): 573–595.

76 Chao, Y.C., Chen, P.H., Su, W.S. et al. (2022). Effectiveness of different root-end filling materials in modern surgical endodontic treatment: a systematic review and network meta-analysis. *J Dent Sci.* 17 (4): 1731–1743.

77 Plotino, G., Abella Sans, F., Duggal, M.S. et al. (2020). Clinical procedures and outcome of surgical extrusion, intentional replantation and tooth autotransplantation – a narrative review. *Int. Endod. J.* 53 (12): 1636–1652.

78 Dhillon, H., Kaushik, M., and Sharma, R. (2016). Regenerative endodontics – creating new horizons. *J Biomed Mater Res B Appl Biomater* 104 (4): 676–685.

79 Murray, P.E., Garcia-Godoy, F., and Hargreaves, K.M. (2007). Regenerative endodontics: a review of current status and a call for action. *J Endodont* 33 (4): 377–390.

80 Sedgley, C. (2004). Root canal irrigation – a historical perspective. *J. Hist. Dent.* 52 (2): 61–65.

81 Arias-Moliz, M.T., Ordinola-Zapata, R., Baca, P. et al. (2015). Antimicrobial activity of chlorhexidine, peracetic acid and sodium hypochlorite/etidronate irrigant solutions against enterococcus faecalis biofilms. *Int. Endod. J.* 48 (12): 1188–1193.

82 Basrani, B. (2015). *Endodontic irrigation chemical disinfection of the root canal system*. [XVII, 316 pages 152 illustrations, 114 illustrations in color]. ebook. Cham: Springer Available from: https://ezaccess.libraries.psu.edu/login?url=http://dx.doi.org/10.1007/978-3-319-16456-4.

83 Basrani, B.R., Manek, S., Sodhi, R.N. et al. (2007). Interaction between sodium hypochlorite and chlorhexidine gluconate. *J Endodont* 33 (8): 966–969.

84 Wang, N., Lin, P.Y., Yang, J.C. et al. (2025). Micro-CT evaluation of a nanodiamond irrigant for hard-tissue debris removal during sonic agitation. *Int. Endod. J.* 58 (2): 346–356.

85 Hanaei, S.B., Murugesan, R.C., Souza, L.P. et al. (2024). Multifunctional gallium doped bioactive glasses: a targeted delivery for antineoplastic agents and tissue repair against osteosarcoma. *Biomed. Mater.* 19 (6): 1–16.

86 Silva, E., Pinto, K.P., Torabinejad, M. et al. (2025). Overall success rate of permanent teeth pulpotomy using ProRoot MTA: a systematic review and meta-analysis of randomized clinical trials. *PLoS One* 20 (4): 1–19.

87 Worthington, H.V., Khangura, S., Seal, K. et al. (2021). Direct composite resin fillings versus amalgam fillings for permanent posterior teeth. *Cochrane Database Syst. Rev.* 8 (8): CD005620.

9

Directly Restoring Coronal Anatomy

Dentists directly restore tooth structure (coronal anatomy) that was destroyed by caries or broken due to trauma. Before a direct restoration is placed, a dentist uses instruments and abrasive rotary instruments to remove some dentin and enamel, and perhaps an older restoration. A space is created for the dental restorative to be situated and adhere the restorative material; the locations of direct restorations were depicted in Figure 3.2. A direct restorative product is applied, shaped, and cured on the tooth, replacing the dentin and enamel; the materials restore the form, function, and esthetics of the tooth and ideally seal the cavitated area to prevent secondary caries. This chapter describes the contributions ceramic materials have made in direct dental restoratives; that is, those directly fashioned and cured by the dentist on the tooth in the operatory.

Direct restorative materials need to be easy to place and fast-setting at body temperature, particularly for treating children. Durability and prevention of the ingress of bacteria (microleakage) are the most problematic issues for the direct materials. Microleakage is the passage of bacteria through or around dental materials, particularly at the edges abutting natural tooth tissue (margins). Other desirable features for direct restorative materials are listed in Table 9.1; many features are common with dental materials described in other chapters. As discussed below, ceramic powders, especially glasses, have been the key to meeting the objective of esthetic, durable, direct restorative materials.

"Silicate" Restoratives

In the late 1800s, silicate restoratives were invented that combined a partially soluble glass powder with a phosphoric acid solution, which hardened and had a tooth-like appearance (1). When the powder and liquid were mixed, the

Ceramics in Dentistry: Materials, Manufacturing, and Clinical Applications,
First Edition. Carolyn M. Primus.

Table 9.1 Some requirements for direct restorative materials.

Characteristic	Preferred property
Tooth-colored	Tooth shades or be chameleon-like
Suitable for direct placement	Fast-setting and easy to place in moisture
Adhere to enamel and dentin	Achievable with etching and other adhesives
Thermal expansion	Similar to teeth from 0 to 100 °C
Biocompatibility	At a minimum, should be non-cytotoxic, non-irritating to mucosal membranes, non-genotoxic, non-sensitizing
Insoluble	Resistant to dissolution by acids of foods
Wear-resistance	Durable for more than 5 years
Radiopaque	Components with a high atomic number, for x-ray imaging
Prevent secondary caries	Marginal sealing at enamel and dentin interfaces

self-setting paste was directly applied to a tooth, hardening into a translucent and fairly durable material called a silicate restorative or silicate cement. The silicate cements were a big advancement because they were esthetically better as a direct restorative for anterior teeth, compared to the alternatives of gold or amalgam. The name silicate cement is too generic for materials scientists to embrace, since hundreds of silicate glasses are used in dentistry, and many glass formulas are suitable for direct restoratives.

The success of the silicate restoratives depended on the glass formulas melted and ground into powder by the manufacturers. The glasses contained silica and significant amounts of alumina – see Table 9.2 for examples. Aluminum phosphate ($AlPO_4$) was a raw material used in melting these glasses because it adds alumina and phosphate to the glass. Fluoride was incorporated by including sodium fluoride (NaF), calcium fluoride (CaF_2), or cryolite (Na_3AlF_6) in the raw materials; after melting, a silicate restorative glass contained 12–25% fluoride (3). Some of the silicate restorative glass formulas also contained beryllia, nickel oxide, strontia, iron oxide, zinc oxide, magnesia, or lithia as minor components (<10%).

The liquids for silicate restoratives were concentrated phosphoric acid solutions (40–66% acid). When the powder and liquid were mixed, an exothermic setting reaction occurred. The acidic liquid dissolved Al, Na, Ca, and F ions from the glass particle surfaces. The liquid in the matrix would become saturated with phosphate and fluoride ions, which would gradually precipitate, creating a silica–phosphate matrix surrounding the partially dissolved glass particles. Depending on the manufacturer, phosphates of zinc, magnesium, or aluminum (<20%) and water (balance) were also dissolved in the acidic liquid to slow the setting speed,

Table 9.2 Silicate, glass-ionomer, and megafiller restorative glass compositions after melting (weight percent unless noted).

	Silicate restoratives		Ionomers	Fuji II LC, RMGIC (2)	Resin composites*								ß-quartz megafiller (mol%)	Leucite-glass mega filler
					Jia									
Component	Range	Typical	Range		C	E	S2	Chadwick	Kunert	Grabowski	Hoeschler	Bowen	Range	Typical
SiO_2	30–47	39.7	35–36	34.4	65–72	52–56	64–66	28	20–45	55–70	75–97	48	56–60	60
B_2O_3					<8	5–13			<10		<5	14		2
Al_2O_3	21–33	35.8	7.5–12.5	25.0	1–7	12–16	24–25		5–35		<5	8	16–21	15
CaO	3–13	3.2	0–43		4–11	16–25		<0.1	<8		<5			
Li_2O										<15			6–8	
Na_2O	2–9	6.5	1–11		9–13	<0.8	<0.2		1–10	10–25				6
K_2O									<8	<15				11
F	6–15	11.0	5–17	3.3 (NaF)				11	7–20	3				
P_2O_5	3–24	3.9	0.5–6	4.5					2–7				0–3	
ZnO					<6	<6			2–20				5–20	
MgO			0–1		<5			9.5–10		<5	<5		3–6	
TiO_2				0.2									0–6	
ZrO_2									2–10	10–25	3–30		0–4	
Sr, Ba La oxides			0–20	32.5				45 (Ba)	<20(Sr) <10(La)		<30 La	<5(Sr) <5(Ba)	30 (Sr)	
CeO_2													0–2	
Yb_2O_3								20						
Fe_2O_3							<0.1						0–0.2	

* Names of inventors of glasses for resin composites are listed. Jia used C, E, and S2 commercial glasses.

allowing enough working time for the dentist to apply and shape the materials. Zinc oxide powder was sometimes combined with the silicate powder as a hybrid zinc phosphate–silicate restorative. Mixing on a cool glass slab was recommended so the paste would not be too hot for the tooth; a similar recommendation is made for mixing zinc phosphate cement described in Chapter 11. The mixed but unset silicate paste could not be placed near the pulp because its acidity would injure the pulp. Therefore, a base or cavity lining material – Chapter 8 – was imperative before placement of the silicate cements in deep cavity preparations. The silicate restoratives had an initial setting time of 3–8 minutes. Petrolatum was placed over the silicate restorations to protect the silicate cement from dehydration between the initial and final setting times. The silicate restoratives strengthened over about seven days as the setting reaction slowly progressed; therefore, finishing (shaping) of the anatomy of the restoration was usually delayed a few days after placement, to allow the silicate's compressive strength to improve, as high as 170 MPa.

Besides the esthetic benefit of the silicates over amalgam, the silicate restoratives were known to reduce caries around the restoration. This anti-cariogenic effect was attributed to the slightly soluble fluoride in the glass and matrix. The fluoride ions may have exchanged ions with the enamel to form fluoroapatite near its margins, creating more acid-resistant enamel, as discussed in Chapter 13. However, acidic foods tended to dissolve this restorative (4), and staining was also a problem over time. Silicate cements had a thermal expansion higher than that of teeth and were relatively "soft" – having a hardness similar to dentin but lower than enamel – contributing to lower durability than would be ideal.

Silicate cements were the starting point for modern, tooth-colored, direct restorative dental materials. Over the last century, the silicate's glass powders and liquids have been modified to create better dental restoratives and cement, particularly the glass ionomers (GIs) and resin-based composite restoratives described below.

Glass Polyalkenoate/Glass Ionomers

Glass polyalkenoate dental restoratives, known to dentists as glass ionomer cements (GI or GIC), were invented in the 1950s, evolving from the silicate cements (5). The goals for these restorative materials were to have superior esthetics, stain resistance, and durability compared to the prior silicate cement restoratives. Modified glass formulas and an acid other than phosphoric were combined. The glass ionomer powders are fluoroaluminosilicate glasses, and the liquids are solutions of polycarboxylic, itaconic, polyacrylic, and tartaric acids. The slightly acid-soluble fluoroaluminosilicate glass compositions contain silica, alumina, calcia, fluoride, and strontia or baria; the latter two oxides impart radiopacity.

Table 9.2 has a range of compositions for such glasses, which are similar to the earlier silicate glasses. The glasses are ground to a particle size of 0.02–4 µm and have a surface area of 2.5–6 m^2/g to achieve a usable setting rate reaction for dentistry (US Pat. 6,136,737). Nonreactive ceramic powders may be included for rheological, setting speed control, or as pigments.

GIs undergo an acid–base hardening reaction that has several stages. The reaction begins with the attack of the acidic liquid on the surface of the glass particles, causing partial dissolution and release of calcium, aluminum, and fluorine ions. The next stage is gelation (freezing phase) when the calcium ions cross-link to the polymeric acids. Dissolution of the aluminum ions from the glass is slower than other ions, which then cross-link to the polymeric acid chains in the final "maturation phase." Sometimes, dry tartaric acid is blended with the powder, not the liquid, to reduce the speed of setting and achieve a "snap-set"; that is, a sudden increase in reaction speed occurs when the tartaric acid surface coating on the powder is penetrated by the liquid.

Some glass ionomer products – and other dental materials such as cements or endodontic sealers – have required hand mixing by the dentist or assistant of drops of liquids and scoops of powder. Mixing the precise proportions is always an issue in dentistry; therefore, some GIs have been packaged in a dual-chamber capsule with premeasured amounts for a unit-dose. The capsule is "activated" by breaking the barrier between the powder and liquid compartments and then mixing the powder and liquid capsule in an automatic mixer called an amalgamator or trituration device. The GIs have a brief working time of 1–3 minutes after mixing. The mixed glass and acid are often sticky, and placement must be done quickly while the cement has a glossy surface, indicating that the carboxylic ions are unreacted and can bond with the tooth. A wonderful advantage of GIs is that the COOH of the hydrophilic acid groups form hydrogen bonds to the hydroxyapatite crystals of the teeth through ion exchange. The calcium or other alkaline earth ions released from the glass also bond to the tooth via the polycarboxylic acid (COO^-) (Figure 9.1).

Fluoride ions dissolved from the glass powder exchange with the tooth's hydroxyapatite ($Ca_5[PO_4]_3OH$), form fluoroapatite ($Ca_5[PO_4]_3F$), which reduces the tooth's vulnerability to acid and provides a clinical benefit akin to the silicate restoratives. GIs are suitable for patients at high risk for caries, such as children with rampant caries. The GIs are also useful where proper isolation of the restoration from saliva and moisture/blood is difficult to achieve; the cements include water to wet the tooth surface. After setting, the GI cements contain 11–24% water as part of the matrix around residual glass particles.

Another advantage of the glass ionomer materials is that they can be placed in a wet field (on a moist tooth), but they must be kept moist during setting to bond. The surface of a glass ionomer restoration is often coated with petrolatum to

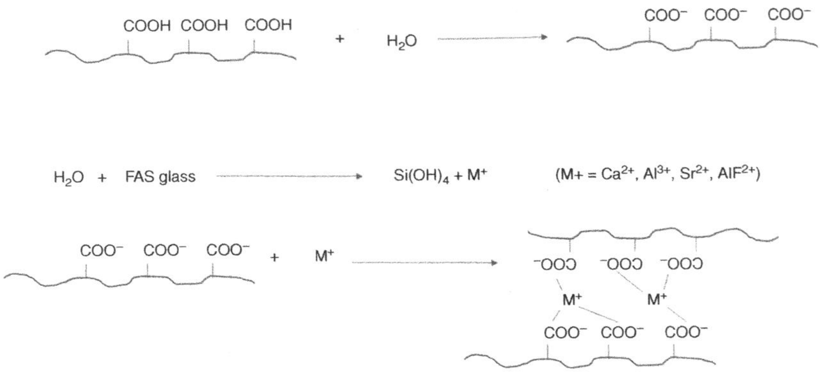

Figure 9.1 Schematic of setting reaction of glass ionomer materials with water, acrylic acid, and fluoroalumino silicate glass (FAS). *Source:* Courtesy of Solventum Company.

prevent drying of the surface during the final setting to avoid cracking or debonding. After setting, the material will normally not dehydrate although patients with xerostomia (dry mouth) may have durability issues with GIs. In another situation, drying of glass ionomer cements can be used to advantage. When glass ionomer cement (Chapter 11) is used to bond orthodontic bands, the cement can be desiccated with air from the clinician's air gun, loosening the cement's bond to the band for removal after treatment is completed.

The esthetics of glass ionomer restoratives are superior to silicate restoratives and amalgam, and the durability is greater than the silicate restoratives. The hardened GIs are biocompatible when set, durable, inhibit caries by fluoride release, and are strong and wear-resistant enough for long-term dental use. However, the GI restoratives are rather opaque. Opacity occurs because the indices of refraction of the polyacid solution and the glass have an inherent mismatch, scattering light at the interfaces of the particles, as described in Chapter 4. A few shades of glass ionomer restoratives are available from manufacturers to maximize their esthetics.

Glass ionomer cements are classified according to their clinical use, in the ISO 9917-1 and ADA 96 standards. They enjoy wide indications as luting cement (Chapter 11), base or liner for vital pulp therapy (Chapter 8), direct restorations, or pit and fissure sealing as a thin coating on the occlusal surface to prevent caries (Chapter 11). The GI cements are used for luting (cementing) metals to teeth such as pediatric stainless steel crowns, orthodontic bands, and orthodontic brackets. As a base, GI cements can prevent postoperative sensitivity under a deep resin-based composite restoration in permanent teeth. The GICs are used as restoratives in Class III and V restorations in permanent teeth for teeth with a high risk for caries (refer to Figure 3.2 for these locations). Other "restorative" indications are repairs of prior composite restorations and the margins of crowns, use as short-term temporary restorations or long-term interim restorations, and buildup of the coronal anatomy to hold a crown.

However, the GI cements are not as strong in compression, flexure, or tension as some other materials, such as amalgam, or resin composites (discussed below); therefore, other formulas have been developed to compete whose nomenclature is given below:

- Conventional GI (discussed above)
- Reinforced GIs
- High-viscosity GIs
- Giomers
- Glass carbomers and
- Nano-ionomers.

Additions have been made to increase (reinforce) the strength of conventional GIs, including ceramic powders – alumina, titania, and zirconia – and fibers of alumina, glass, and carbon. Metal particles have been added as well, using the silver alloy used in amalgam. "Cermet" GIC is the term used for glass and metal particles, usually silver-containing, that have been sintered together and then ground into a powder for inclusion in the glass ionomer with the goal of improving the cement's hardness and wear resistance. The esthetics are lessened but remain more pleasing than amalgam.

High-viscosity glass-ionomer cements use larger particle sizes and higher powder-to-liquid ratios than conventional GIs to increase the compressive strength for restoring posterior teeth. Conventional GIs use a powder:liquid ratio of 3:1 or 4:1; high viscosity GIs use a 6:1 or 7:1 ratio (by weight). The high-viscosity GIs have been used for "Atraumatic Restorative Treatment." This technique requires no electrical equipment because no drilling is performed to complete the tooth restoration, which makes it suitable for use in developing countries and on dental missions. Beneficially, the high-viscosity GIs are less affected by moisture. Zinc oxide has been added to some glasses in the high-viscosity GIs for strengthening, but the esthetics are not as good as the conventional GIs.

Giomer is a proprietary tradename that the Shofu company uses for GIs made via with their proprietary formula and processes to create fluoro-boro-strontio-aluminosilicate glass particles. They expose their glass particles to polyacrylic acid, which partially dissolves the glass and creates a gradient in the composition from the outside to the core of the glass particles; this powder is denoted as surface-pre-reacted glass (SPRG). Giomer resin-based materials are available for all restorations of primary and permanent teeth (classes I, II, III, IV, and V shown in Figure 3.2), pit, and fissure sealants. "Giomer" and "SPRG" are marketing terms used for the Shofu-patented glass formula and processing techniques, not a scientific term.

"Glass carbomers" denote a GI material that includes a hydroxyapatite powder. A curing light is used to accelerate the setting by warming the cement. Nanoionomers contain nanosized (<100 nm, <0.1 μm) fillers, which have allowed a greater proportion of filler and higher strength GIs.

An array of glass ionomer materials and modifications are used for adhesive and restorative purposes, combining the anticariogenic benefits of GI's fluoride release, tolerance of moisture, lack of shrinkage, thermal expansion similar to dentin or enamel, and biocompatibility with teeth and oral tissues.

Resin-Based Composites

Although GIs are advantageous over the silicate restoratives, the quest for durability and better esthetics motivated researchers to investigate alternatives using resins. Epoxy resins were evaluated in the 1950s for restoratives (6); their polymerization shrinkage and coefficient of thermal expansion were too high compared to that of enamel, so quartz powder was added. The epoxy resin with filler had to be mixed with a "curing agent" to harden into an insoluble thermosetting solid. The adhesion, insolubility, and color stability were favorable, but setting was hindered by moisture, ever present in operative dentistry. Epoxies for restoratives were superseded by a hybrid resin containing methacrylate and an epoxide, the Bis-GMA monomer (bisphenol A glycidyl methacrylate) of Bowen (US Pat. 3,066,112). "Bowen's resin" was more esthetic, stronger, stiffer, had less polymerization shrinkage, and its thermal expansion coefficient was more similar to that of enamel. The original Bowen resin-based composites had two components to mix, that would react and set. The first commercial resin-based composite was a two-part material from the 3 M company, Addent, followed by Adaptic from the Johnson & Johnson company. Mixing had to avoid incorporation of air, which created pores and weakened the resin-based composite.

The first methacrylate resin was used in dentistry after 1937 with limited success, but by the 1950s, resin composites (resin reinforced with glass powders) (5, 7) and their subsequent refinements revolutionized the practice of dentistry (8). Resin composite materials are now the most common and important class of direct restoration because they are tooth-colored and versatile; they have good clinical properties, good durability, and a reasonable cost. Resin composites, colloquially called composites by dentists, are the strongest of the current esthetic direct restorations although not stronger than amalgam; however, less tooth structure needs to be removed for composites compared to amalgam, which needs undercuts in teeth for retention – bonding is poor.

Modern composite materials are comprised of three main components: polymerizable resin (monomers), powdered ceramic fillers, and initiator components. The properties fundamentally depend on the volume fraction of each phase and the interfaces between them. Resin monomers are usually clear viscous liquids chosen from these resins: dimethacrylate (Bis-EMA), urethane dimethacrylate (UDMA), and cross-linking diluents (to adjust the viscosity of mixtures) such as triethylene glycol dimethacrylate (TEGDMA), decanediol dimethacrylate (D3MA), and 2-hydroxyethyl methacrylate (HEMA). The larger monomer molecules undergo less polymerization shrinkage than the original monomethyl methacrylate resins of the early 20th century, a benefit for their performance.

Resins alone are not durable enough for use in restoring teeth; therefore, ceramic powders are essential to the success of the resin composite filling materials. The monomer matrix is bonded to the ceramic fillers via a silane coupling agent, creating a strong and durable solid after curing. The ceramic powders strengthen the cured composite, reduce long-term wear by mastication, and can be polished to a luster that mimics teeth. The powders' characteristics and loading percentage influence the mechanical, optical, handling, and tribological (wear) characteristics of the cured composite resin. Furthermore, the ceramic powders add to the esthetics by mimicking the surrounding tooth structure and imparting translucency, opalescence, and UV fluorescence. The esthetics of resin composites are superior to the GIs because the fine particles of glass and other ceramic filler powders in resin composites achieve a more natural luster when polished than GIs. Refractive indices are also closer between the resin and glass fillers. Resin-based composites are cured by photoinitiation, by a chemical reaction initiated by mixing two pastes, or a combination thereof. Initiators and curing are described later in this chapter.

The ISO 4049 standard for polymer-based restorative materials – composites – has these classifications based on indications for use:

- Type 1: suitable for restorations involving occlusal surfaces
- Type 2: luting materials and materials used on non-occlusal tooth surfaces
  - Class 1: Self-curing, achieved by mixing two components
  - Class 2: External energy starts curing, such as blue light or heat
    - Group 1: Curing done intra-orally
    - Group 2: Curing done extra-orally, known as indirect composites. These materials require a separate cement to affix to a tooth.
  - Class 3: Dual-cured material, where curing occurs by mixing and an external source.

The ISO 4049 standard for resin-based composite materials requires a minimum 3-point flexural (bend) strength of 50 MPa for a Type 2 "luting" cement (Chapter 11) but more than 80 MPa for use as a Type 1 direct restorative. Resin-based composites for restorations typically have flexural strengths of 130–200 MPa, higher than GIs (40–50 MPa).

The desirable features of the resin-based direct restoratives composites are their biocompatibility, polish-ability, flexural strength, radiopacity, and translucency; the latter contributes to shade matching and blending with adjacent teeth. Resin-based composites require curing after placement on the tooth, a process that transforms the liquid monomers into hard, solid polymers that surround and bond to the ceramic particles. A lack of stickiness to an instrument is favored for ease of convenient insertion of the paste into the cavity before curing. Because of their strength and esthetics, resin composites are considered the best direct restorative material, and hundreds of products are available worldwide from many manufacturers.

Ceramic Powders in Resin-Based Composites

The ceramic powders in composites are specialized silicate glasses and may contain heavier oxides to impart radiopacity higher than 1 mm of equivalent Al, as required in ISO 4049. Common glass compositions are based on silica and alumina with baria or strontia, the latter two for radiopacity. Table 9.2 shows examples of the wide variety of glass formulas patented for use in resin composites. The original composite patent by Bowen (US Pat. 4,215,033) disclosed a glass that included silica, boron oxide, alumina, and strontia, with one or more from the group of calcia, zinc oxide, tin oxide, and zirconia. Grabowski's formula (US 5,641,347) had more silica and zirconia without baria or strontia, but included lanthana, yttria, tantalite, or niobia or gadolinium oxide (*archaically*, gadolina) to create radiopacity. Kunert (US 6,297,181 Bl) patented a glass with strontia, not baria. The glass in Chadwick's patent (US 7,175,700 B2) was made radiopaque with baria and ytterbium oxide. Hoescheler's glasses (US 2008/0255265 Al) were higher in silica than others and contained zirconia, alumina, or boron oxide along with components selected from the group TiO_2, HfO_2, Y_2O_3, Sc_2O_3 La_2O_3, CeO_2, or other lanthanum-series oxides (metal oxides with atomic numbers from 58 to 71); some alkali and alkaline earth oxides (Columns IA and IIA on the periodic table) were included. Glass flakes were disclosed by Jia (US 2006/0241205 Al) of standard, commercial C and E glasses – containing silica, boron oxide, calcia, and alumina as well as S2 glass fibers containing silica and alumina. Jones (2005/0256222) disclosed fascinating doughnut shapes of glass fillers for higher filling, adhesion, polishing, and retention in a resin rather than angular ground particles. The breadth of compositions in Table 9.2 for the glass fillers shows that each manufacturer and inventor has a proprietary approach to fillers to achieve their marketing or product improvements. Fluoride salt powders of yttrium (YF_3) and ytterbium (YbF_3) may also be included with the glass particles in the resins to augment the radiopacity. Silica and silica/zirconia mixed oxide nanoparticles are also used in some products.

Physical and esthetic properties of dental resin-based composites are determined by the ceramic filler: percent, size distribution, shape, hardness, index of refraction, and surface coating. The refractive indices of the resin and ceramic fillers need to be close in value to achieve the translucency needed for esthetic restorations, especially at the more transparent incisal edges of teeth; light scattering at the particle/resin interfaces creates opacity (as described in Chapter 4). Nano-sized particles are useful because they are smaller than the visible wavelengths of light and create less opacity.

Minor amounts of pigment powders such as alumina or titania (white), iron oxide (red, black), or iron hydroxide (yellow) are blended with the glass and resin to create individual shades. The refractive indices of these pigments are higher than the resins, which adds opacity. Organic, fluorescent pigments and dyes may be included; opalescent pigments or dyes are another option (US Pat. 8,722,759). Alternatively, opalescence and fluorescence may be created with phase-separated glass filler particles. Fumed silica (Figure 7.1) is a common component in composite resin materials for raising the viscosity of the uncured paste and for easy polishing of the cured surface.

Ceramic-Resin Interfaces

Resin composites succeed because of the "coupling" of the glass filler with the resin mixtures, as identified by Bowen. The ceramic powders are coated with an organo-silane liquid before compounding with the resin in manufacturing. A common silane coupling agent is 3-methacryloxypropyltrimethoxy-silane, whose formula is depicted in Figure 9.2. The coupling agent allows the hydrophobic resin to wet and spread on the hydrophilic ceramic particles when they are blended. The silane compound covalently bonds the filler and the resin via a hydrolysis and condensation reaction on the ceramic powder during curing; that is, the silane (condensation) portion of the molecule (Figure 9.3) attaches to the ceramic powder surface. This improved contact of resin and ceramic allows more ceramic filler to be included in a resin-based composite, resulting in higher

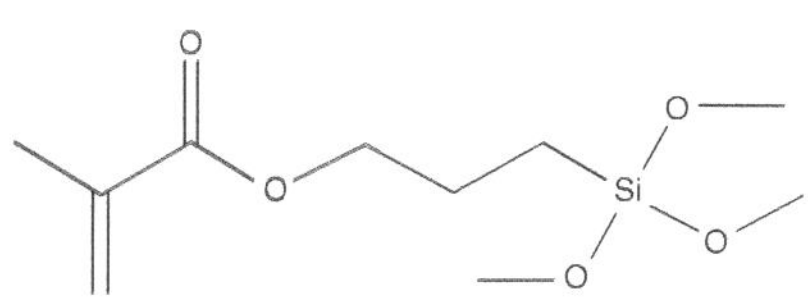

Figure 9.2 Structure of the coupling agent 3-methacryloxypropyltrimethoxy-silane. *Source:* Courtesy of Solventum Company.

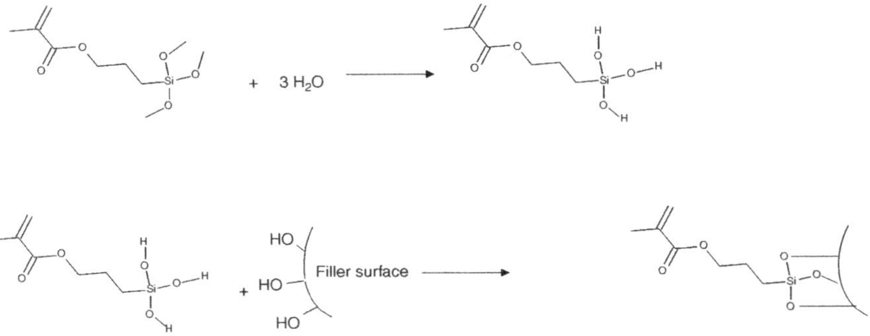

Figure 9.3 Silane hydrolysis and condensation reaction on a ceramic powder (filler) surface. *Source:* Courtesy of Solventum Company.

strengths and better wear resistance. The free-radically reactive methacrylate end of the silane molecule will co-polymerize with the resin during the monomers' chain growth polymerization during curing by the dentist.

Some manufacturers have developed organo-metallic, polymeric complexes analogous to silanes (ORMOCER® technology, organically modified ceramics) for their resin-based composites. These materials contain three-dimensionally cross-linked copolymers and ceramic filler particles, bonded via a hybrid, organo-metallic polymeric condensation reaction. The monomer–polymer matrix has a carbon backbone and pendant-free, radically-reactive groups for bonding. The monomers react with the inorganic fillers, similar to silane coupling agents. When cured, the polymers have a "backbone" of SiO_2 with methacrylate side-branches to ensure cross-linking with conventional resin compounds; they have the advantages of lower shrinkage and toxicity (9) compared to some other resin combinations. Sol–gel methods are used for ORMOCER manufacture. Systematic reviews have not shown a superiority to other monomers in clinical performance.

Resin-Based Composite Classifications

The resin composites are also categorized other ways than in ISO 4049: (1) ceramic filler loading and viscosity, (2) size of ceramic fillers, or (3) indications. Each set of categories is described below.

Viscosity of uncured composites ranges from medium to high, analogous to as low as honey and as high as cold butter. Higher viscosities are denoted as "universal"; lower viscosities are "flowable." The clinician will choose a higher or lower viscosity product based on the cavity's location. The thick, putty-like universal composites are dispensed from a screw syringe or unit-dose capsules with a large

1–3 mm orifice. Universal composites are indicated for the stress-bearing, cavity designs for Class I to IV (refer to Figure 3.2) because their thick viscosity, with 70–85 wt.% of ceramic filler is suitable to be packed, shaped, and sculpted in a cavity preparation prior to curing. The densities of the resins are low (~1 g/cc), and the density of the filler is higher (>3 g/cc), which when converted means that the volume percent of filler is about 60%. The high ceramic filler percentage increases the flexural strength and elastic modulus (stiffness) and reduces wear. Flexural strengths as high as 200 MPa make them well-suited for occlusal surfaces.

The flowable composites have less ceramic filler (60–70 wt.%) than their universal counterparts and lower viscosity for easier dispensing from a smaller orifice syringe. Some flowable composite resin pastes are so low in viscosity that they slump under gravity before curing, which allows for excellent adaptation in a tooth cavity, filling the roughness, imperfections, and undercuts. However, with less filler and more monomer, the flowable materials are "stickier" than universal composites before curing. When cured, flowable composites have lower strength, less stiffness, and less wear resistance; they are typically used in "non-occluding" indications (no tooth-to-tooth contact) such as in a cervical, Class V cavity (Figure 3.2), or as the bottom layer in a cavity preparation, or to cover a layer of calcium silicate/aluminate cement for vital pulp therapy. A few flowable composites have higher filler and viscosity for use on occlusal surfaces.

Alternatively, composites – flowable or universal – can be characterized by the ceramic filler's characteristics, such as composition, particle size, shape, or morphology. The four primary categories of composites determined by their filler type are (1) hybrid, (2) microhybrid, (3) microfill, and (4) nanocomposite or nanohybrid. Notably, all current composites have smaller particles than the original composite materials in the 1960s, which were as large as 150 μm.

Hybrid and microhybrid composite materials contain fine powders of glasses and polycrystalline ceramics, created by grinding and distinguished by filler size. Hybrid composites have a mean particle size of a few microns, and microhybrid composites have a smaller mean particle size, about 0.4 μm. Both types of composites contain a broad particle size distribution of irregularly shaped glass particles, which enables the composite to up to about 80 wt.%. The interstices among larger particles are filled with smaller particles. However, the larger ceramic particles can be "plucked out," when the composite is abraded by food, toothbrushes, toothpaste, or opposing teeth, generating a rougher surface, which may be detectable with the patient's tongue. A rougher surface scatters more light, dulling the luster and reducing the esthetics over time. The microstructure of a microhybrid composite is shown in Figure 9.4a with its broad particle size distribution of irregularly shaped particles. The hybrid and microhybrid composites are strong, wear-resistant, and useful for load-bearing areas, such as posterior Class I and Class II restorations, but are less esthetic over time than alternatives.

(a)

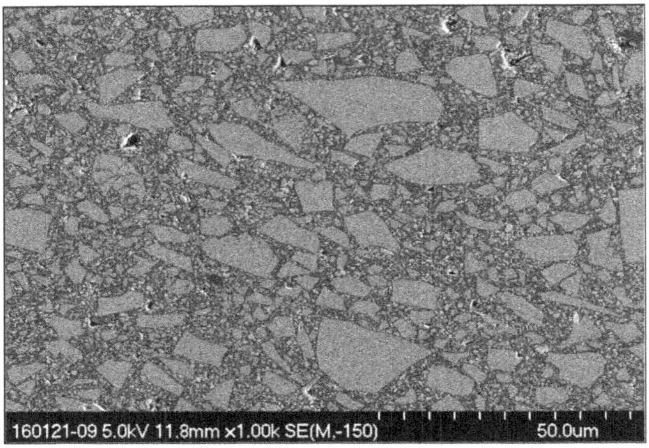

(b)

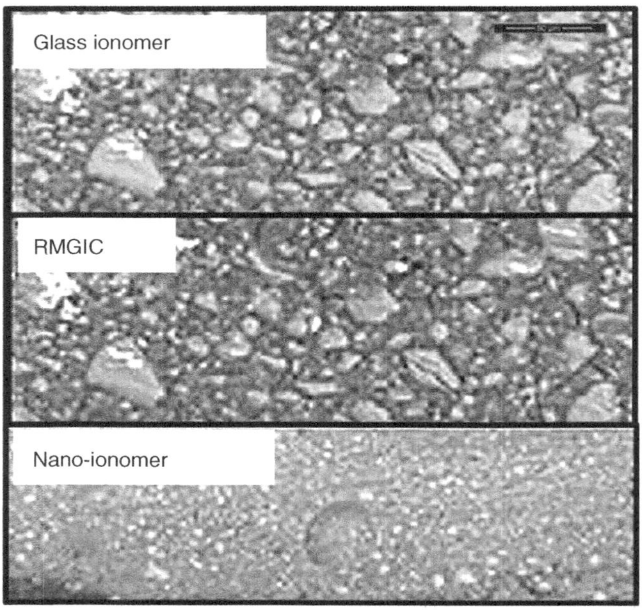

Figure 9.4 (a) Scanning electron micrograph image of a polished surface of a cured microhybrid composite showing ground filler particles of two size distributions. Image courtesy of Solventum Company. (b) Scanning electron micrograph image of a polished surface of a glass ionomer, resin-modified glass ionomer (RMGIC), and a nano-ionomer, showing the white filler particles. Note the difference in the 50 µm scale between 9.4a and b for making comparisons. *Source:* (41) / Georg Thieme Verlag KG / CC BY NC ND 4.0.

Microfill composites contain as much as 40 vol.% fumed silica; the amount of fumed silica is limited (<40) by the fumed silica's low density (<0.2 g/cc), very high surface area (200–600 m^2/g), and its branched structure (Figure 7.1). Fumed silica powder is treated with silane and blended with monomers to form a high viscosity, thixotropic (shear-thinning) resin paste before curing. That is, an uncured microfill composite will respond quickly under the stress of an instrument during its application to a tooth; without stress, the uncured composite is firmer and remains in place without slumping. Microfill composites can be polished to a high gloss because the silica particles are so small, making them especially esthetic for anterior restorations. The microfill composites are weaker than universal composites and therefore less suitable for posterior teeth.

When only nanometer-sized ceramic fillers are blended with resins, the dental material is designated a "nanocomposite," the newest composite resin category. The nanocomposites contain discrete and clustered nanoparticles (Figure 9.5), which enable the amount of filler (loading) to be high, up to 80% by weight and confer other advantages. The nanoparticles are smaller than selected wavelengths of visible light, preferentially scattering only the shorter wavelengths, which makes the composite opalescent, mimicking natural teeth. The nanocluster particles fracture under occlusal stress and abrasion, resulting in more uniform wear than the hybrid, microhybrid, or microfill composites (10, 11) because the whole particle is not dislodged. Such materials combine the strength and wear resistance of microhybrid or nanohybrid composites, with the polishability equal to or better than microfills. Nanocomposites are highly esthetic and strong, making them suitable for restorations in the anterior and posterior teeth.

Nanohybrid resin composites combine nano-sized (<100 nm) fillers and the coarser glass particles used in the hybrid or microhybrid composites. The

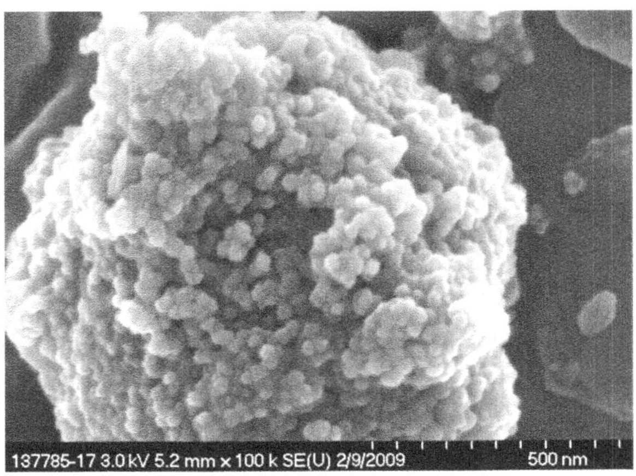

Figure 9.5 Scanning electron micrograph image of a nanocluster ceramic filler. Note the particle size of less than 1000 nm composed of the aggregated grains smaller than 100 nm. *Source:* Courtesy of Solventum Company.

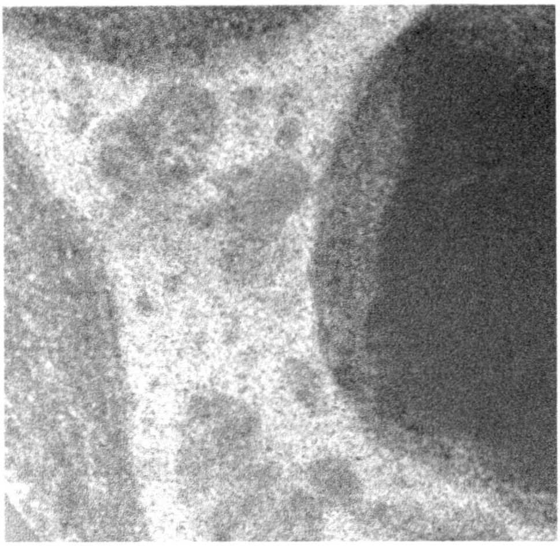

Figure 9.6 A transmission electron micrograph (TEM) image of a composite containing nanocluster and nanoparticle fillers. Lighter gray particles are silica; darker areas are zirconia. *Source:* Courtesy of Solventum Company.

nanofillers reinforce the resin matrix, reduce resin wear, and slightly improve polishing compared to hybrid or microhybrid material. Nanohybrid resin composites are also suitable for use in both anterior and posterior applications. The microstructure of glass ionomer, resin-modified glass ionomer, and nano-ionomer are shown in Figure 9.4b for comparison to the microhybrid in Figure 9.4a.

"Suprananocomposite" composites have been developed to include silica, alumina, or zirconia to particles, 200–250 nm. See Figure 9.6 for a transmission electron image showing the fine ceramic microstructure of a combination of silica and zirconia nanoparticles. These variations in filler illustrate composite products' the goal to ever-increase the polishing, handling, and durability without losing the ease of placement and fast curing.

Specialized-Indication Composite Materials

Composite resins have usually been cured in 1.5–2.5 mm layers to maximize conversion of the monomers and reduce polymerization shrinkage stresses. A recent trend in direct restorative dentistry is the use of "bulk-fill" composites. These composites are designed to be cured in thicker layers (3–5 mm) to increase the speed of the procedure by requiring fewer layers (curing increments) in deep cavities. Faster filling reduces the possibility of wet or bacterial contamination. To cure thicker layers, the more transparent composites are needed so fewer pigment particles are included bulk-fill composites to achieve the greater transparency. Fewer shades of bulk-filled composites have been available than for the universal composites; some are available at a flowable viscosity.

Experimental fiber-reinforced composites have been investigated (12) in contrast to particulate-filled composites, to enhance fracture toughness. S- or E-glass fibers (13) and E-fibers with barium borosilicate glass (14), zirconia, and "silica" (15) fibers have been tested. The fibers varied from 0.05 to 6 μm diameter and 100–300 μm long. Fibers do increase fracture strength and have limited commercialization (15); glass fibers may be more beneficial than polycrystalline ceramic fibers. The percentage and the elimination of voids in the uncured fiber-reinforced pastes are crucial to the durability and smooth surface finish needed for future successful clinical use.

Glass Ionomer and Resin Combinations

The clinical success of both GIs and resin composites has prompted the development of combined products, both resin-modified glass ionomer cements (RMGICs) and polyacid-modified composite resins (Compomers).

Since 1989, products have been developed by combining GIs with a modest amount of resin composite to exploit the best properties of both. The RMGICs contain fluoroaluminosilicate (FAS) glass, polyacrylic acid, photoinitiators, hydroxyethyl methacrylate monomer (HEMA), and water. The glass powders in RMGICs are similar to those in conventional GIs although the glass composition may be altered to match the refractive index of the resin system. The acid–base reaction of the glass and polyacrylic acid contributes to setting; the GI portion does not set before use because the monomer dispersion prevents reaction of the glass and polyacrylic acid in the paste. RMGICs have a higher compressive strength, abrasion resistance, working time, and are less sensitive to moisture than conventional GIs. However, the HEMA content makes them less biocompatible. The RMGICs were first used as material for a cavity base and later as a cement, direct restorative and pit/fissure sealant. The higher transparency makes RMGICs suitable for anterior and primary teeth. The RMGICs are especially popular with pediatric dentists for restoratives and as a cement for pediatric crowns. The RMGICs are available as a powder–liquid, paste–paste, and single syringe formats, depending on the initiators used.

The resin component of RMGIC products reduces the elastic modulus and fluoride release compared to GICs but increases the strength, transparency, and speed of setting. The elastic modulus is lowered to 3–5 GPa from 15 to 20 GPa for conventional GIs. The lower modulus can durability for Class V restorations that are subject to flexing during chewing or speaking. Flexural strengths can be increased to approximately 70 MPa, compared to 40–50 MPa for conventional GIs. The dual-curing of RMGIC is faster than conventional GIs. A primer material (see Chapter 11) may be applied to the tooth prior to the RMGIC for enhanced bonding.

Compomers, “polyacid modified resin materials,” are also a combination of GIs (~30%) and light-curable resins (~70%); they were introduced in 1991. Their curing reaction begins with photopolymerization of the resin in the material, as with the RMGIC materials. The curing depth and compressive strength are higher than RMGIC, but the bond strength to dentin and enamel and the fluoride release are lower because more monomer is used in compomers. Compomers are popular in pediatric and orthodontic dentistry because of the combination of their fluoride release, easy application, and esthetic appearance (better than conventional GIs). Compomers are used as pit/fissure sealants, for bonding orthodontic bands, and as a restorative for Class II and V cavities (Figure 3.2). Their popularity has been limited because their slightly higher fluoride release compared to composites has not been clinically shown to be advantageous for caries prevention. Primer-adhesive systems should be used before placement of compomers, which add cost and time.

Adhesion and Curing of Resin Composites

Unlike the GIs, the dental acrylic resins do not adhere to tooth structure; therefore, the resin-containing restorative materials need a bonding system (Chapter 11) applied before the resins are placed on the tooth. Michael Buonocore introduced of etching/roughening of tooth enamel with phosphoric acid (85%) in 1955 (16) – this changed the course of restorative dentistry. Acid etching allows interdigitation of resin into the enamel microporosities created by the phosphoric acid (17). The higher surface area can be filled by the adhesives to bond the tooth and composite restorative. More dilute phosphoric acid is now used (~37%). Acid etching is very effective with enamel but when dentin is etched, the hydroxyapatite component is dissolved but collagen fibrils remain. Adhesives have been developed to infiltrate the wet fibrils to create a bond; however, infiltration may be incomplete. Since the advent of enamel etching, bonding systems have improved and been simplified. The original three-step process (called the total etch technique) required the etching with phosphoric acid, rinsing, application of a hydrophilic primer, followed by a hydrophobic resin. Now, one-component, self-etching adhesives are common, and acids other than phosphoric are used. Adhesives are discussed in Chapter 11. Adhesion to enamel and dentin is imperative because un-etched enamel doesn’t have adhesion, and unprotected, un-infiltrated dentin collagen fibers can harbor bacteria, leading to secondary caries infection.

Chemical curing was first used for composites. Around 1970, ultraviolet light – below 400 nm wavelength – began to be used to initiate light curing for composites; the initiators contained benzoin methyl ether or similar UV-sensitive compounds (e.g. 1-phenyl-1,2-propanedione, bisacylphosphine oxides, triacylphosphine oxide, and the germanium-based Ivocerin). Initiating polymerization with exposure to light eliminated the need to mix two pastes for a chemical curing reaction

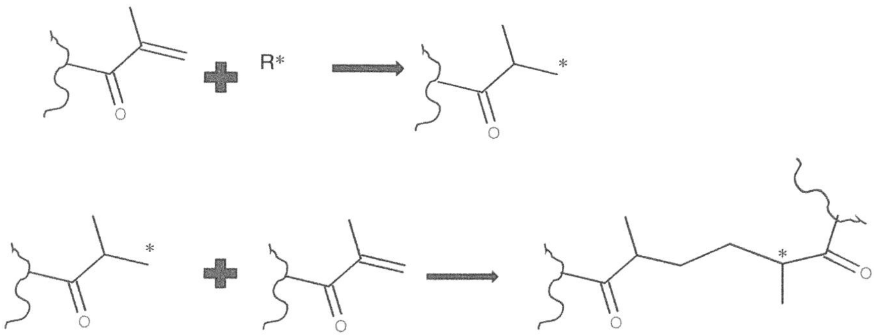

Figure 9.7 Free radical chain propagation reaction scheme. *Source:* Image courtesy of Solventum Company.

and created the concept of extended working time and "curing on demand" (when the material was exposed to a strong light). However, UV light was limited in its depth of penetration, and safety concerns about the intensity arose for the patient and dental professionals' eyesight. Blue-light activators, sensitive at about 468 nm wavelength, replaced UV activators in late 1970s for composites; camphorquinone (CQ) and a tertiary amine activator (co-initiator), and sometimes diphenyliodonium hexafluorophosphate are used. Blue light activates the photoinitiators, which cleave and form a free radical, donating free electrons, causing the monomers to polymerize as depicted in Figure 9.7. Iodonium salts (halonium ions, such as H_2I^+or R_2I^+, open-chain or cyclic) are incorporated in some light-cured systems to extend the radical's shelf life and improve the degree of double-bond conversion (polymerization) of the resin. Two-paste, dual-curing resin composites include both chemical and photo-sensitive initiators. Dual curing is useful for darker resin shades and when resin cement is used to affix a crown, which inherently have less light penetration.

The first (blue) visible curing lights had tungsten-halogen filled glass bulbs with blue light filters, standardized under ISO 10650-1 and ADA 48. These curing lights had intensities up to 800 mW/cm^2, and the cure times were 20–40 seconds; the bulbs were effective but inefficient and hot. Since the beginning of the 21st century, light-emitting diode bulbs (LED lights) have become commonly used, as they don't require wavelength filters and emit less heat. The first LED devices had low output, but intensities are now as high as 2000 mW/cm^2. The LED curing lights use a gallium nitride-based semiconductor for blue light emission, which has shortened cure times to as little as eight seconds to adequately cure composite materials of a lighter shade or low opacity; more curing time is needed for darker opaque shades and thicker layers (>1 mm). Some multi-LED curing devices emit multiple wavelengths. Plasma-arc curing lights are another high-intensity light source using a fluorescent glass-enclosed bulb that creates an intense light from the plasma in the bulb. Its intense light accelerates the polymerization process; however, the high light intensity generates heat in the composite and tooth. Too much heat will injure the pulp and cause cell death; this is a risk factor for deep restorations that are close to the pulp. Manufacturers' recommendations for curing times and intensities should always be followed when placing a composite restoration.

No matter which curing equipment or mechanism is used or what material is cured, the conversion of monomers to polymers is never 100% and is commonly less than 75%. Furthermore, composite resins shrink 1% to 4% linearly as the monomers form polymers. As the resins are cured, they exert shrinkage stress at the interface with the tooth. Ideally, the composite resin should not pull away from the tooth structure as it shrinks during curing because bonding to the tooth is key to success. The bulk-fill composites can be cured in 4 mm increments (18). The depth of cure of all composites is enhanced by higher irradiance ($\geq$1000 mW/cm^2) and longer exposure times ($\geq$20 seconds) (19). The adaptation, bonding, and curing processes are crucial to preventing bacterial ingress, which would allow caries to form and necessitate more treatment. Ongoing objectives for composite manufacturers is to reduce curing shrinkage, improve the bonding, and maximize the conversion of the monomers to polymers.

Indirect Resin Restorations

Direct composites never reach 100% conversion of the monomers to polymers when cured in the mouth, even with modern LED curing lights especially in deep cavities (20). To improve the performance of the composite restorative materials, laboratory fabrication of direct composites has been used – this has been dubbed the indirect resin restoration or indirect resin composite.

An indirect restoration requires an impression (Chapter 14); then a model is fabricated by the dental laboratory. A separating medium (oil) is placed in the cavity preparation of the model, which allows the cured composite in the next step to be removed. A composite material is condensed into the cavity preparation for curing with light, heat, steam, pressure, vacuum, nitrogen, or combinations thereof. Special equipment for heat-assisted-curing under nitrogen gas was the first method used to improve the mechanical properties (21) by enhancing the degree of polymerization. Multiple curing cycles can be performed to perfect the fit. The cured composite device/restoration is returned to the dentist, who cements the "fully cured" indirect composite into position. Shrinkage and stress on the tooth are obviated by this technique; the only shrinkage is that of the thin cement layer. This method does require two appointments.

An alternative is the "semi-indirect" resin restoration. For this method, a separating medium (oil) is placed directly in the patient's cavity preparation, and then a composite material is condensed into the preparation and partially cured. Next, the partially cured composite is removed from the tooth and cured in the dental laboratory of the dentist's office at about 110 °C for less than 10 minutes in a special curing apparatus from the manufacturer. After curing, the semi-indirect composite is cemented into its tooth position. This approach does not need an impression and enables a one-appointment visit. The extraoral curing process makes it possible to use materials and methods that clinicians would not favor for in vivo direct placement.

These indirect curing techniques increased the degree of conversion of the monomers, leading to higher values for the flexural strength, the elastic modulus, and hardness (20). The materials for semi-indirect and indirect composite restorations can contain greater filler content, and some include pre-polymerized particles. Pre-polymerized particles contain polymer and ceramic filler and have been polymerized and then ground by the manufacturer; these particles are blended with monomers. The resulting combination has less monomer to cure, which reduces shrinkage. Lower wear resistance, better marginal adaptation, and reduced microleakage at the margin were the goals. Even so, these methods and materials are less common than direct composites.

Ceramic "Megafillers" for Direct Restoratives

The shrinkage that occurs during the curing of resins creates problems for bonding and ensuring complete adaptation at the margins to prevent caries recurrence. Indirect composite resin techniques from above are one approach to improve adaptation and curing; another approach was to use small glass inserts, megafillers, in a direct dental restoration, placed in a pool of uncured resin composite. Bowen suggested the use of ceramic inserts to reduce the amount of polymer in a restoration, thereby reducing polymerization shrinkage and stress (22). Ceramic inserts such as ebony, glass, or crystalline gemstones have been used historically and may have been both decorative and functional to fill a cavity (imperfectly). Megafiller dental inserts were several millimeters in size and suitably shaped and pigmented for insertion in conventional Class I or II cavity preparations: some inserts were cylindrical, others conical. They functioned as a noncustomized ceramic inlay to reduce wear and improve the marginal adaptation. Two megafiller ceramics were commercialized, made of beta-quartz and "leucite glass" (22).

These inserts lowered the coefficient of thermal expansion of the restoration and included a ceramic material with an elastic modulus more like teeth.

The beta-quartz inserts were a type of glass–ceramic. The small glass items were heat treated just above their annealing temperature to nucleate crystals and then further heat treated between 750 and 1000 °C to grow fine crystals of beta-quartz, the high-temperature, hexagonal crystal of silica. Other crystals also formed: beta-eucryptite ($LiAlSiO_4$), beta-spodumene (high-temperature tetragonal $LiAlSi_2O_6$), and keatite (tetragonal silica). These phases were usually solid solutions, meaning that the crystals did not have the stoichiometric formula listed, and included substitutions such as titania (TiO_2). Colorants were added: iron oxide (Fe_2O_3) at about 0.1 mol% and ceria (CeO_2) up to 2%. The crystals were microscopic, and few enough were present that light was transmitted through the dental inserts to allow light curing of the composite around and beneath the insert. The manufacturers coated the inserts with 3-methacryloxy-propyltrimethoxy silane to enable them to adhere to the composite resins in which they were placed.

The leucite glass inserts were made by several companies in various shapes and colors. Some were nearly transparent, relying on blending with the color of the surrounding tooth by internal reflections from the leucite crystals. Because of their transparency, the percentage of leucite crystals is suspected to be lower than that used in the dental porcelains described in Chapter 10. Presumably, these inserts were made by heat treating potassium feldspar to transform its orthoclase crystals into a glass with dispersed leucite crystals. The leucite-glass inserts were etched with hydrofluoric acid (HF) to roughen the glass and then coated with silane by the manufacturer for the dentist.

Megafillers were individually packaged for the dentist to choose the size, shape, and shade before placement in the uncured composite resin lining a cavity preparation. After curing the composite, the surface had to be contoured and polished to create the proper occlusion. Silicon carbide (SiC) and diamond burs were used for shaping, and alumina was used for polishing (Chapter 17). Invented in the 1980s, their clinical acceptance was meager in the 1990s and has been surpassed in performance by newer composite resins.

Impact of Ceramics in Direct Dental Restorations

Direct restorative dentistry has improved tremendously, especially since the 1950s. A schematic depiction of the continuum of direct restoratives advancements discussed in this chapter is shown in Figure 9.8, from GIs to resin composites. Each direct restorative filling material has advantages and disadvantages. GIs offer the benefit of fluoride release, relative insensitivity to moisture, and bonding

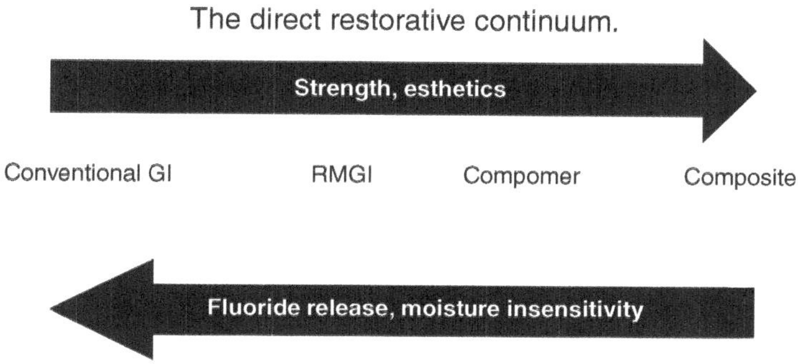

Figure 9.8 The continuum of direct dental restorative materials, illustrating the trade-off between strength and esthetics versus fluoride and moisture tolerance. *Source:* Image courtesy of Solventum Company.

to the tooth, but have lower strength, are less esthetic, and more difficult for the dentist to place. Composite materials provide better esthetics, higher strength, less wear over time, and are easier for the dentist to place compared to GIs. However, composites are much less tolerant of saliva or other contamination during placement, lack fluoride release, and require a separate adhesive to bond them into or onto the tooth structure, which can be vexing for the dentist and a source for secondary decay. The RMGICs and compomers are hybrids of these two chemistries with properties that lie in between. Each patient's restoration is a unique situation where the clinician must determine which material may be best suited to the case.

Acrylic polymers, adhesive dentistry, and ceramic powders have been key to these advances. The glass and ceramic powders for ionomers and resins are as important as the polymers because the ceramics provide the esthetics, form, and durability for direct restoratives. The ability of manufacturers to create fine particle sizes of glasses by various milling techniques has been the basis for ever-better direct restorative materials. Higher glass contents in composites have reduced interoral wear (increased durability) and created better esthetics.

The glasses used for these restorative materials have different requirements depending on the curing matrix; therefore, many glass formulas have been used. In general, glass formulas for ionomers have lower silica content and higher alumina that used in composite resins. Fluoride is needed in the GIs but is less common for the glasses in composite resin. Radiopacity is achieved with ceramic powders blended in the resins or with higher atomic number components in the glasses.

Table 9.3 has a summary of properties for the groups of direct restorative materials extracted from Table 6.1. The values for mechanical properties always vary

Table 9.3 Tooth and direct restoratives.

Material	Thermal expansion coefficient (ppm/K)	Hardness (GPa)	Fracture toughness (MPa-$m^{1/2}$)	Flexural strength* (MPa)	Compressive strength (MPa)	Elastic modulus (GPa)
Tooth enamel (23–31)	7.8–17	~4	0.5–2.1	478–493	62–386	54–120
Dentin (23, 24, 26, 27, 29, 32, 33)	8.3–11	1.3	1.1–3.1	51, 164	194–340	11–28
Resin composites, indirect comp (20)	16–94 (27) 16–21	0.8–1.2	1.0–2.3	60–200 77–150	320–400 136–500	2–20 (34) 3–22
Glass ionomers	10.2–11.4	0.4–0.8 (35)	0.4–1.0	40–50 (36)	60–300	15–20
Resin-modified glass ionomers		40–124 (37)	0.3–1.5 (38)	20–70		3–5

* May be 3- or 4-point bending, or biaxial flexural strength tests.
Source: From reference (39), Chapter on Crystallography and Engineering Properties of Ceramics, or (7, 40) unless noted.

among the cited testers, hence the range. The lack of durability (high solubility) of the silicate restoratives caused their replacement despite their fluoride release and their thermal expansion and elasticity similarities to dentin. The GIs are not as strong as dentin or enamel but have a thermal expansion similar to teeth and the stiffness of dentin. The composites have compressive strengths in the range of enamel and dentin and are as stiff as dentin but not enamel and have higher thermal expansion than teeth. The resin composites are the most commonly used restoratives, with an abundance of brands and formula variations. The elastic moduli of direct restoratives are similar to dentin but lower than enamel. None of these restorative materials have hardness like materials in Chapter 10, and their fracture toughness is low.

Sometimes a tooth has suffered severe trauma, repeated direct treatments, or endodontic interventions that necessitate more than a direct restorative filling. The next chapter describes ceramics that have been used to fulfill the needs for crowns and bridges that are cemented onto teeth, which are called fixed prosthodontics, or indirect restorations.

Ceramics in Chapter 9

The following ceramics and other inorganic materials were mentioned in this chapter:

- alumina
- aluminum phosphate
- aluminum sulfate (alum)
- aluminum phosphate
- baria
- ß-quartz
- ß-eucryptite
- ß-spodumene
- beryllia
- boron oxide
- calcia
- calcium sulfate and its hydrates
- calcium carbonate
- calcium chloride
- calcium fluoride
- ceria
- cryolite
- diamond
- ferric sulfate
- fluoroapatite
- gadolinia
- gallium nitride
- hafnia
- hydroxyapatite
- iodonium salts
- iron oxide, iron hydroxide
- keatite
- lanthana
- leucite
- lithia
- magnesia
- magnesium chloride
- magnesium phosphate
- nickel oxide
- niobia

- phosphoric acid
- potassium sulfate
- scandia
- silica: fumed, cristobalite, diatomaceous earth, quartz
  - fluoroaluminosilicate glass
  - fluoro-boro-strontio-aluminosilicate glass
  - C, E, and S2 commercial glasses
- silicon carbide
- sodium fluoride
- strontia
- tantalite
- tin oxide
- titania
- yttria
- yttrium fluoride
- ytterbium fluoride
- zeolite
- zinc acetate
- zinc oxide
- zinc phosphate
- zirconia

References

1 Wilson, A.D. and Batchelor, R.F. (1967). Dental silicate cements. I. The chemistry of erosion. *J Dent Res* 46 (5): 1075–1085.
2 Teimoory, F.S., Rezaie, H.R., Yekta, B.E. et al. (2024). Enhancing mechanical strength of Sr-based oxyfluoride glasses in glass ionomer cement through phase separation. *Ceram Int* 50 (14): 24970–24978.
3 O'Brien, W.J. (2008). *Dental materials and their selection*, 4the, 425. Hanover Park, IL: Quintessence Pub. Co.
4 Pulver, J.C. and Rossington, D.R. (1970). Solubility of a silicate cement. *J Dent Res* 49 (6) Suppl: 1530–1536.
5 Smith, D.C. (1968). A new dental cement. *Br Dent J* 124 (9): 381–384.
6 Bowen, R. (1956). Use of epoxy resins in restorative Materials. *J Dent Res* 35 (3): 360–369.
7 Bayne, S.C. (2013). Beginnings of the dental composite revolution. *J Am Dent Assoc* 144 (8): 880–884.
8 Ferracane, J.L. (2024). A historical perspective on dental composite restorative materials. *J Funct Biomater* 15 (7): 1–13.

9 Van Landuyt, K.L., Snauwaert, J., De Munck, J. et al. (2007). Systematic review of the chemical composition of contemporary dental adhesives. *Biomaterials* 28 (26): 3757–3785.

10 Mitra, S.B. (2012). Nanoparticles for dental materials. In: *Emerging nanotechnologies in dentistry* (ed. K. Subramani and W. Ahmed), 15–33. William Andrew.

11 Mitra, S.B., Wu, D., and Holmes, B.N. (2003). An application of nanotechnology in advanced dental materials. *J Am Dent Assoc* 134 (10): 1382–1390.

12 Petersen, R.C., Reddy, M.S., and Liu, P.-R. (2018). Fiber-reinforced composites: a breakthrough in practical clinical applications with advanced wear resistance for dental materials. *EC Dent Sci* 17 (5): 430–459.

13 Garoushi, S., Vallittu, P., and Lassila, L. (2022). Development and characterization of ion-releasing fiber-reinforced flowable composite. *Dent Mater*: official publication of the Academy of Dental Materials 38 (10): 1598–1609.

14 Alshabib, A., Silikas, N., and Watts, D.C. (2024). Properties of model E-glass fiber composites with varying matrix monomer ratios. *Dent Mater*: official publication of the Academy of Dental Materials 40 (3): 441–450.

15 Albergaria, L.S., Scotti, C.K., Mondelli, R.F.L. et al. (2023). Effect of nanofibers as reinforcement on resin-based dental materials: A systematic review of in vitro studies. *Jpn Dent Sci Rev* 59: 239–252.

16 Buonocore, M. (1955). A simple method of increasing the adhesion of acrylic filling materials to enamel surfaces. *J Dent Res* 34 (12): 849–853.

17 Perdigao, J., Araujo, E., Ramos, R.Q. et al. (2021). Adhesive dentistry: current concepts and clinical considerations. *J Esthet Restor Dent*: official publication of the American Academy of Esthetic Dentistry [et al] 33 (1): 51–68.

18 Aggarwal, N., Jain, A., Gupta, H. et al. (2019). The comparative evaluation of depth of cure of bulk-fill composites – an in vitro study. *J Conserv Dent* 22 (4): 371–375.

19 Lima, R.B.W., Troconis, C.C.M., Moreno, M.B.P. et al. (2018). Depth of cure of bulk fill resin composites: a systematic review. *J Esthet Restor Dent* 30 (6): 492–501.

20 Nandini, S. (2010). Indirect resin composites. *J Conserv Dent* 13 (4): 184–194.

21 Miara, P. (1998). Aesthetic guidelines for second-generation indirect inlay and onlay composite restorations. *Pract Periodontics Aesthet Dent* 10 (4): 423–431.

22 Federlin, M., Thonemann, B., and Schmalz, G. (2000). Inserts – megafillers in composite restorations: a literature review. *Clin Oral Investig* 4: 1–8.

23 Zhang, Y.R., Du, W., Zhou, X.D., and Yu, H.Y. (2014). Review of research on the mechanical properties of the human tooth. *Int J Oral Sci* 6 (2): 61–69.

24 Chun, K., Choi, H., and Lee, J. (2014). Comparison of mechanical property and role between enamel and dentin in the human teeth. *J Dent Biomech* 5: 1–7.

25 Bechtle, S., Ozcoban, H., Lilleodden, E.T. et al. (2012). Hierarchical flexural strength of enamel: transition from brittle to damage-tolerant behaviour. *J R Soc Interface* 9: 1265–1274.

26 Banks, R.G. (1990). Conservative posterior ceramic restorations: a literature review. *J Prosth Dent* 63 (6): 619–626.
27 Fei, X., Li, Y., Zhang, Q. et al. (2024). Novel pit and fissure sealant with nano-CaF(2) and antibacterial monomer: fluoride recharge, microleakage, sealing ability and cytotoxicity. *Dent Mater J* 43 (3): 1–13.
28 Stifler, C.A., Jakes, J.E., North, J.D. et al. (2021). Crystal misorientation correlates with hardness in tooth enamels. *Acta Biomater* 120: 124–134.
29 Ismail, H.S., Morrow, B.R., Ali, A.I. et al. (2024). Effect of different storage media on elemental analysis and microhardness of cervical cavity margins restored with a bioactive material. *Restor Dent Endod* 49 (1): 1–16.
30 Arola, D.D., Gao, S., Zhang, H., and Masri, R. (2017). The tooth: its structure and properties. *Dent Clin N Am* 61 (4): 651–668.
31 Cui, B., Li, J., Wang, H. et al. (2017). Mechanical properties of polymer-infiltrated-ceramic (sodium aluminum silicate) composites for dental restoration. *J Dent* 62: 91–97.
32 Iwamoto, N. and Ruse, N.D. (2003). Fracture toughness of human dentin. *J Biomed Mater Res A* 66 (3): 507–512.
33 Chen, Y., Maghami, E., Bai, X. et al. (2023). Which dentine analogue material can replace human dentine for crown fatigue test? *Dent Mater*: official publication of the Academy of Dental Materials 39 (1): 86–100.
34 Cho, K., Rajan, G., Farrar, P. et al. (2022). Dental resin composites: a review on materials to product realizations. *Compos Part B* 230: 1–22.
35 Bala, O., Arisu, H.D., Yikilgan, I. et al. (2012). Evaluation of surface roughness and hardness of different glass ionomer cements. *Eur J Dent* 6 (1): 79–86.
36 Lohbauer, U. (2009). Dental glass ionomer cements as permanent filling materials? – properties, limitations and future trends. *Materials* 3 (1): 76–96.
37 Osiewicz, M.A., Werner, A., Roeters, F.J.M., and Kleverlaan, C.J. (2022). Wear of bulk-fill resin composites. *Dent Mater*: official publication of the Academy of Dental Materials 38 (3): 549–553.
38 Daabash, R., Alshabib, A., Alqahtani, M.Q. et al. (2022). Ion releasing direct restorative materials: key mechanical properties and wear. *Dent Mater*: official publication of the Academy of Dental Materials 38 (12): 1866–1877.
39 Gauthier, M.M. (ed.) (1995). Crystallography and engineering properties of ceramics. In: *Engineered materials handbook desk edition*, 691–1188. ASM International.
40 Bowen, R.L. (1963). Properties of a silica-reinforced polymer for dental restorations. *J Amer Dent Assoc* 66 (1): 57–64.
41 El Wakeel, A.M., Elkassas, D.W., Yousry, M.M. (2015). Bonding of contemporary glass ionomer cements to different tooth substrates; microshear bond strength and scanning electron microscope study. *Eur J Dent* 9 (2): 176–82.

10

Indirect Ceramic Restorations

Indirect restorations are made in a dental laboratory and cemented onto teeth by the dentist. Figure 3.2b shows examples of the shapes of the indirect dental restorations, which are also known as fixed prosthodontics. Crowns, bridges, inlays, onlays, and veneers are indirect restorations.

Crowns, colloquially known as caps, are prescribed by dentists to protect the integrity of a tooth compromised by decay or breakage. Crowns cover teeth that have missing coronal anatomy, have recurrent caries, one or more fillings, or have had a recent root canal treatment; crowns are also needed over a dental implant. A prescription means the dentist has "prepared" – shaped the tooth or teeth – for a fixed prosthodontic device. The impression of the preparation, physical or electronic, is conveyed to a dental laboratory to custom-make a device that is later cemented by the dentist onto the patient's teeth. The methods of duplicating the tooth preparation via an impression to create the precise shape of the indirect restorative are in Chapter 14, and the cements for adhesion of indirect restorations are described in Chapter 11. Pediatric dentists also place crowns over primary teeth that are so badly decayed that a filling (direct restoration) is insufficient protection, particularly while the child's jaw is growing and developing, and the primary tooth should preferably not be extracted. These pediatric crowns are available in various sizes but are not custom-made; no impression or dental laboratory is needed.

Bridges are needed to span the space where a tooth has been extracted; a bridge is anchored (cemented) on the adjacent teeth via abutment crowns. Between the two abutment crowns are pontics that have the form of the missing tooth's crown. Bridges can span several missing teeth, depending on the strength of the material used. Inlays and onlays are made when only the occlusal surface needs covering, but these are less common in modern dentistry. Veneers are thin ceramic "shells" that are cemented over the facial surface of anterior teeth, usually for esthetic

Ceramics in Dentistry: Materials, Manufacturing, and Clinical Applications,
First Edition. Carolyn M. Primus.

reasons such as loss of incisal anatomy, or for improving alignment and occlusion or masking discoloration. Veneer has another meaning in European dentistry: it describes the coating on a metal substructure.

The dentist and especially the dental laboratory technician require skills to design the shape of the restoration, considering the specifics of the patient's occlusion and teeth alignment, as well as the potential forces of tooth-to-tooth contact during eating, bruxing, and parafunctional habits of the patient. Proper restorative design minimizes cracks and abrasion of the opposing teeth or the restoration to ensure the device is long-lasting. In addition, the desired shade must be communicated to the dental technician to create. All these factors influence the choice of the indirect restorative material.

Ceramic substances were always recognized to have the esthetic potential to serve as beautiful, indirect dental materials, but their realization required the confluence of new technologies during the Industrial Revolution. The development of indirect ceramic restorations lagged that of denture teeth (Chapter 15) because in the 1800s dentists lacked a good drill for shaping teeth for crowns, a precise impression material, a suitable ceramic to create strong esthetic crowns, a good porcelain enamel for precious metals, a reliable cement, a small enough furnace for easy firing of tooth-sized ceramic crowns, and the techniques for forming custom, indirect, ceramic restorations. Unique formulas and manufacturing methods were invented to create the durable, tooth-imitative, ceramic restorations described herein.

Inventors have developed many ceramic materials for fixed prosthodontics having these beneficial traits: inherent biocompatibility; low thermal conductivity to protect the pulp; chemical durability for acidic diets; good strength for chewing; wear resistance from eating or bruxing; and the ability to be precisely custom-fabricated by dental lab technicians with esthetics that blend with the remaining teeth. These dental ceramics are categorized in ISO 6872/ADA 69 (Dental Ceramics). Type 1 includes powders, pastes, or aerosol sprays, and Type 2 is all other ceramics, such as ceramic ingots for hot pressing or machining. Separately, the standard lists six classes of dental ceramics distinguished by their indications; see Table 10.1 for the descriptions and minimum flexural strength requirements, from 50 to 800 MPa. Three methods are allowed in this standard for flexural strength tests: three- or four-point bending, and biaxial (piston on three balls). Oddly, the minimum strengths are the same for all methods, even though they are known to yield different values. Indirect ceramic restorations that fall under ISO 6872 have been made of porcelain, porcelain fused over a metal substructure, glass-ceramics, polycrystalline ceramic materials (alumina, magnesia, and zirconia), and sometimes polymer-infused.

Ceramic indirect restorations are not without failures. Ceramic crowns have been known to fracture from flaws initiated on the intaglio. Some fractures occur

Table 10.1 ISO 6872 classes of dental ceramics.

Class	Clinical indications	Examples	Minimum flexural strength (MPa)
1	a) Coverage of a metal or a ceramic substructure b) Single-unit anterior prostheses, veneers, inlays, or onlays	Porcelain enamel on metals or ceramic copings Porcelain	50
2	a) Adhesively cemented, single-unit, anterior or posterior all-ceramic b) Adhesively cemented, single-unit, anterior or posterior enameled ceramic	High-leucite porcelains or lithium disilicate	100
3	a) Up to 3-unit prostheses (not molar) b) Up to 3-unit prostheses (not molars), or etching the metal. These methods fully enamelled adhesively or non-adhesively cemented	Lithium disilicate	300
4	Substructure for 3-unit restoration with molars posterior prostheses, partially or fully covered	Very high alumina, glass-infiltrated alumina, veneered lithium disilicate, zirconia	500
5	Substructure for prostheses involving four or more units	Zirconia	800

soon after seating of the restoration on the tooth; later fractures are attributed to fatigue. High hoop stresses may cause fracture of ceramic crowns if an expansive cement has been used to affix a crown or onlay. Chipping may occur when the thermal expansion mismatch is too large between porcelain coating and material. Stresses induced by the rapid cooling of zirconia have caused its porcelain to chip. For all-ceramic bridges, e.g., zirconia bridges, the unsupported joints between teeth are a common source for fracture, caused by the repeated flexure of the pontics from mastication or bruxing. The connections between the abutments and pontics need to be large enough in cross-section to support the forces but small enough to create the anatomical esthetics and allow flossing.

Indirect restorations require strength, which has been achieved in ceramic restoration by (1) using metal reinforcement (substructures for enameling);

(2) dispersing crystals in glasses (porcelains), including "whiskers" (filamentary, single crystals, known for having very high tensile strength); (3) high percentage of crystals in a glass (glass-ceramics); (4) ion exchange on the surface of a glass (surface toughening); and (5) use of low-porosity crystalline ceramics without an interstitial glass phase (alumina and zirconia). The following sections are in historical order, but also in order of increasing strength.

Porcelain enamel on dental alloys (porcelain-fused-to-metal [PFM]) has been very successful in creating beautiful, durable, indirect restorations since the 1950s, as discussed below. PFMs are an important option for longer span bridges and when the vertical separation of the maxillary and mandibular teeth is limited; all-ceramic crowns and bridges require greater thickness and more tooth removal. Metal substructures provide strength for long-span bridges and for patients with a severe bruxing habit. Various ceramic coping materials have been used, but currently, dental laboratories primarily make crowns and bridges out of zirconia and lithium disilicate; PFM accounts for only about 10% of today's indirect restorations.

Porcelains

Porcelain items contain primarily glass with embedded crystals. Traditionally, porcelain was formed from minerals: sodium feldspar, quartz, and kaolin. For medical devices today, ceramics, including porcelains or dental glasses, are created from high-purity oxides or purified minerals to produce specialized glass formulas. Porcelain has greater strength, transparency, and whiteness than earthenware or stoneware pottery; it may be glazed and "decorated."

Porcelains have been classified by their required firing temperatures in Table 10.2 based on normal radiant heating, not any special newer sintering technique described in Chapter 7. Any porcelain restoration made in a dental laboratory is formed by heating to fuse glass and crystalline powders. The first porcelain veneers, inlays, and crowns were made in the late 19th and early 20th century by Dr. Charles Land (1), using the same high-fusing porcelain as was being used for artificial teeth for dentures (Chapter 15). Land recognized the benefits of porcelain over amalgam and gold foils for protecting and preserving tooth structure. He evaluated about 12 formulas of porcelain and favored the higher fusing porcelains used for artificial denture teeth, adding ceramic pigments to enable crowns to match adjacent teeth. Land's crowns were fashioned by making a platinum or platinum–iridium foil "impression"; he allowed the foil to remain under some inlays to improve the conformity of the restoration in the cavity and protect its margins. He fired the porcelain in a gas-fired furnace in air

Table 10.2 Dental porcelain firing ranges.

Designation	Firing temperature range (°C)	Uses
High	1200–1400	Alumina coping, denture teeth
Medium	1050–1200	Dental alloy enameling, porcelain veneers or inlays
Low	850–1050	Dental alloy enameling on lower melting dental alloy, porcelain veneers

(using two firing cycles) and achieved a high gloss; his esthetic crowns were beneficial for the prevention of decay and were durable. Porcelain inlays were not as successful as desired because of fractures – the weakness of the porcelain, imperfect fit, and lack of resilient cements; they were less successful than gold inlays that more intimately conformed to the tooth.

Land also described "enameled metal caps" – crowns with high-fusing porcelain over platinum/iridium foil. He had clever methods to improve retention of the foil, which had a thermal mismatch to the porcelain. He used platinum pins embedded in the porcelain, or notches or pockets formed in the foil; a lower-fusing porcelain was fired first, to lock the ceramic layer over and onto the metal. Later developments included platinum foil electroplated with tin to create a tin oxide surface for chemical bonding to a high-fusing porcelain, even those with alumina crystals. Porcelain crowns have been manufactured on other metal foils, electroplated gold, or burnished and sintered gold powder; such metal layers were approximately 0.1 mm thick.

Land performed extensive rehabilitations, placing crowns on anterior and posterior teeth of adults and young adults, and reported that the restorations lasted at least 20 years. Dr. Land is also known for other dental innovations in medicaments and cements and had patents in the United States and Canada. He designed crowns to improve the shape of "peg" (undersized) lateral anterior teeth, invented an improved cementing method to overcome the "washout" or erosion of zinc phosphate cement (Chapter 11), and was aware of the importance of vital pulp preservation (Chapter 8).

Prior to the 1950s, dental porcelains were fired in air in small kilns designed for dental laboratories, but that has been superseded by low vacuum-firing (minus 29 in. of Hg, which is equal to 10 Torr or 1 kPa) kilns. Vacuum-firing was a huge advancement for porcelains for indirect dental restorations and the ceramic artificial teeth in Chapter 15 because it reduced the number of pores in porcelain, created better esthetics (less opaque), and increased the porcelain's strength. Finer particles were suitable for vacuum-firing because the pores were more readily removed during vacuum firing, unlike firing fine particles in air. The exception to vacuum-firing in a dental laboratory is the final firing step with a thin outer glaze (glass coating), which is conducted at atmospheric pressure. Glazing – and polishing – is performed to create a smooth surface, which strengthens ceramics, reflects light, is biomimetic to the surface of tooth enamel, and reduces the tendency to accumulate dental plaque.

All-porcelain restorations are not common now, except as veneers, but porcelain coatings are used on ceramic and metal "copings" cores. Ceramic coping materials – glass-bonded alumina, high-purity alumina, magnesia, lithium disilicate, and zirconia – each require its own porcelain coating to match its thermal expansion. What follows is a synopsis of the evolution of ceramic crowns after Dr. Land, beginning with glass-bonded alumina.

Alumina Coping Restorations

The first "alumina porcelains" were made by combining powders of clay, feldspar, and flint; this means the starting powders contained hydrous aluminosilicates, with sodium, calcium, or potassium aluminosilicates, and silica, respectively. Small amounts of ceramic pigment powders (e.g., iron oxide, manganese oxide, and chromium oxides) were blended with the powder to facilitate shade matching to the surrounding teeth after firing. This technique required a model of the prepared tooth that was created from an impression (Chapter 14). The alumina porcelain powders were mixed with water and shaped on the model of the prepared tooth to create the tooth form, usually a crown. Hand tools or brushes were used for placement, and then the porcelain was "condensed" to remove moisture. The condensation step relied on a skilled dental artisan who gently vibrating and blotting the porcelain on the model to remove the water but maintain the anatomical shape of the tooth with the ceramic powder. These skills are also used in making PFM crowns and bridges, described later. The porcelain was then dried and fired in air in an oven at temperatures less than 1200 °C. Metal foils were used to support the porcelain during firing, which helped confine the shrinkage to the thickness of the porcelain so the crown would fit the original, prepared tooth. Later, "refractory die" materials were developed (Chapter 18) that supported the porcelain during firing, which also limited the shrinkage to create a good fit. The clay, feldspar, and silica powders would react during firing and form crystals, including alumina, which strengthened the porcelain restoratives. Multiple layers and repeated firings were usually needed to obtain the desired shape and shade (color). Later developments eliminated the minerals and used pre-fired glasses and dispersed alumina crystals. The pre-made aluminous porcelain was ground into powder that could be fired on a foil.

The alumina porcelains evolved into all-ceramic crowns called "jacket" crowns, consisting of a glass-bonded alumina coping that was veneered, by firing, with a lower melting, more transparent porcelain, having a thermal expansion to the underlying coping. Jacket crowns were just strong enough for the anterior teeth, and only when the occlusal clearance was greater than 0.8 mm. They were unsuitable for the teeth with greater biting force, such as molars. It's a mystery why the jacket crowns with alumina were less successful than Land had claimed, but the microstructures and compositions have not been compared.

Stronger ceramic copings were developed containing more (~50%) and finer alumina particles. Incorporating more alumina required a higher firing temperature and made the coping more opaque. An esthetic compromise used larger alumina particles (about 25 μm) blended with a finer glass. Next, to increase the alumina but keep a firing temperature as low as possible, alumina was pre-sintered with a glass frit and then ground into a powder. This intermediate powder was blended with another glass for making a coping. The resulting porcelain, having 50% or more alumina, had fewer pores than just blending 50% alumina and glass powders. This concept of pre-firing an intermediate powder combination and adding a third powder is often repeated in dental porcelains or other ceramic items. Alumina whiskers – needle-like single crystals – have also been blended with glasses to strengthen alumina-based porcelains, but these whisker-reinforced porcelains have not been commercialized. These higher alumina coping required a top layer of translucent porcelain for esthetics.

Higher strength alumina with less glass was developed industrially after World War II. Finer powders and less glass created finer alumina grains after firing that had a smaller aspect ratio (length to width) and were less-needle-like; this reduced the stress created by the anisotropic thermal expansion of hexagonal alpha-alumina. In the 1970s, the alumina content of dental jacket crowns was increased to about 75% (2). These higher-alumina crowns were formed and fired into copings upon which thermal expansion "matching" porcelains were fired. Good contact (low surface tension for "wetting") between the porcelain and coping was achieved at higher temperatures. Later, hot-pressing was used to make the alumina porcelain copings with fewer pores. Making higher-alumina crowns required a more expensive platinum-wound electric furnace to achieve the firing temperature – higher than 1200 °C, the maximum achievable in a conventional Kanthal® wire oven. Metal heating wires, either the FeCrAl alloy or platinum, are wound in the spiral raceways of a cylindrical aluminosilicate ceramic tube. The metal wires are electrically heated and they radiate heat inward; the wires and oven chamber are insulated with a fibrous ceramic "blanket."

Very high purity alumina powder, with minimal silica and about 0.5% magnesia (MgO), was developed; when sintered, the alumina had higher fracture toughness and strength compared to the earlier glass-bonded alumina materials and was much less opaque, having few pores and fine grains. Lucalox® high-purity alumina was used as the envelope for high-pressure, sodium-vapor streetlights (3). Based on these advances with alumina, several techniques were commercialized to make high-purity alumina (>99%) dental crowns in the 1990s.

High-purity alumina crowns have been made by CAD-CAM techniques. The software was used to design oversized alumina crowns that were machined from a dry-pressed and partially sintered alumina. The oversized alumina crowns were sintered at about 1550 °C for one hour (4), during which the alumina would shrink to the desired size crown with low porosity for good strength and appearance. At first, the design of the crowns had to be transmitted digitally to manufacturer who machined and sintered the crowns for the dental laboratory. Later, the laboratories could buy the alumina and machine it themselves because the Procera® alumina had reproducible shrinkage to create a good fit of the crowns after sintering. These fired alumina crowns had a small grain size (~4 µm) and higher strength (up to 700 MPa in flexure (5)) than earlier alumina crowns because glass was not present. See Figure 10.1 showing the Procera microstructure. It was not as transparent as Lucalox but was suitable for dental crowns. This microstructure, and other dense ceramic microstructures in later photos, illustrates the polygonal patterns of sintered grains (7). Porcelain was fired on the exterior of the crown to finish the esthetic appearance.

"Non-Shrinking" Alumina Crowns

A "non-shrinking" method of making alumina copings for crowns was developed by Coors Porcelain Company (US Pats. 4,265,669 and 4,585,417) and marketed by Johnson & Johnson Company as Cerestore material (8). Its compressive strength

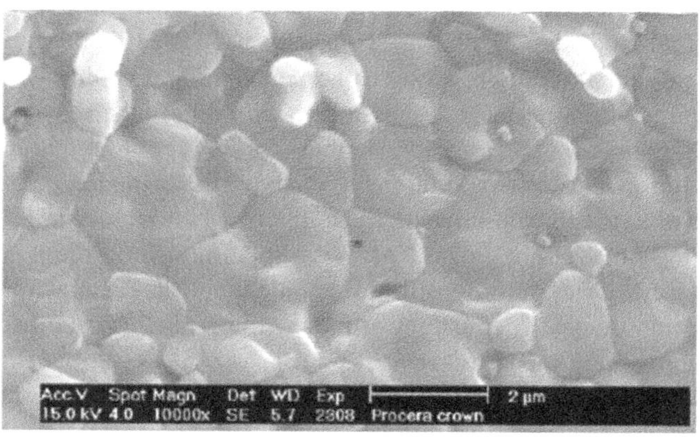

Figure 10.1 Microstructure of etched Procera high-alumina crown material (6) / American Association for Science and Technology.

was reported as about 400 MPa and a flexural strength of about 170 MPa. The Cerestore coping material primarily contained 60% alumina, with 9% MgO, 13% of a high baria glass, and 4% kaolin clay; about 43% of the alumina in Cerestore was a coarse alumina (<100 µm) powder. These ceramic components were supplemented with some organic materials: 12% silicone and 2% wax compound. The minor clay and binder additions contributed to the moldability of the Cerestore material during the pressing step, below.

This dental laboratory process started by forming the desired crown shape in wax on a unique epoxy die material. A butt or chamfer design (not tapered) was required for the margins. The die and coping were "invested" (completely cast in) in dental stone (plaster). The dental stone was boiled, which removed the wax. Next, the Cerestore material, available as a disc, was warmed to 160 °C and uniaxially pressed into the plaster mold to make a "green" unfired (coping), using special equipment provided with the system. The plaster mold was cooled and removed, leaving the epoxy die and the "green" Cerestore material. The die, with the overlying Cerestore material, was fired in air in a programmed Cerestore furnace; the firing cycle required about 10 hours, including a hold at 500 °C (for wax and silicone decomposition), and a peak temperature of about 1300 °C.

During firing, the magnesia component reacted with the finer alumina particles, forming spinel crystals ($MgO.Al_2O_3$) and expanding about 8% in volume (2.4% linear). The spinel crystals were partially dissolved in the high-baria glass. Also, the glass component precipitated some crystals of barium osumilite ($BaMg_2Al_3[Si_9Al_3O_{30}]$), a rare mineral with a lower thermal expansion coefficient than alumina or spinel. The fired Cerestore copings contained primarily alumina and spinel, with a lesser amount (<10%) of the osumilite and glass. The multiphase microstructure (8) included glass, interspersed with alumina grains up to about 100 µm and some pores. Energy-dispersive x-ray analysis confirmed the presence of silica, baria, and calcia (9).

The non-shrinking aspect of Cerestore was cleverly created by the inclusion of the silicone resin (binder), which decomposed during the firing of the Cerestore material, leaving residual silica. This residual silica became incorporated into the glass phase of Cerestore to obviate some of the shrinkage that would have occurred had non-silicone organic binders been used that do not leave an inorganic residue.

The Cerestore crowns were considered to have a good fit and esthetics. Four shades of the coping materials were available, but the system included a variety of accessory porcelains to finalize the esthetic match to adjacent teeth; these porcelains had a thermal expansion equal to the fired coping material (~5.6 ppm/K). Unfortunately, the Cerestore crowns had an unacceptably high fracture rate (~18% over 4 years) (10). The patent acknowledged the presence of pores, which contributed to Cerestore fractures. Zinc phosphate cement (Chapter 11) was used to affix the Cerestore crowns to teeth; resin cements were not common at that time. As with the Dicor glass-ceramic crowns described later, a contemporary resin cement would have reduced Cerestore fractures by providing better support and greater flexibility (elasticity) of the resin cement to reduce interfacial strain at the tooth surface. The Cerestore product was discontinued.

Porcelain-Fused-to Metal

Precious metal alloys of gold, platinum, palladium, ruthenium, rhodium, iridium, and osmium, frequently including silver and other minor metals, have been used in dentistry for eons for their lack of corrosion and biocompatibility. These metal alloys are very desirable for dental use because many are strong, malleable, durable, corrosion resistant (biocompatible), and non-abrasive. The alloys can be melted with an oxy-acetylene torch for casting via the lost-wax technique. Certain precious alloys are used for all-metal (no porcelain) restorations. Other alloy formulas, with higher melting ranges, were developed so that porcelain enameling at about 900° could be performed. Base alloys of nickel-chrome and cobalt-chrome are also used for lower-cost.

Dozens of noble, semi-precious, and base metal alloys are available worldwide. The alloys vary in their castability, hardness, percent elongation, oxide color, resistance to discoloration of porcelain, yield and tensile strengths, and cost. Every alloy has its advantages and disadvantages (i.e., high-cost platinum versus the low-cost nickel-chrome (NiCr) alloys); notably, the NiCr alloys may cause a nickel allergic reaction at the gum line and may contain beryllium, which has its own toxicity issues. The metal alloys used for fixed and removable restorations (Chapters 10 and 15) are standardized in ISO 22674 and ADA 134 – Metallic Materials for Fixed and Removable Restorations and Appliances – having requirements and test methods for metals with or without a ceramic coating.

Porcelain enamel on such metals was an early idea to make fixed prosthodontics, but large differences in thermal expansion plagued the early dental enameling of these metals. The thermal expansions of the available porcelains were too low, and the porcelain cracked and spalled from the metals. Most glasses and ceramics have a thermal expansion greater than zero but less than about 8 ppm/K, significantly lower than the precious metal dental alloys (~13–15 ppm/K); therefore, the “conventional” glasses and porcelains were unsuitable for enameling. The chemically durable, borosilicate glasses were out of the question, because these glasses do not expand when heated (zero coefficient of thermal expansion). Their low expansion is what makes the Pyrex® formula (also known as Duran®) – 80.6% SiO_2, 12.6% B_2O_3, 4.2% Na_2O, 2.2% Al_2O_3, 0.1% CaO, 0.1% Cl, 0.05% MgO, and 0.04% Fe_2O_3 – unsuitable for metal enameling but excellent for cookware and labware. A new porcelain was needed for enameling of the precious metal alloys to create chemically durable, porcelain coatings on metal crown and bridge copings. Such a porcelain needed to have a firing temperature below the melting point of the candidate alloys to avoid distortion of the metal but have a thermal expansion similar to the alloys.

Serendipitously, Dr. Abraham Weinstein, a dentist, discovered and patented a high-expansion porcelain in the 1950s, based on potassium feldspar (US Pats. 3,052,982 and 3,052,983), which began the successful era of "feldspathic" porcelain used for enameling dental metals. He used potassium feldspar mineral ($KAlSi_3O_8$), which is unique because when it incongruently melts above 1100 °C, the feldspar crystals decompose and precipitate leucite ($KAlSi_2O_6$) crystals in a silicate glass containing potassia and alumina. That is, the crystalline feldspar mineral is transformed into a glass-ceramic, a glass matrix with embedded crystals of leucite. Figure 10.2 shows the binary phase diagrams illustrating the equilibrium phases of leucite, potassium feldspar, and silica. The fortuitous finding was that the leucite crystals have a high thermal expansion, about 20–25 ppm/K, and the glass surrounding the crystals has a lower expansion; together, the frit (porcelain powder) made from the potassium feldspar has an expansion of about 18 ppm/K.

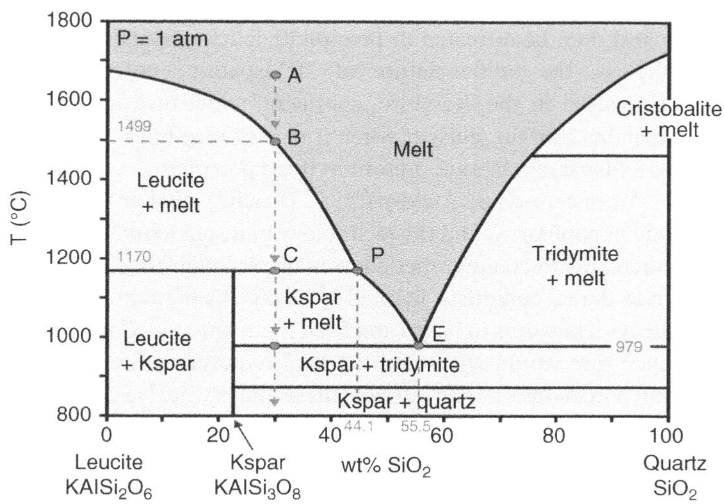

Figure 10.2 Binary phase diagram depicting phase relations of leucite, potassium feldspar (Kspar), and silica crystals (cristobalite, tridymite, and quartz). At temperature A, potassium feldspar is molten; at temperature B, leucite crystals will form in the molten, glassy material and will increase in amount to temperature C. Below temperature C, the feldspar crystals could precipitate from the leucite and glass; however, if the material is quenched from temperature higher than 1170 °C, leucite crystals and glass will be retained. P is the peritectic temperature of incongruent melting of potassium feldspar; E is the eutectic temperature for silica crystals and potassium feldspar.

Weinstein noted that lithium or potassium carbonate were useful for making the higher thermal expansion frit from the potassium feldspar, probably by accelerating the incongruent melting reaction to form leucite. Weinstein never mentioned "leucite," but he did describe how to create dental porcelains by combining the heat-treated feldspar powder with other frits (powdered glasses) to manufacture a dental porcelain with a suitable high thermal expansion for the precious metal alloys. These alloys and the leucite dental porcelain changed mid-20th century dentistry. Porcelain enameled crowns or bridges, also known as porcelain-fused-to-metal (PFM) indirect restorations, combine the strength of the metal substructure that functions as a strong foundation, stronger than alumina copings.

Leucite crystals had been identified in the 1800s in igneous minerals but were not recognized for their thermal expansion. The unique character of leucite is appreciated when compared to the other common feldspar minerals, anorthite or albite (Ca and Na feldspars, $CaAl_2Si_2O_8$ and $NaAlSi_3O_8$); they do not form a similar high expansion phase akin to leucite. Other feldspar phases exist, such as nepheline syenite and sanidine, but they have low thermal expansion, about 4 ppm/K, emphasizing the inventive success of using potassium feldspar. Later, inventors recognized that potassium feldspar was not necessary as a starting material; a glass could be melted having the approximate composition of potassium feldspar and then heat-treated to precipitate leucite crystals (US Pat. 4,455,383). Nevertheless, the nomenclature of "feldspathic" porcelain has persisted and been misused in the literature, confusing many researchers into thinking dental porcelains contain feldspar when it may or may not have been a raw material and no feldspar crystals are present in these porcelains.

The "Ceramco" (Weinstein-type) "feldspathic" (leucite) dental porcelain enamels quickly grew in popularity, and the technology matured to include many other specialized porcelains to create esthetic layers of porcelain fired on metal. Technicians, known as dental ceramists, learned special skills to manually apply combinations of porcelain powders in layers and fired them onto metal substrates. Alloys were developed that would withstand the heat required to fire (enamel) low-to-medium firing porcelains on their surface; these alloys were based on gold, palladium, platinum, and later nickel-chrome to be specifically thermally compatible with the Ceramco porcelain.

Dental porcelain has been manufactured from mining high potassium feldspar rock, which has few accessory minerals like other feldspar or mica. The rock is crushed and sent through a magnetic separator to remove iron oxide particles that would discolor the porcelain. The crushed feldspar rock, perhaps with some alkaline earth additions, is loaded into refractory ceramic containers (often called "saggers") that can withstand an extended heat treatment above 1150 °C to form leucite-glass from the feldspar. The heating rates, peak temperature, duration, and cooling create a unique percentage and distribution of leucite crystal sizes. If the heat-treated feldspar is cooled too slowly or held for extended times at temperatures just below the incongruent melting temperature, the leucite crystals can transform to monoclinic sanidine feldspar ($K[AlSi_3O_8]$) crystals, having an undesirably lower thermal expansion. As with any high temperature process, the results of the heat treatment depend on the manufacturer's furnace size, its rate of heating, the batch size, the additives, and how the feldspar is packed in the oven. These feldspar heat treatment procedures are proprietary because they create to product advantages, particularly the thermal stability of the leucite porcelain when fired repeatedly on dental alloys. The resulting bolus from each container is usually reheated and then quenched in water to facilitate crushing and grinding it into a powder.

The next step in making dental porcelains is to blend the high-leucite content frit (powder) with other glass powders and pigments having a lower thermal expansion. The other frits are usually made by melting, quenching, drying, and grinding glass powders. As many as eight glasses are combined with the leucite frit, depending on the manufacturer. The non-leucite glass powders usually have fluorescent materials and other qualities and the heterogeneous blend with the leucite frit has an average thermal expansion in the realm of the precious metal alloys, 13–15 ppm/K, depending on the manufacturer. Certain characteristics are imperative for each type of dental porcelain for metal (or ceramic) copings: thermal expansion equal to or slightly lower than the alloy (or ceramic coping), adhesion to the underlying layer, softening temperature below the softening or melting range of a metal or ceramic coping, chemical resistance to the acidic oral environment, surface hardness to resist but not cause abrasion, resistance to heat or thermal shock (such as might be imparted by ice cream followed by hot coffee), tooth-like color, translucency, and fluorescence. Dental porcelains ideally wet (spread) and bond to its substrate during fusion from 800 to 1100 °C. Overall, the dental enamel porcelains contain more than 50% silica with lesser amounts of alumina, potassia, soda, and lithia. Minor amounts of other glass network formers are used and vary with the brand; they include calcia, magnesia, boron oxide, and phosphorous pentoxide. Figure 10.3 shows an example of the leucite porcelain microstructure, showing the dispersion of leucite crystals ($<10\,\mu m$) in a glass matrix.

Dental manufacturers create porcelain "kits" that include multiple shades and assortments of powders to create the most esthetic restorations. The types of porcelains needed in a set of porcelain products are "opaque," "shoulder," "body," and "incisal" (to create the anatomy), "add-on" porcelains for anatomy corrections, plus accessory materials including stain, glaze, and "modifiers" (for color adjustments) porcelain powders. These porcelain groups differ in their firing temperature and opacity.

A porcelain-enameled indirect restoration – either crown or bridge – starts with making a metal substructure, customarily formed via the lost-wax technique. The

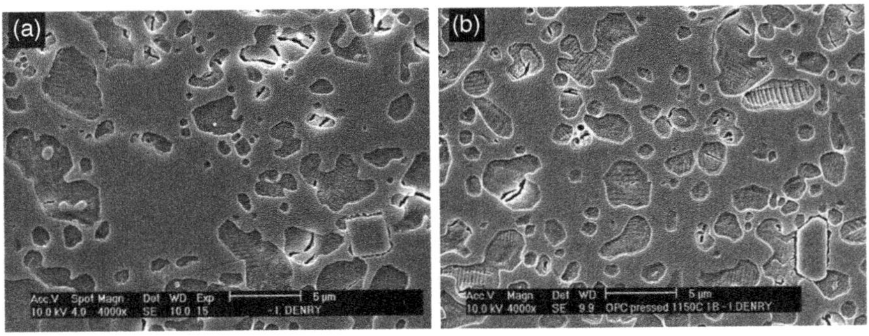

Figure 10.3 Microstructure of HF-etched leucite porcelain for fusing to metals (a) and for hot-pressing (b) from (11) / MDPI / CC BY 3.0, illustrating the greater number of leucite crystals in B.

dental alloys are melted in a ceramic crucible with an oxyacetylene torch, which has a flame temperature of 3480 °C; the molten metal is dispensed using a centrifugal casting machine into a custom, refractory investment mold (ceramic mold, Chapter 18). The cavity of the mold has the desired shape for the metal, crowns, or bridges which had been formed in wax, which was "burned out" of the mold. After the cast metal is cooled, it is "devested" from the refractory. Other specialized methods can be used to form the metal substructures for enameling, such as sintering of metal powders, electroplating, selective laser melting, and milling. Stronger metal alloys are used for multi-unit bridges (spanning several teeth) and for removable partial dentures (Chapter 15). The metal surface that is to be enamel coated is roughened to help with mechanical adhesion by sandblasting. The metal substructures are heated in air to create a thin oxide coating that serves as a transition zone between the metal alloy and the glass, at least one molecule thick for chemical adhesion. Precious metals form a thinner oxide layer than the non-precious metals. Oxide layers on base metal alloys are less adherent than other alloys to the underlying metal although they are adherent to the porcelain. The margins (edges) of metal copings may be festooned with gold by applying a fine gold powder and firing it. The gold powder creates a yellow color at the margin, where the porcelain is thinnest, which adds to esthetics. For tooth preparations with sub-gingival margins, a metal "collar," without porcelain, may be maintained on the crown, because those margins won't be visible.

The dental porcelain enameling steps are performed using a dental furnace, a relatively inexpensive, low-vacuum furnace having a maximum temperature of 1200 °C. These compact, electric dental ovens/kilns have FeCrAl alloy (Kanthal) heating elements surrounded by insulating refractory ceramics. Several crowns or bridges can fit in a compact chamber of less than 20 cm in diameter and about 5 cm high. Usually, the prosthesis is poised for firing on a light-weight honeycomb made of cordierite ($2MgO.2Al_2O_3.5SiO_2$, $Mg_2Al_4Si_5O_{18}$), the same material used in catalytic converters. The cordierite kilnware, commonly with metal pegs stuck in the honeycomb to support the prostheses, is placed on the ceramic platform that is part of the bottom plug of the furnace. The lighter weight of the honeycomb contributes to faster, more uniform heating and cooling with less energy consumption than the older dental kiln-ware made of solid mullite ($3Al_2O_3.2SiO_2$).

Modern dental furnaces are programmable and have mechanisms to automatically lift the platform into the oven (or lower the furnace over the device), start the vacuum, heat at a controlled rate, hold at a peak temperature and cool quickly or gradually; these features are wonderfully convenient for the dental technician. Dental ovens, like all kilns or ovens used for firing and sintering ceramics, have thermocouples for determining the temperature. However, furnace designs – chamber, insulation, power, programming of temperature rise, and thermocouple placements – vary among manufacturers and give differing reports of the temperature. Even with identical external digital readings of temperature, the degrees of firing may vary among dental furnaces, which can be identified by the dental technicians. The ISO 13078-2/ADA 164 standards are used to assess the degree of firing via visual methods for evaluating reproducibility or comparing dental furnaces. The visual assessments are "correctly fired, underfired, or overfired." Underfired dental porcelain has visible porosity, low translucence, indistinct color, milky to gray/white opaque, and a rough, non-lustrous surface. Overfired dental porcelain appears dense and has a high luster, but the edges of a crown are too rounded. Correctly fired porcelain crowns and bridges do not have apparent porosity, the surface is translucent, and the edges of the anatomy are only slightly rounded. The ISO 13078/ADA 163 standards have a test method for the calibration of dental furnaces in the temperature range of 600–1050 °C; ISO 13078-3/ADA 209 is used for calibrating dental furnaces that require higher temperatures, such as sintering zirconia, using a separate thermocouple.

Porcelain enameled crowns and bridges are created by successive firing of a series of porcelains from a manufacturer, each having a thermal expansion suitable for the chosen alloy per ISO 9693 and ADA 38 for metal-ceramic dental restorative systems. The layering of dental porcelain on a metal crown is depicted in cross-section in Figure 10.4. Multiple steps are needed for firing porcelain – drying, preheating (as the restorations are gradually moved near the furnace's entrance), controlled heating, usually at about 10 °C/min in a low vacuum, a brief hold at peak temperature (less than 1 minute), release of the vacuum, and quick removal of the copings from the oven. Rapid cooling contributes to creating a compressive stress on the leucite porcelain enamel, a benefit for strengthening this relatively weak ceramic on the metal. Although rapid cooling is used for dental porcelain on metal, slower cooling is used for porcelain fired on zirconia, as described later.

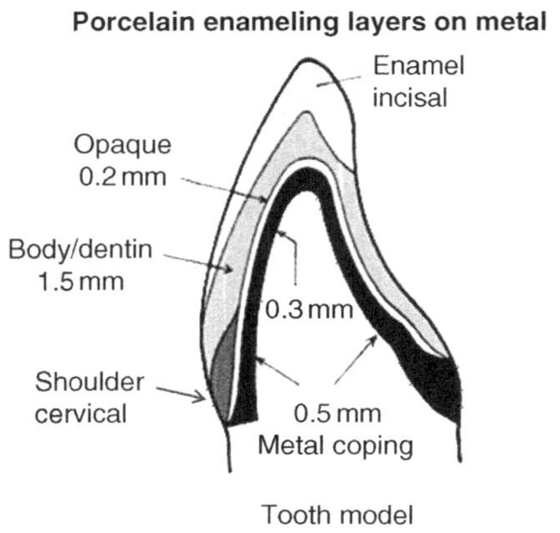

Figure 10.4 Cross-section of the layers of dental leucite porcelain fired with a metal coping and shown on a tooth model.

The first porcelain fired on a metal substructure is always an opaque porcelain (that is, the base coat) to obscure the color of the metal. The opaque porcelains are composed of a leucite frit, other glass powders, and an oxide – as much as 30% of ceria, alumina, titania, or tin oxide; the high percentage of oxide crystals impart the opacity and hiding power in a thin layer without being dissolved in the glass. This base coat has very fine particles, less than 10 μm, so it does not add any anatomical features. Some opaque porcelains are supplied as a powder; others are available as a paste containing the opaque porcelain powder dispersed in an organic liquid such as butylene glycol. The opaque porcelain is applied manually to the metal copings (substructure), such as with a narrow, flat artist's brush to make a thin coating, but spray coating has also been used to apply opaque porcelain powder. The copings with the opaque porcelain are carefully dried to avoid craquelure (a surface network of drying cracks) and then fired to a temperature to soften glass in the porcelain and establish adherence to the metal understructure by bonding to the metal oxide ("scale"). Two thin coatings and two firing steps are usually required to create sufficient coverage, about 100 μm thick.

Next, the anatomical form of the crown and pontics, if present, are created with shoulder (margin), body (dentin), and incisal (enamel) porcelains. The shoulder, body, and porcelains have lower opacity, larger particle sizes, and slightly lower firing temperatures than the opaque porcelain. Generally, these porcelains have a mean size of about 40 μm. Particle packing is a science that porcelain manufacturers have explored to make "condensation" and porcelain "build-up" easier. Bimodal particle fractions may be combined for denser packing, such as combining particles 40–60 μm with others ranging from 10 to 16 μm. Most manufacturers remove the particles coarser than about 75 μm (+170 mesh) and particles finer than 10 μm; this particle size range facilitates the anatomical build-up of porcelain powders, other than the opaque layer, using the condensing technique. Finer particles are omitted because they sinter too quickly and trap tiny bubbles (pores) that create internal reflective interfaces of porcelain with air, making the porcelain appear whiter, opaque, and less tooth-like. Coarse particles are excluded because they do not create a smooth surface.

After the opaque porcelain is fired, a "shoulder" porcelain may be applied and fired at the edges of the copings to further mask the metal at the margin and create a good fit that is maintained during successive firings. The fit of crowns at the margin of the restoration is critical to preventing bacterial invasion underneath and secondary caries, which require new dental interventions. The shoulder porcelains are slightly more opaque and higher fusing than the subsequent body and incisal porcelains, but lower firing than opaque porcelain.

The body and incisal porcelains are fired together because they contain the same percentage of component glass powders; they differ by less than 1% in their pigment content. The body porcelains have slightly more color and opacity than incisal porcelains to create the prescribed shade. Incisal porcelains are placed at the biting edge of the crown. The skilled ceramist technician chooses the combination and placement of the body and incisal porcelains to create the esthetic appearance of natural teeth.

The shoulder, body, and incisal porcelain powders are applied with a spatula or more artistically applied with a moist pointed brush; these powders are mixed with water or a water-based "modeling liquid." Water-based modeling liquids may have surfactants to create a lower surface tension and assist with condensing the porcelain using paper tissues and dry brushes to create a more compact powder before firing. Condensing is akin to slip casting, where a ceramic slurry is thickened (condensed) by water absorption into a plaster mold. Condensing reduces the shrinkage and avoids steam formation during firing, so that the porcelain has fewer pores, although the dental porcelain crowns may contain about 1% pores, preferably tiny. The moist powders are built up oversized because these powders will shrink by about twenty linear percent during firing.

Auxiliary powders may be used with or mixed with the body (dentin) and incisal (enamel) powders to create the best visual match to the surrounding teeth. The auxiliary powders – denoted as modifiers (various colors to modify the body porcelain shade) or "opacious" body/dentin porcelains – are made of the same glass combinations as the body or incisal powders but with different pigments. "Opacious" body porcelains are more opaque than the body porcelains but less opaque than shoulder porcelains. Choosing the auxiliary porcelains and their placement is part of the expertise and artistry of the dental ceramist.

A final porcelain enameled crown or bridge must have the anatomy and shade as prescribed, which may require small additions of the body, incisal, or auxiliary porcelains; a lower firing "add-on" (corrective) porcelain may be used to corrections. The technician may use rotary hand tools to adjust the anatomy or appearance of fired enamel. The glaze firing is performed last, and this may include special "stain" porcelains that create unique effects or alter the shade of the tooth as needed to meet the prescription. Glaze firing is usually performed without a vacuum because the glaze and stain powders are applied in a thin layer of very fine particles, like the opaque porcelains, smaller than 10 μm. The final, enameled crown or bridge should be appreciated as a miniature work of art that recreates the anatomy and esthetic characteristics of a tooth to mimic – or improve – the appearance of the natural crown it replaces.

The ceramic pigments and rare earth oxides used for fluorescence were described in Chapter 6. Urania (uranium dioxide, UO_2) was the first fluorescent used in dental porcelains but was replaced by other fluorescing oxides with more natural appearing fluorescent colors, such as terbia (Tb_2O_3) or combinations of lanthanide oxides. In the 1990s, a limit of 1,000 Bq/kg (1 Bq/g) of U^{238} was imposed in the ISO 6872 standard for dental ceramics, including porcelains for enameling. A becquerel (Bq) is the unit of radioactivity in the International System of Units (SI) defined as one decay per second. For applications relating to human health, this is a small quantity. The urania used in dental porcelain was always lower than this limit.

Silver is a common ingredient of gold, palladium, and platinum alloys to reduce the melting point (and cost); technically, silver is not a precious metal. For instance, palladium-silver alloys have good resistance to deformation during firing and a higher elastic modulus (stiffer) than other similar dental alloys, but silver is known to discolor some leucite-containing porcelains, creating a greenish or yellowish discoloration at the margins of crowns where the porcelain enamel is thin. The silver ions from the metal may diffuse into the opaque layer of porcelain and coagulate as colloidal silver; this may be visible at the thin layer of porcelain at the margin of a crown. Colloidal silver in glass is well known as a colorant to produce a yellow to green-gray color (12). Earlier alloys for porcelain enamel contained copper, which also caused discoloration. The addition of tin oxide to porcelain frits is helpful in reducing discoloration by silver.

The thermal expansion "fit" or match of porcelains and alloys is crucial; otherwise, the stress between the enamel coating and the alloy will cause cracking or spalling after firing. Ideally, the porcelain enamel will have a thermal expansion that is modestly lower than the metal alloy, a difference of about 1 ppm, between room temperature and the porcelain's softening point temperature. With this small difference, the porcelain enamel coating will be in slight compression when cooled, which strengthens the enamel surface slightly. The stability of the leucite crystals during the enameling firing cycles is also important so that variations in firing temperatures and the number of firing cycles do not jeopardize the thermal compatibility with the underlying metal by dissolving or precipitating more leucite crystals. Porcelains having thermal compatibility with many dental alloys are desirable. Unique porcelain systems have been developed for certain thermal expansion ranges of alloys; some alloys with lower melting ranges require lower fusing porcelains. The hazard of low-fusing porcelains is the potential for higher glass solubility.

Dental porcelain is sometimes additionally strengthened by an ion exchange treatment, which entails a heat treatment in a salt without sodium. Potassium, cesium, or rubidium salts have been used – chlorides, carbonates, sulfates, or some phosphates, per US Pat 4,546,006 – and are applied to the surface of the porcelain for heating at about 400 °C for less than one hour; this temperature is lower than the melting point of the salt or the glazing temperature of the porcelain. The dental porcelain surface undergoes ion exchange to release sodium and replace it in the porcelain with the larger alkali metal ions to create a surface layer in compression. The atomic radii are 1.9, 2.66, 2.96, and 3.38 Å for sodium, potassium, rubidium, and cesium ions, respectively). The resulting porcelain strengthening is modest, from about 20 to 120 MPa, and the highest flexural strength reported has been about 220 MPa for an 11-hour treatment in potassium nitrate (13). Salt-bath ion exchange – Ca/K-nitrate salts at 400 °C – can also strengthen the lithium disilicate materials (14) discussed later.

Nickel-chrome, cobalt-chrome, and titanium alloys have also been used as substrates for dental porcelain veneering. The nickel-chrome alloys have thermal expansion like the precious metals, and the same porcelains can be used for both precious and non-precious metals. The Co-Cr alloys require a slightly higher thermal expansion porcelain because the alloys have an expansion of about 16 ppm. Titanium copings for fixed prosthodontics were extensively investigated in the 1970s (15), when pure titanium became more available, it presents a unique set of obstacles to enameling. Titanium metal requires melting in an inert atmosphere because it is easy to oxidize; also, the metal transforms from a close-packed hexagonal α-phase to a body-centered cubic-ß phase at 882 °C. For casting, calcium zirconate is used as an investment material. The lower expansion of titanium (~10 ppm/K) compared to the precious metal alloys requires a lower expansion and lower sintering porcelain enamel.

The "press-over-metal" method has also been developed for the efficiency of making PFM restorations. A metal coping is cast, then wax is formed over the metal in the shape of the desired crown, including a sprue. The metal and wax are embedded in a refractory material, which is "burned-out" to eliminate the wax. The refractory assembly is placed in a specialized uniaxial hot-press oven; a dental porcelain ingot is heated in the oven and then a piston gradually compresses/deforms the ingot through the sprue into the mold where the wax had been, onto the metal. After cooling and removal of the refractory, the finishing touches of shaping and polishing the crown are completed. The pressing process takes less than an hour. The advantage of hot pressing is the ability to form the ceramic to a near-net (accurate) shape in just one firing step with fewer pores. Fewer firings of porcelain mean faster production of crowns although they are less artistically characterized to match the surrounding dentition.

PFM crowns and bridges are a strong, reliable fixed prosthodontic that can be beautiful and indistinguishable from adjacent teeth. However, the metal margins may be undesirably visible if they are supragingival or if gum recession occurs, and the porcelain may chip over time in the mouth.

The compressive strength of leucite porcelains is about 80–100 MPa (16), which is too low to withstand the usual forces of occlusion and mastication without a metal substructure. However, leucite porcelain has been successfully used for veneering anterior teeth. Veneers (Figure 3.2b) are thin shells (<1 mm) that are cemented on the facial side of anterior teeth to modify the shape or shade. In Europe, "veneer" may mean any coating on an underlying substrate, such as the polymer-coated devices discussed above; here, veneers are used to denote a thin shell cemented on anterior teeth. When a dentist prepares a tooth for a veneer, very little to no enamel is removed from the facial side, and then an impression is made. A dental ceramist creates a model from the impression and builds porcelain powder on the model for the veneers. The first porcelains for ceramic veneers were the leucite-containing body and incisal porcelains for enameling metals. These porcelains have an intermediate transparency that could be used effectively to improve the appearance of teeth. The veneers are made by applying and condensing porcelain powder on either on a platinum foil or a refractory die material that has the shape of the underlying tooth (a model). Body, incisal, and auxiliary porcelains are condensed on the model, followed by firing in the same manner as a PFM crown. Stains and glaze may also be used to create a perfect and beautiful facial covering for the tooth.

After firing, veneers are detached from the underlying foil or refractory investment model, then "gently" sandblasted to create a rough inner surface that will face the tooth. The dental laboratory will etch the intaglio with 5–12% hydrofluoric acid (HF), which roughens the surface by dissolving some of the interstitial glass. Thorough rinsing is required before a silane coating is applied by the dental lab. The completed veneer is returned to the dentist to bond with a resin cement (Chapter 11) to the facial surface of a tooth. Resin cement is used to support the ceramic "shell" via intimate contact with the underlying tooth, making veneers very durable, despite using the relatively low-strength porcelain. Light-curable or dual-curing resin composite cements are used for bonding because the translucency of veneers will allow the light to penetrate to the cement. The color of the cement contributes to the esthetics of the veneer after bonding. Selection of the cement requires skill and experience because the cements do not necessarily match the veneer's shade, and the veneers are translucent. The resulting color match depends on the underlying tooth, the cement, and the veneer in combination. Veneers are popular for esthetic purposes, such as masking discoloration and altering the size and shape of the anterior maxillary and mandibular teeth. The benefit of veneers is that they require less tooth removal than a crown does to make esthetic improvements.

Higher Expansion Porcelain Restorations

In the late 1980s, slightly higher-strength veneer porcelains were introduced; these porcelains contained more leucite crystals than the porcelains for metals. The higher leucite content increased their strength, opacity, and thermal expansion. The extra leucite content adds opacity, but these porcelains were still esthetic. The higher thermal expansion – more leucite – was immaterial since veneers were not fused to metal. Higher leucite added stiffness and incremental flexural strength to as high as 150 MPa.

Uniaxial hot-pressing, developed in the 1990s, was useful for forming higher leucite content, anterior crowns. This technique is akin to the press-over-metal technique described for porcelain enamel and also uses a refractory mold. Manufacturers made shaded ingots of a leucite glass ingot for specialized furnaces. The ingots were heated to the softening point, about 920 °C (17) and the piston applied pressure on the ingots to fill a heated refractory mold as described before. Pressure was needed because the higher crystal content raised the firing temperature of the porcelain; pressure enabled the softened, but viscous porcelain to fill the refractory mold's cavity. The method was designed to reduce the number of pores, also contributing to higher strength. However, incisal porcelains were needed to create the best esthetics after hot-pressing and divesting the all-ceramic porcelain crowns. High leucite incisal porcelains were applied in a conventional dental furnace. These high leucite porcelains had success as the hot-pressed Empress crown by Ivoclar Vivadent and Optec by Pentron Corporations.

All these leucite-based porcelains contain glass and crystals but are not strictly a glass-ceramic; those described later in this chapter.

Magnesia Copings

A magnesia (MgO) coping material was invented in the 1980s (US Pat. 4,576,922) known as MagCor. MagCor contained about 40–60 wt.% of coarse (larger than 50 μm) magnesia particles and a silicate glass containing 58% silica, 10% soda, 9.5% boron oxide, 6% zirconia, and 5% each of titania, potassia, and fluoride, with about 1.5% alumina (18). The coping material was fired at about 1150 ° C for as long as two hours; firing formed a fine dispersion of forsterite ($MgO.2SiO_2$) crystals in the glass matrix phase. Magnesia-titania ($MgO.TiO_2$) or magnesia-zirconia ($MgO.ZrO_2$) crystals were also formed at the interface of the glass and residual magnesia grains. The method of making the copings was not described in the patent but is presumed to be similar to the powder condensation method used for dental porcelains. The white MagCor material had a strength of about 125 MPa in bend tests, higher than leucite porcelains. Magnesia has a high thermal expansion, about 15.5 ppm/K, and the glass used for MagCor had a thermal expansion of about 9 ppm/K. MagCor had a high enough thermal expansion that the leucite dental porcelains for enameling metals could be used to veneer the copings (18). Precipitating more magnesium silicate (forsterite) crystals (up to 40%) raised the flexural strength (~ 140 MPa in three-point bending) (18). However, forsterite has a decidedly lower thermal expansion (~4 ppm/K), and the combination of magnesia and forsterite could have caused the thermal incompatibility of the leucite porcelains. This invention was not commercialized.

Glass-Infiltrated Restorations

Another clever method of making dental crowns and bridges was invented in the 1990s based on creating a porous ceramic coping, followed by a heat treatment to infiltrate the interconnected pores with glass (US Pat. 5,695,337). The concept was commercialized as the InCeram product line from Vita Corporation. The ceramic powders were alumina (Al_2O_3), spinel ($MgAl_2O_4$ or $MgO.Al_2O_3$), or alumina-zirconia (Al_2O_3 and ZrO_2) that were partially sintered into porous frameworks as distinct phases. The crown or bridge copings were infiltrated with glass. The indications varied with the strength of the material, the strongest being those with alumina-zirconia for 3- or 4-unit bridges; strengths were reported from 235 to 800 MPa (19).

The InCeram copings were made in a dental lab using a modified slip-casting technique. Fine powders, 2–10 μm, were suspended in water with a deflocculant. The suspension of powders was applied in layers to a plaster model to create the framework of the intended restoration. The plaster model absorbed enough water, á la slip casting, to create the desired thickness of a "green" ceramic crown or bridge, which was then removed from the model. This green body was dried and then fired in a dental oven at a temperature high enough to cause the ceramic particles to bond but low enough to avoid shrinkage (surface, not bulk sintering mechanisms of Chapter 7). According to the patent, the interconnected porosity had diameters from 0.2 to 20 μm and overall porosity between 15 and 50 vol.% after partial sintering. For the next step, a special, high-lanthana (La_2O_3) content glass powder was applied to the partially sintered coping, which infiltrated the interconnected pores during a second heat treatment at about 1100 °C over a period of three to six hours. The goal was to completely fill the interconnected pores, strengthening the ceramic substructure. See Figure 10.5 for a microstructure showing the high lanthana glass surrounding the alumina crystals. Each

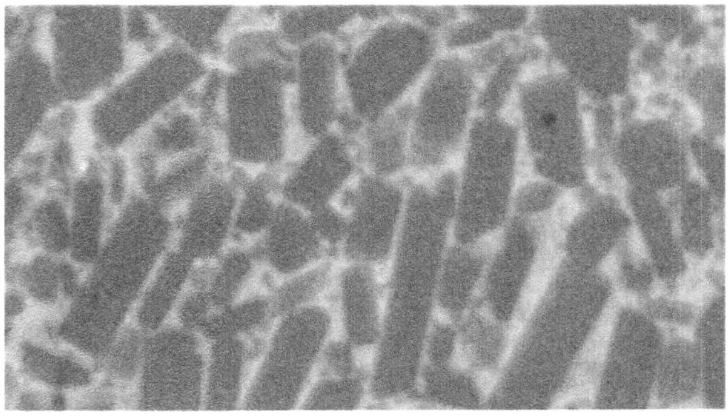

Figure 10.5 Microstructure of an etched InCeram alumina crown material (6) / American Association for Science and Technology. The high lanthana glass is a lighter gray, surrounding the acicular alumina crystals.

crystalline InCeram material requires a different glass formula, with the amounts varying from 25% to 50% lanthana to reduce its surface tension for infiltration. In later adaptations, the ceramic powders for the frameworks were mixed with a thermoplastic material and applied to the model; slow heating was required to decompose the polymer and then partially sinter the coping.

After the infiltration firing, excess glass was removed from the surface, and specially designed porcelains were applied and fired to create the coronal anatomy. These porcelains contained silica, alumina, and boron oxide, with lesser amounts of ceria and calcia and ceramic pigments. The thermal expansions were about 7–8.6 ppm the coping materials and their accompanying glasses (20).

The InCeram alumina/zirconia material contained about 67% alumina. The zirconia was partially stabilized with 10–12 mol% of ceria or 2–3 mol% of yttria per US Pat. 5,695,337. Up to 1% of transition metal oxide pigments were part of the InCeram coping powders to create various shades. Later, a simplified approach was marketed for this material – "soft machining" (21). For the machining innovation, porous (partially sintered) ingots were made by the manufacturer, which the dental technician milled to the desired coping shape using CAD-CAM software and milling equipment, described in Chapter 4 and later in this chapter. Coping were infiltrated and veneered in two heating steps. Another adaptation was to infiltrate the porous ceramic copings with resin (US Pat. 11,622,918) for milling polymer-infiltrated ceramic crowns described later in this chapter. InCeram systems were discontinued because of its lower strength compared to all-zirconia crowns discussed later.

Glass-Ceramic Restorations

Glass ceramics are made from a cast glass item that is heat-treated to precipitate crystals. They are useful because a complex glass shape can be cast with virtually no pores and then strengthened. The development of glass-ceramics in the potassia–magnesia–silica–fluorine system for dental crowns, not bridges, was undertaken by Corning Glass Works with Peter Adair of Biocor, Inc. (22) and commercialized by Dentsply International (now Dentsply Sirona) as Dicor® glass-ceramic crowns. This glass-ceramic formula was an adaptation of a "machinable" glass-ceramic composition containing fluoride-tetrasilicic mica crystals patented by Grossman (US Pat. 4,652,312) in 1972 (23). The Dicor glass after melting contained 45–70% SiO_2, 13–30% MgO, 5–20% K_2O, 0–2% Al_2O_3, 0–7% ZrO_2, 4–9% F, and 1–4% BaO (wt.%). Zirconia was included to improve chemical durability. The fluoride content was contributed by MgF_2 or other fluoride compounds in the glass's raw materials, which were dissolved in the glass during melting at about 1300–1450 °C. One to two percent of "coloring oxides" could be included, such as oxides of the transition metals V, Cr, Mn, Fe, Co, Ni, or Cu. Rare earth compounds – cerium oxide (CeO_2) and terbia (Tb_2O_3) – were included to create fluorescence akin to natural teeth (US Pat. 5,387,558). An important issue was identified in the patent – the "cerammed" surface of the crowns would adsorb moisture; this moisture would evaporate during the firing of the outer surface stain, creating bubbles and weakening the crown. Baria reduced this moisture adsorption although it slightly increased the opacity. Corning melted, cast, and annealed ingots of glass for dental laboratories to cast into dental crowns.

The Dicor laboratory technique (24) required a wax pattern of the desired crown form, including a sprue, to be cast with (encased in) a unique phosphate-bonded investment material. The investment mold was heated to decompose the wax, and then placed in the Dicor casting machine. The casting equipment had a platinum-wound furnace for melting and centrifugal casting of the 4-g glass ingots (at 1360 °C) (24). The cast glass crowns were devested (removed) from the refractory investment. Then, the crowns were re-imbedded on the intaglio with another refractory material, which supported the crown to prevent deformation during the next ceramming step.

The crowns were "cerammed" – heat-treated – in a pre-programmed Dicor oven via a two-step process for crystal nucleation and growth of fluormica crystals. According to the patent literature, crystals nucleation occurred between 750 and 850 °C and required one to six hours. Next, the temperature was raised to 1100–1150 °C for the growth of the nucleated crystals; the total ceramming time was about eight hours. The Dicor ceramming process formed sheet-like crystals of synthetic fluorine mica known as fluorophlogopite ($KMg_{2.5}Si_4O_{10}F_2$), which were dubbed tetrasilicic because no aluminum or boron was present in the composition to displace the silicon in the sheet-like crystals. After heat treatment, the Dicor crowns contained about 55 vol.% tetrasilicic fluormica crystals in a glass matrix. However, a thin, opaque surface layer (~45 μm) that formed by contact with the ceramming investment material did not have tetrasilicic fluormica crystals; this layer was sometimes removed. As noted in Chapter 5, crystal nucleation and growth in glasses are time and temperature-dependent; the growth of crystals over time was documented in micrographs in (23). A representative Dicor micrograph is shown in Figure 10.6. The crystals improved the fracture toughness, flexural strength, abrasion resistance, and chemical durability compared to the starting glass, which made the glass-ceramic suitable for a dental crown.

Dicor crowns were available in one translucent color; they were completed by firing a self-glazing, porcelain veneer coating to match the surrounding teeth. Very fine accessory porcelain powders were available to achieve shade matching and esthetics, even for crowns over teeth whose core had been rebuilt with (dark-colored) amalgam. Usually, four layers of thin porcelain were applied by repeated firing to about 940 °C, creating a layer only 125 μm thick. Sometimes, this thin coating would become abraded by contact with the opposing teeth, leaving a lighter spot. Unfortunately, the porcelain was vulnerable to dissolution by acidulated fluoride, which is not a common treatment but was used.

An important feature of the innovative Dicor crowns was that the cast crowns did not shrink or crack during casting and ceramming. Another outstanding feature of Dicor crowns was the unique scattering of light to produce a biomimetic appearance. The flat mica crystals acted as minute mirrors, producing numerous internal reflections and creating visual depth with translucency and color that mimicked tooth enamel.

The Dicor crowns were acid etched and luted to teeth with zinc phosphate, glass-ionomer, and resin cements – see Chapter 11. HF-acid etching of the Dicor intaglio was beneficial for the crown's long-term service. Failures were lowest for

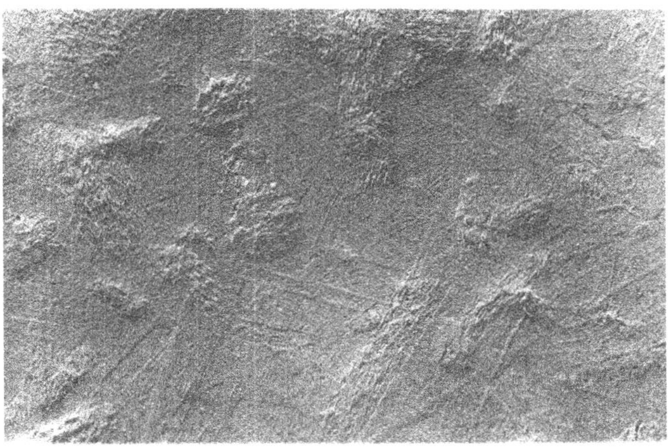

Figure 10.6 Microstructure of an etched Dicor glass-ceramic crown material, illustrating the interlocking sheets of mica-like crystals (25) / Quintessence Publishing Company, Ltd. Crystals are about 1 μm wide.

those crowns placed with resin cement and highest with zinc phosphate cement, the latter being much less flexible. Crowns on molars were more susceptible to fracture than crowns on premolars or anterior teeth, and more failures occurred in men versus women, indicative of their stronger masticatory forces. It appears that the strength of Dicor was just high enough to withstand the oral stresses in the anterior, when supported by a resin cement. The Dicor crowns used familiar techniques for fabrication, were easy to adjust, and were resistant to plaque adherence with excellent marginal accuracy and esthetics. However, the failure rate was too high, so the material was discontinued and later superseded by lithium disilicate glass-ceramic crowns.

In addition to the Dicor material developed as a castable product, a second machinable glass-ceramic denoted as Dicor MGC was developed (1972) for the CEREC CAM system of milling inlays, onlays, and crowns (US Pats. 4,575,805 and 4,663,720). This material contained almost 70 vol.% tetrasilicic fluoromica crystals, up from 55% in the cast crowns. Corning Glass Works used a different heat treatment schedule to create the ingots of Dicor MGC to precipitate more and larger crystals, and the crystals enabled it to be machined with metal-working tools. The Dicor cast material had a three-point bending strength of 150–180 MPa, whereas the machinable version had a higher flexural strength, 210 ± 15 MPa (26). These strengths were higher than for the porcelains and MagCor, but about the same as the Cerestore crowns. More crystals made the MGC material slightly more opaque but acceptable; this material was also superseded by lithium disilicate glass-ceramic crowns.

Dicor was not the only glass-ceramic formula invented for dentistry (25). Denry and Rosenstiel (27) modified the Dicor composition by adding 2.5% lithium fluoride to increase the flexure strength, but the crowns were still subject to failure. A material denoted as Cerapearl from Kyocera was another glass-ceramic that included the precipitation of hydroxyapatite crystals and had a flexural strength of about 150–300 MPa and compressive strength of 870 MPa. This glass-ceramic contained calcia and phosphorus oxide, and less silica and magnesia than Dicor: 44.6% CaO, 34% SiO_2, 16.2% P_2O_5, and 4.6% MgO (28). Cerapearl glass-ceramic was made using similar methods to Dicor, but the melting temperature was higher (1510 °C), and the cast crowns had to be annealed before devesting. The intaglios of the crowns were embedded with a refractory material for support during ceramming, which consisted of crystal nucleation at 800 °C and growth at 900 °C. For esthetics, porcelains were fired on the surface of the Cerapearl cerammed crowns, and resin cements were required for adhesion to teeth. After two years, clinical performance was considered very good, but Kyocera Inc. discontinued this product.

Zirconia has been added to the mica-ceramics, like Dicor, for higher hardness, stiffness, and fracture toughness (29). A new glass-ceramic (IPS d.sign, Ivoclar) has been developed into a product line for enameling metals and contains fluoroapatite and leucite crystals. None of these glass-ceramics seems to be as popular as the lithium disilicate glass ceramics described below.

Lithium Disilicate Glass-Ceramic Restorations

Lithium disilicate was recognized as early as 1971 as a potential glass-ceramic for dental crowns (25); however, a glass-ceramic made solely of silica and lithia has insufficient strength and chemical durability for dental use; alumina and calcia were needed to improve the chemical durability. US Pat. 4,189,325 disclosed a glass, which can form lithium disilicate crystals, having this approximate composition in mole percent: 28–32% Li_2O, 59–69% SiO_2, 1–4% Al_2O_3, and 2–6% CaO. Inventors have added platinum and niobium oxide in minor amounts to reduce cracking during crystallization; these additives induce faster nucleation of finer crystals that create less internal stress. Unlike the Dicor process, this glass could be melted and cast directly into a conventional dental investment material used for casting the metal alloys used for porcelain enameling. The cast glass was heat-treated within the traditional dental investment to form lithium disilicate crowns.

Another method for lithium disilicate crowns was to hot-press a glass ingot above 930 °C, which was quickly cooled to avoid crystallization (US Pats., 5,507,981, 5,702,514, 5,897,885, 6,346,306B1, 6,376,397Bl, 6,485,849B2, and 6,818,573B2). The heated ingot was pressed into the investment mold, under vacuum, using a crushable crucible that would seal around the edge of the mold's cavity as the glass was pressed into the mold's cavity. The glass crown was heat-treated to form 0.5 to 20 μm crystals. The crowns retained 45–55 wt.% of glass for translucency. The glass composition is in Table 10.3; its flexural strength was about 360 MPa after ceramming. The thermal expansion was about 11 ppm/K, suitable for the application of a leucite-containing dental porcelain (29).

Starting in the 1990s, the first lithium disilicate dental crowns were commercialized by Ivoclar Inc. as Empress II. They manufactured "cerammed" ingots containing lithium disilicate crystals that could be uniaxially hot-pressed, similar to the high-leucite porcelain ingots described before. When heated, pressure was used to deform the glass-ceramic ingot, which filled a cavity in an investment material; this was a change from the centrifugal casting of Dicor or metals. The ingots contained about 65% lithium disilicate crystals ($Li_2O.2SiO_2$, $Li_2Si_2O_5$), 1% of pores, and 44% glass by volume. The ingots had an interlocking, plate-like, and needle-like assembly of crystals. The lithium disilicate products surpassed the strength and fracture toughness of the leucite, higher leucite, MagCor, Dicor, Cerestore, or alumina porcelains (29).

Table 10.3 Nominal Porcelain and Glass compositions.

Oxide in weight percent	Leucite -containing opaque[c]	Leucite containing body[c]	Porcelain for alumina	Porcelain for t-zirconia or lithium disilicate[d]	Glass for lithium disilicate crowns[e]	Glass for ceramic-polymer hybrid
Silica	45	59	69.5	60–65	67–71	58–63
Boron oxide	1.5		7.5	3–5	0–2	0.5–10
Calcia			1.8	0–2	0–1.25	<1
Potassia	10	15	8.3	6–9	1.5–3.5	4–6
Soda	7	11	4.8	5–7	1–2	6–11
Alumina	6	7	8.1	10–13	4.5–5.0	20–23
Lithia	1.5	1.5		1–3	14–15	
Baria				2–5	1.25–3.0	
Zirconia[a]	24	<1		<1		
Misc. oxides[b]	5	6.5		5	0–2	<1

[a] Titania, ceria and tin oxide are also used for opacity.
[b] May include terbia, titania, tin oxide, phosphorous pentoxide, ceria, yttria, and magnesia.
[c] From US Pat. 5,713,994.
[d] From US Pat. Application 11,426,332.
[e] From US Pat. 6818,573.

From the early 2000s, lithium disilicate indirect restoration products have blossomed, each having slightly different compositions, as noted in Table 10.4. Several brands of slightly different compositions are available; all contain SiO_2, Li_2O, K_2O, P_2O_5, and ZrO_2 for esthetics, chemical resistance, and toughening. Nucleating agents for the crystals are phosphorous pentoxide, zirconia, or titania, to create a strong, fine-grained, lithium disilicate glass-ceramic. These oxides are added to control the kinetics of crystal growth: Na_2O, ZnO, Al_2O_3, and MgO (30). Shades are achieved with minor amounts of oxides of tin, titanium, manganese, magnesium, cerium, iron, nickel, vanadium, chromium and undisclosed fluorescing oxides (30). Some of the lithium disilicate glass formulas contain oxides not mentioned above, such as boron oxide, calcia, ceria, magnesia, terbia, yttria, zinc oxide, and zirconia. Analyses of five brands and two experimental lithium disilicate blocks are in reference (31), noting that zirconia has been used for "reinforcement" in some materials. The fraction of crystals varies from 50% to 80% leading to variations in strength, toughness, hardness, and modulus. Importantly, all five lithium disilicate materials met the insolubility criteria of the

Table 10.4 Approximate compositions of glass-ceramic restorative materials (19) (weight percent).

Tradename →	Macor (Corning)	Dicor (Corning & Dentsply)	Celtra duo (Dentsply Sirona)	E-Max CAD (Ivoclar Vivadent)	Suprinity PC (Vita Zahnfabrik)	Amber mill (Hass corp.)
Type of ceramic→ oxides present ↓	**Tetrasilicic mica**		**Lithium Disillicate Glasses for Ceramming**			
Silica	47.2	56–64	58.0	57–80	56–64	66 ~ 83
Lithia			18.5	11–19	15–21	9–13
Potassia	9.5	12–18		0–13	1–4	0–1
Soda						0–1
Phosphorous pentoxide			5.0	0–11	3–8	2–5
Zirconia			10.1	0–8	8–12	
Zinc oxide			1.0	0–8		
Alumina	16.7	0–2	1.9	0–5	1–4	2–8
Magnesia	14.5	15–20		0–5		
Calcia						
Ceria	0.06		2.0		0–4	0–3
Boron oxide	8.5					
Fluoride	6.3	4–9				
Zirconia						
Pigments			~ 3.5%	0–8	0–6	0–7

ISO 6872 test method, requiring less than 100 μg/cm^2 solubility in 4% acetic acid at 80 °C for 16 hours for minimum surface area exposure.

Dental laboratories have embraced more affordable CAD-CAM equipment beginning since 2005. This technological advancement provided the impetus for developing machinable (subtractive milling) versions of lithium disilicate that are now the dominant method of making lithium disilicate dental restorations. Manufacturers melt and cast the ingots and then nucleate lithium metasilicate ($Li_2O.SiO_2$, Li_2SiO_3) crystals in the ingots at about 450 °C, followed by crystal growth at about 800 °C. This heat treatment creates ingots with about 40% lithium metasilicate crystals smaller than 0.5 μm, a flexural strength of about 130–150 MPa, and a fracture toughness of less than 1.25 MPa·m$^{1/2}$. Ingots with lithium metasilicate are easier to mill than ingots with lithium disilicate crystals. Dental laboratories use CAD software to design a slightly oversized crown, considering the shrinkage factor. The ingots are milled to the CAD shape, and then the crowns are heat-treated (cerammed) to develop the preferred, stronger lithium disilicate crystals (32). This heat treatment is performed at 820–850 °C, with a hold time of less than 10 minutes (30). During heat treatment, residual glass reacts with the metasilicate crystals to form lithium disilicate crystals via reaction Eq. (10.1) (30). This transformation causes linear shrinkage of about 0.2% (33):

$$Li_2SiO_3 + SiO_2 \rightarrow Li_2Si_2O_5 \quad (10.1)$$

During this heat treatment, the ingots change color from the purplish hue of the finer metasilicate crystals to the desired dental shade achieved with the larger lithium disilicate crystals, increasing the strength to about 360 MPa by the transformation of the metasilicate into disilicate crystals. See Figure 10.7 for a comparison of lithium metasilicate and lithium disilicate microstructures. The microstructure (crystalline identity, percent, and size) of the lithium disilicate products – and all ceramics – depends on the exact composition and heat treatment (32), including the furnace's size and design, the heating and cooling speed, the hold time, and the thickness of the restoration (35). These factors are a tautology for heat treatments of ceramics.

Another heat treatment to develop lithium disilicate crystals begins with a heat soak at 500–600 °C for two to six hours, a slow increase in the temperature to 925 °C, another soak at 925 °C for one to two hours and then cooling. The heat treatments are designed to create the manufacturer's desired distribution of crystals for strength and beauty, characteristics that are intertwined with the primary and minor components of the starting glass formula. For instance, lithium phosphate (Li_3PO_4) and silica (cristobalite) crystals may be formed with lithium metasilicate

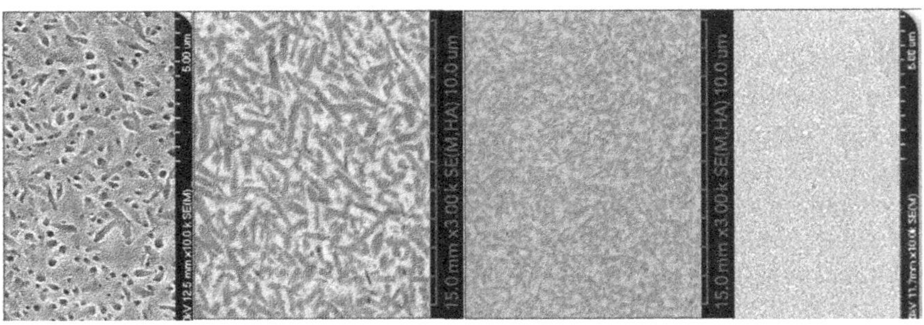

Figure 10.7 Examples of the microstructure of a lithium metasilicate (left), two lithium disilicate microstructures in the center (34) / The Royal Society, and nanoscale lithium disilicate (right) materials.

during the manufacturers' heat treatments used for ingots. Then, lithium disilicate crystals can be nucleated on the lithium phosphate crystals during the post-milling heat treatment. The combination of crystals and their orientations changes the thermal expansion. The variations in thermal expansion are known to range from 3.5 (cristobalite) to 15.4 in ppm/K for the c-axis of lithium metasilicate, compared to 10.1–10.8 in ppm/K for crystalline lithium disilicate. This disparity highlights the criticality of the formulas and the heat treatments performed by the manufacturers and dental laboratories to avoid deformation and cracking.

The molar ratio of SiO_2 to Li_2O in lithium disilicate products has diverged from 2.0; the ratio may be as low as 1.6 to or as high as 3.0 (29, 32); the SiO_2 to Li_2O ratio influences the crystals formed during heat treatment, and the reported percentage of crystals varies from 45% to 80%. Clearly, the lithium disilicate restorative products vary, which clinicians may not realize when they send a prescription to a laboratory. Variations of the lithium disilicate compositions have been studied for mechanical properties. The lithium disilicate ceramic dental materials have three-point flexural strengths of 200–360 MPa, biaxial strengths from 380 to 670 MPa, fracture toughnesses of 1.4–3.3 MPa-$m^{1/2}$, Young's moduli of 77–80 GPa (30), and thermal expansion coefficients of about 10.6 ppm/K (36). Experimental materials have had strengths as high as 1,000 MPa and a fracture toughness of about 6 MPa-$m^{1/2}$. Some lithium disilicate blocks for CAD-CAM are marketed as being "100%" crystallized, which may be after ceramming. Other lithium disilicate brands, such as Amber Mill from Hass Corporation, create finer crystals with less glass by controlling crystal growth with secondary crystalline phases (29). Strengths as high as 450 MPa were reported with nanocrystal formation (37). See Figure 10.7.

Lithium disilicate dental products are strong enough to be processed into anterior and posterior crowns, inlays, onlays, and three-unit bridges for the anterior and premolar regions; the lost-wax/hot pressing or the CAD-CAM/heat treatment methods are used; additive manufacturing is envisioned for future commercial products. The ingots for pressing or milling are available in multiple shades, and the resulting crowns are translucent enough to be esthetically acceptable. The versatility and the variety of lithium disilicate products have been a boon for dentistry and a benefit for patients. The manufacturing and the dental laboratories' processing requires careful control of the heat treatment schedules to achieve a crystal dispersion – composition, size, and percent – having high strength balanced with esthetics: shade, translucency, and fluorescence.

To minimize the need for porcelain after machining, "multi-colored" CAD/CAM blocks are available that combine different degrees of chroma (color intensity) and transparency along their length. This enables a crown to be machined that has less chroma and more transparency at the incisal edge than at the opposite gingival region. Using such blocks reduces the need for applying incisal porcelain for esthetics although fine-tuning of the esthetics or anatomy is possible using the same porcelains used for veneering metals.

Lithium disilicate crowns should be etched (roughened) on the intaglio in a dental laboratory with HF (~8% for 20–30 seconds) and thoroughly rinsed before the dentist "tries in" the prosthesis. After the "try-in" (fit check) on the tooth, the interior of lithium disilicate restorations should be cleaned with phosphoric acid or a hydroxide solution to remove saliva remnants; alcohol and water rinsing are not sufficient for this cleaning step, and sandblasting is not advised because it obliterates the etched surface and weakens the lithium disilicate material.

CAD-CAM Indirect Restorations (Subtractive Manufacture)

Computer-aided design and computer-aided manufacture (CAD-CAM) are methods of manufacturing materials adapted for dentistry since the 1990s and broadly adopted in the 21st century. The dental CAD-CAM methods differ from industrial CAD-CAM because every dental crown or bridge is individually customized for the patient – no two cases are the same, and every crown or bridge requires its unique .STL, .PLY, or. OBJ file for machining. CAD replaces the manual work of forming a wax model of the desired dental restoration; CAM replaces processes such as hot-pressing or the lost-wax casting of metal or glass.

The CAD/CAM technology offers several benefits. In some cases, this technology allows dentists to provide a single-visit (albeit two sessions in one day) experience for a patient to receive an indirect dental restoration. CAD-CAM indirect devices made in the dental office may also require fewer resources and improve communication with an off-site dental laboratory. Several CAD/CAM systems are available, so the issue of transferring the prescription (impression and shading information) must be coordinated with a dental laboratory for data transmission, design, and manufacturing processes. The ISO 18618/ADA 145 standards specify an extensible markup language (XML) format to transfer dental case data (impressions and designs of prostheses) to machining software, and the ADA 146 technical report refers to machining of abutments (Chapter 16) using DICOM software. Abutments of zirconia have been cleared by the FDA since 2006.

Early machining equipment used a copy-milling CAM technique like that used to replicate brass house keys (Mikrona Corporation's CELAY® copy milling system). For this equipment, a dental technician cast a model of the prepared tooth, created a light-cured composite model on the tooth of the restoration that was needed, which was transferred to the CELAY machine that copied the model by direct contact and milled a ceramic crown, veneer, inlay, or onlay. This equipment was compact enough to be housed in the laboratory within dental offices.

Manufacturers started making small blocks of ceramic on metal posts that could be inserted into the milling machines. These blocks – made by the manufacturers – are less likely to have pores than hand-condensed ceramic formed by dental technician. The first blocks were made of high-leucite porcelain, alumina, or Macor® glass-ceramic. Later, the porous InCeram ceramics were milled before the framework was infiltrated with glass.

Lithium disilicate and zirconia milling blocks and disks are now available. Blocks are available with a metal base to enable the zirconia to be easily grasped in a CAM apparatus and can be milled to the desired shape in less than 10 minutes and then finished without the metal stem with fine polishing adjustments. Disks as large as 98.5 mm in diameter and thickness up to 18 mm are available for CAD-CAM manufacture of multiple restorations, even long-span bridges or dentures.

Hybrid polymer-ceramic materials are also available for machining; these are more quickly milled than 100% ceramics. Like the other CAD-CAM materials, several shades are available for single tooth restorations: inlays, onlays, veneers, partial crowns, copings, and telescopic crowns – an inner crown used to attach removable dentures. One brand of the resin-based hybrid materials allows crown indications if a circumferential reduction of 1.5 mm is completed for the tooth. Surficial organic stains may be applied, but porcelain cannot be used because firing would destroy the methacrylate in the hybrid material.

The CAM systems differ in the number of axes (up to six) and the ability to mill materials in the “green” or the fully dense state. As many as seven steps for CAM may be required, with several tools operated at speeds, feeds, and increments recommended by the manufacturer. The materials may be milled wet (with water) or dry, depending on the product. Sophistication keeps increasing for more convenience in milling, including touchscreens for programming, tool detection, and automatic cycles.

Various ceramic blanks are used in machining systems of different chemical and microstructural characteristics but encounter common machining and performance issues – machining damage, minimum machined thickness, and machining tolerances. Most CAD-CAM-suitable ceramic materials require sintering or heat treatment after machining. After milling, pre-set and custom firing programs are used to sinter a zirconia restoration or crystallize a lithium disilicate crown.

Zirconia and alumina as green or partially sintered blanks have shrinkage values of 20–35 vol.% when sintered into a fully dense restoration. Before machining, the green density or shrinkage factor must be known so that oversized crowns/bridges are designed and machined with CAD/CAM software and will fit accurately when sintered. Homogeneity of the blocks is important to avoid differential shrinkage and warping. Glass-ceramics (e.g. lithium disilicate) usually require crystallization after machining. Lithium disilicate glass-ceramic has less shrinkage than sintered oxides as noted before. If crystallization is not required, machining damage that causes surface and subsurface damage must be avoided. The ISO 18675/ADA 131 standards include guidance for evaluating the effects of machining on ceramic materials and the dimensional changes occurring after crystallization or sintering, as well as assessing machining damage.

As mentioned above, the CAD-CAM restorations may need finishing porcelains, stains, or glazes applied to the exterior to complete the anatomical shape or shade to match the underlying teeth. However, less porcelain is needed than in the earlier methods because the CAM crowns or bridges are closer to the final restoration design, near net shape.

3D Indirect Restorations (Additive Manufacture)

Three-dimensional printing was first patented in 1986; ceramics were tested by 2000, and zirconia for dentistry was investigated for 3D printing by 2009 (38). Crowns and implants have been made using 3D printing techniques (39), but the process is nascent. The dominant printing techniques are stereolithography, direct light processing, and direct inkjet printing (40). The reported strengths have not been as high for 3D printed zirconia crowns compared to the CAM (subtractive milling) technique, perhaps because the 3D printing methods impart flaws, which can introduce inaccuracies and defects. Additive manufacturing of ceramics for fixed prosthodontics does not waste crown material, unlike machining, but 3D manufacturing requires the removal of the organic printing aid, which is always a complicated heat treatment.

The powders for 3D printing should be smaller than 5 μm. After printing, the removal (burnout/decomposition) of approximately 60 vol.% of a light-cured binder must be carefully performed in air with multiple dwell times and heating rates between 0.1 and 30 °C/min; otherwise, pores will be created by the release of the organic binder decomposition gases. The composition of the powder and binders, and the printing parameters, are crucial for success, which subsequent heat treatments cannot undo or correct. Shrinkage occurs from a printed object to a sintered object of about 40 vol.% (~13% linear shrinkage). The post printing is not a fast process for ceramics, unlike the all-polymer 3D printing of items like nightguards.

Additive manufacturing has been tested for lithium disilicate (41, 42). In one case, sintering and crystallization were performed at 900–940 °C with a hold time of about 20 minutes, and the heating rate was slower than 5 °C/min. In another 3D-printed report, the heat treatment was 1325 °C for 10 hours. In one report, the flexural strengths were less than 300 MPa, less than some CAM results, indicative of flaws introduced by the printing method or a dearth of crystals after heat treatment. Research regarding porous lithium disilicate made by 3D printing (digital light processing) showed promise for osseointegration as a lumbar spine implant (43) and is a concept for dental bone graft innovation.

Additive printing parameters using the digital light processing method were comprehensively explored for a combination of zirconia and dicalcium silicate (44), for a potential dental implant. Selecting the printing parameters is complicated and interactive; the burn-off and sintering sequences are equally challenging and do not achieve the same strength of tetragonal zirconia as with other methods.

Future 3D printing (described later) may combine leucite porcelain, lithium aluminosilicate, and lithium disilicate crystalline powders. After burn-out of the printing material, limited heat treatment will be needed as the ceramic powders are crystalline before 3D printing.

Zirconia Restorations

Zirconia (ZrO_2), particularly tetragonal zirconia, is the strongest all-ceramic indirect restorative material currently available. Zirconia is not as strong as dental alloys, but its off-white! Zirconia crowns have been prescribed for the anterior or posterior teeth – including on implants – and they are suitable for inlays, onlays, veneers, resin-bonded bridges, and bridges that span up to 14 teeth (with no spans exceeding two missing teeth) (45). This is a much wider set of indications than for the indirect ceramic restorations discussed in the earlier parts of this chapter. Zirconia fixed prosthodontic devices are not made by sintering in a dental laboratory; no delicate condensation and layering of powders is needed, unlike porcelains. Zirconia fixed prosthodontics have always been made by machining discs or ingots supplied by a manufacturer. CAD-CAM equipment is required, although 3D additive methods are being developed (46).

Dense, fully sintered, partially stabilized magnesia-doped zirconia was marketed for "hard-machining" (47). This zirconia consisted of tetragonal grains within a cubic crystal matrix, but it was plagued by issues of pores and large grains. Although machinable, this product was not as strong as yttria-stabilized tetragonal zirconia, and the product was discontinued (21). From 2000 onward, 3 mol% yttria-stabilized tetragonal zirconia (3Y-TZP, 5.35 wt.% Y_2O_3) became a common material for fixed prosthodontic devices (48). The success of 3Y-TZP is based on its high strength and toughness, the development of partially sintered ingots or pucks (disks) for milling, the availability and affordability of the CAD-CAM equipment, sintering furnaces to finish densifying the zirconia after milling, and its acceptable esthetics. At least two journal articles (49, 50) have lists of commercial zirconia materials suitable for machining crowns and bridges.

Contemporary zirconia crowns and bridges are machined from partially sintered discs or ingots of yttria-stabilized zirconia. The partially sintered (bisque) zirconia materials became successful when the manufacturers created homogeneous partially sintered blocks that had a reliable shrinkage factor provided by the manufacturer. At first, the manufacturers milled and sintered the crowns from CAD files provided to them by a dental laboratory and returned the machined and densified crowns to the dental laboratory for porcelain application. Later, the milling and sintering were released to the dental laboratories because manufacturers could make their partially sintered products very consistent in shrinkage, and they provided shrinkage factors for each batch to use in the CAD calculations before milling. This shrinkage factor enables the design and machining of oversized crowns in the partially sintered state that achieve a reliable fit of the prosthetics after sintering.

The porosity and density of the partially sintered zirconia products are not public and the pre-sintering (bisque firing) cycles of the manufacturers are trade secrets. Studies of the partial sintering of zirconia have used a firing sequence of 2 °C/min to 600 °C, hold for two hours, heat at 5 °C/min to between 1000 and 1150 °C, hold for about two hours, and cool at about 10 °C/min (51). Interparticle necking began above 950 °C, and the porosity started to close above 1200 °C, which gives insights into dental product manufacture. The uniformity of the bisque zirconia ingots or pucks is crucial for the final sintering and achieving excellent-fitting fixed prosthodontics; greater uniformity is likely if the zirconia powder is cold isostatically pressed. Figure 10.8a is a photomicrograph of the microstructure of a partially sintered zirconia.

Each manufacturer's final, après milling, sintering schedule must be closely followed to achieve the highest percentage of theoretical (full, pore-free) density for the highest strength. Some brands of milled zirconia are sintered using a 20-minute heating cycle; other zirconia products may require sintering over seven hours up to 1600 °C. The heating schedules depend on the composition, pre-sintered state, and specialized furnace of the company. Generally, higher temperatures and longer times will lead to slightly larger crystals ($> 1\,\mu m$), which is a tautology for sintering. Examples of sintered zirconia microstructures are in Figure 10.8b for 3% and 5% yttria-stabilized zirconia.

Interestingly, the zirconia crowns are sintered with the margins up, opposite of the porcelain fused-to-metal crowns, which are supported with pegs on the intaglio. A calibration method is given in ISO 13078/ADA 164 standards for furnaces heated to 1700 °C, which is useful for precisely firing zirconia prostheses.

Modern patients want uniform, white teeth. Uniformity means less color variation (characterization) is needed for the restoration; plainer, whiter restorations require less porcelain and less artistic skill by the dentist, or the dental technician compared to PFM crowns. About half of zirconia crowns are placed without any

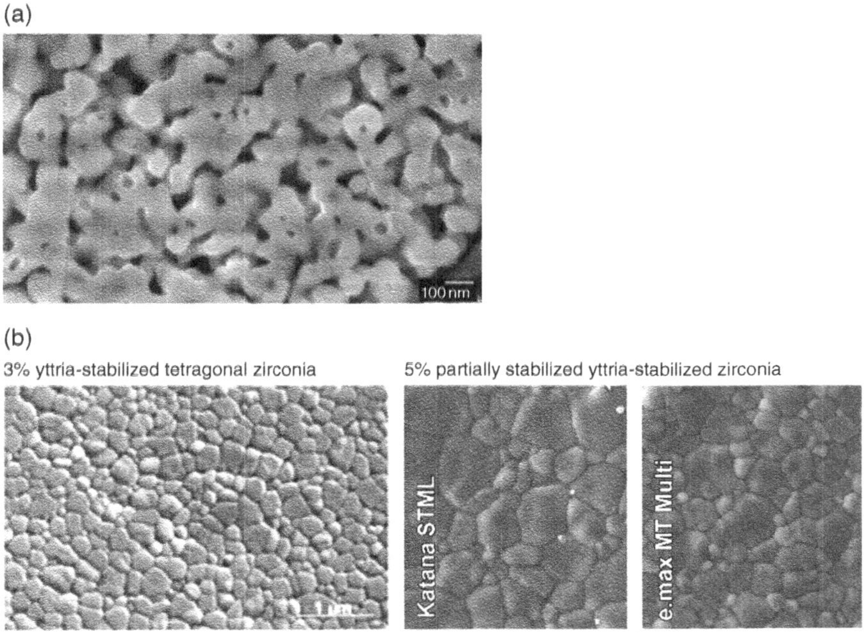

Figure 10.8 (a) Microstructure of partially sintered 3 mol% yttria-stabilized tetragonal zirconia material (51) / with permission of Elsevier. Note the interconnected porosity and the sintered interparticle necks and the fine microstructure in nanometers. (b): Microstructure of a sintered 3% yttria-stabilized tetragonal zirconia material from (52) / John Wiley & Sons (left), and two examples of microstructure of 5% yttria-stabilized zirconia (middle and right) from (53) / MDPI / CC BY 4.0. Note the presence of the larger cubic grains in the samples with 5% yttria.

porcelain layer on top, which is often acceptable for posterior restorations. Yet, the 3Y-TZP materials are verging on too opaque and not the best esthetic choice for the anterior teeth. Dental laboratory technicians have used their skills to dab on the color modifier liquids – which soak into the partially sintered zirconia – on the surface of machined, but not sintered, crowns to enhance the biomimicry of the restoration. Sometimes, a surface porcelain, stain, or glaze is used to scumble the underlying opaque zirconia and soften its difference from adjacent natural teeth. Porcelain can improve the esthetics of 3Y-TZP, hiding its inherent white, opaque, "snow-cone" appearance. Both porcelain and extrinsic stains (colored glazes) have been fired on the surface to achieve the best color match (50). The porcelain and glaze materials require temperatures of less than about 940°C. The zirconia porcelains are unique because of the relatively high thermal expansion of zirconia, 19.5 ppm/K. A slower cooling time after firing is used compared to PFMs; slower cooling has avoided cracks and chipping (54). Porcelain for zirconia is available both as a powder and as ingots for hot, uniaxial hot-pressing on a sintered zirconia crown. Press-over-zirconia (POZ) is a technique that uses uniaxial hot-pressing of a high-leucite porcelain ingot as a coating on a sintered zirconia crown; it merges porcelain, zirconia, hot-pressing, and CAD/CAM for esthetics and strength. Some technicians have removed a thin facial layer of machined zirconia and, after sintering, they fired a layer of porcelain to create a more natural and translucent facial surface. These techniques combine the knowledge of the modifier colors and the artistic skills of dental technicians they have used for PFM crowns.

Translucency at the incisal edge is important for blending the restoration with natural teeth. To meet this esthetic demand, the yttria content has been increased in some zirconia products from 3 to 5 mol% of yttria (55); the latter achieves a translucency similar to the more esthetic (more transparent) lithium disilicate materials. However, 5 mol% yttria in zirconia creates a partially stabilized zirconia, PSZ, that contains cubic and tetragonal crystals. See the composition on the phase diagram in Figure 10.9, which confirms that both crystal forms will be present. The cubic crystals are slightly larger, isotropic, without birefringence, which makes them more transparent (less opaque) than 100% tetragonal zirconia crystals. However, yttria content is inverse with strength; therefore, 5 mol% yttria-containing zirconia is not optimal for bridges spanning four teeth (57).

Zirconia blocks for machining have been commercially available in as many as 19 shades, depending on the brand. Shades of zirconia ceramics are produced by

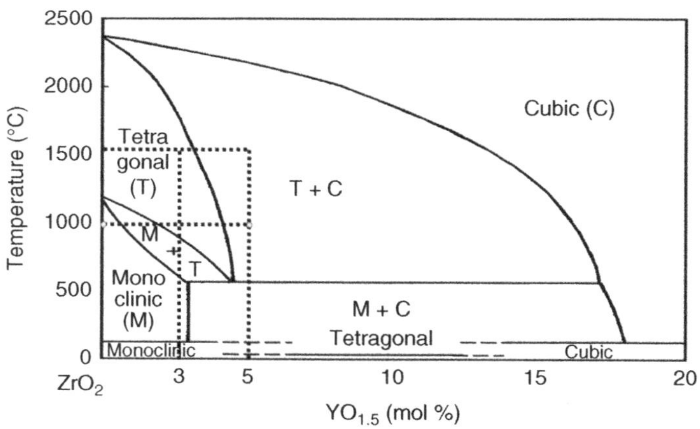

Figure 10.9 Binary phase diagram depicting phase relations of yttria-stabilized zirconia. Yttria, Y_2O_3, is denoted as YO1.5. The tetragonal phase regions are delineated with dashed lines for 3% and 5% yttria. When sintered between 1000 and 1500 °C, the dominant phases will be tetragonal (T) (~3% YO1.5) or predominantly tetragonal (T) with some cubic (F) crystals (~5% YO1.5). Adapted from (56).

blending the tetragonal zirconia powder with metal oxides such as Fe_2O_3, CeO_2, and Bi_2O_3 before firing. Alternatively, shading has been performed by dental laboratories by infiltration of the porous, partially sintered zirconia using metal salt solutions. The salts, such as cerium acetate, cerium chloride, or bismuth chloride, decompose to oxides during final sintering and add the desired tooth color.

Layered zirconia discs have been made to achieve a variation in the translucency of a crown from the gingival to the incisal edge. The manufacture of these layered blocks uses various formulas of Y-TZP from 3 to 7 mol% yttria, compressed on one another before partial sintering (21). The higher yttria layers are partially stabilized zirconia with a mixture of cubic and tetragonal zirconia crystals. See the larger grains in Figure 10.8b for 5% yttria-zirconia. Products with as many as four layers of graduated yttria contents and pigmentation are available that decrease in opacity and chroma from the cervical to the incisal edge. As with any ceramic forming technique, the powder size distribution, binders, and compaction pressure influence the integrity of the interface and must be developed by manufacturers to minimize defects and delamination. Manufacturing a perfect interface between the layers is critical to the strength of the sintered zirconia device. The incisal edge of layered zirconia is millin in the higher yttria, less opaque, but slightly weaker zirconia which is confounding to engineers who want the strongest material at the thinner, biting edge; alas, in dentistry, esthetics sometimes trumps durability. Importantly, zirconia bridge connectors should be designed and milled in the strongest (3Y-TZP) zirconia in these functionally graded disks; technicians must be aware of the thickness of the layers because they differ among the manufacturers. The variations in composition are subject to warpage during firing, so no deviations should be made from the manufacturer's firing instructions.

The ISO 18675 and ADA 131 standards have requirements for machinable blanks – ingot or disk-shaped materials from the manufacturer – as to the materials shrinkage, homogeneity, flexural strength, low temperature degradation, fatigue, thermal expansion, solubility, and radioactivity. The ISO 18675 document considers ceramic machinability more broadly than the ADA 131 standard, which is only for zirconia.

If a zirconia prosthetic is "tried in," it needs to be cleaned before the final cement application to ensure adhesion. Phosphoric acid, alcohol, and water rinsing are ineffective in removing saliva remnants on zirconia; see Chapter 12 on cleaning pediatric dental crowns; KOH or NaOH solutions help remove the adherent proteins as do some lanthana solutions. Sand-blasting of the intaglio of zirconia prosthetics is necessary before bonding, using 0.2–0.3 MPa pressure with 50–100 μm alumina grit for 5–10 seconds. Notably, when a zirconia surface is ground or sandblasted, some tetragonal to monoclinic transformation (transformation toughening) can occur, avoiding cracking. Zirconia restorations are secured on the teeth with a light-curing or dual-curing resin composite cement (Chapter 11).

Zirconia dental crowns and bridges are devilish to "adjust" in the mouth to perfect the occlusion and equally difficult to drill through if a root canal is needed to be performed. Occlusal adjustments are not easy, even with diamond instruments. Alumina polishing discs can help eliminate diamond scratches on zirconia. Ultrashort-pulse lasers and transient/selective lasers are used industrially to machine zirconia with high power (58) but have not been adopted for dentistry due to cost.

Tetragonal crystals of zirconia transform and expand, forming the monoclinic phase under external stress to inhibit crack propagation. This transformation toughening may be induced by grinding, sandblasting, or firing veneer porcelain. Expansion creates a compressive stress on the surface, which increases the flexural strength and fracture toughness. However, the monoclinic grains can be susceptible to being pulled out – creating surface roughness – and potentially forming a micro-crack. This degradation of strength, exacerbated by the presence of water and elevated temperature, is called low-temperature degradation (LTD); it is tested in an accelerated manner in a steam autoclave (~135 °C) for about 40 hours (59) per the method in the ISO 13356 standard. The transformation is more likely if the grains are larger, which depends on the stabilizer type and content and the microstructure created after sintering. Lower sintering temperatures and the presence of a minor amount of alumina decrease the susceptibility of 3Y-TZP to form monoclinic grains (59). Low-temperature degradation has been documented for zirconia in vitro, but significant low-temperature degradation has not been reported clinically or in simulations (57). Ceria-stabilized zirconia is less vulnerable to this strength degradation, but it is not as strong as yttria-stabilized tetragonal zirconia before aging.

As noted previously, zirconia powders inherently contain hafnia, and the hafnia has minimal radioactivity. The radioactivity of surgically implanted, yttria-stabilized zirconia is limited to 200 Bq/kg per the ISO 13356 standard, which is 20% of the amount allowed for porcelain enamel. One study reported the radioactivity of zirconia dental products to be 11–35 Bq/kg (60), well below the limit. Some patients want zirconia dental implants because they are allergic or averse to metals; they may not know about the radioactivity to consider versus the potential for elution of metal ions.

Hybrid Ceramic-Polymer Indirect Restorations

An alternative to high-strength and high-toughness zirconia is to include more flexible materials, achieved by combining ceramic powders with polymer for fixed prosthodontics; such combinations are hybrids available for CAD-CAM fabrication of indirect restorative devices. For such hybrids, either the resin is the matrix, or the ceramic is the matrix.

Some commercial materials use the resin as the matrix and rely on light, heat, and pressure to cure and strengthen a restoration. Clusters of nanoparticles 0.6–10 μm are part of the filler; the particles are well-dispersed, silane-coated, 20 nm silica particles, and 4–11 nm zirconia particles. These indirect composites are more highly cured, than the light-cure or self-cure direct composites (61) discussed in Chapter 9. Flexural strength of these hybrids is about 200 MPa with an elastic modulus more like teeth (11 versus 43 GPa) than, for instance, lithium disilicate. Their fracture toughness is up to 2 MPa-m$^{-1/2}$, and compressive strength about 370 MPa. Materials scientists don't accept these as ceramic restorations.

An alternative approach has been to infiltrate a partially sintered ceramic with resin, a polymer-infiltrated ceramic network (PICN), where the ceramic network is filled with a polymer to deflect cracks. US Pat. 5,843,348 describes a process to create a hybrid material ingot starting with a colloidal suspension of glass, alumina, zirconia, or porcelain powders. The green state of the ceramic is densified by centrifugal casting or other methods to remove the water from a colloidal suspension and form a powder compact. The disk is sintered to less than 1400 °C to achieve a stronger but porous powder compact by surface diffusion sintering. The porous ceramic is infused by the manufacturer with a silane solution, followed by soaking in a monomer liquid, which may include fumed silica. The ceramic/resin combination is then cured by light or heat (e.g., less than 75 °C, for less than 24 hours). Ingots or pucks of this composite may have a gradation of color to imitate dentin and enamel per US Pat. 11,622,918B2.

Some CAD-CAM blocks purport to be a combination of lithium disilicate and resin in an easier-to-mill material that is esthetic and can be repaired with composite (Directa Ceramir). The product information states that a laser sintering process is used, which may be partial sintering of ceramic particles, perhaps for reducing pores, but is not well described. The ceramic network for another brand of hybrid ceramic-polymer materials includes a silica-alumina glass that is infiltrated with a methacrylate resin – see Table 10.3 for the glass formula. The microstructure (Figure 10.10) shows about 70% glass with a minor amount of zirconia (62) and a minor amount of polymer. The reported flexural strengths are less than 200 MPa and fracture toughness of 1.5 MPa-m$^{-1/2}$ which is less than the lithium disilicate materials; such low strength and toughness limit the indications for these materials compared to zirconia or lithium disilicate.

The wear resistance (loss of gloss or chipping), the wear of the opposing teeth, adhesion, fatigue strength, and indications for use, such as limitations for anterior placement or not in bruxing patients (63), are important to consider for prescribing hybrid materials for restorations.

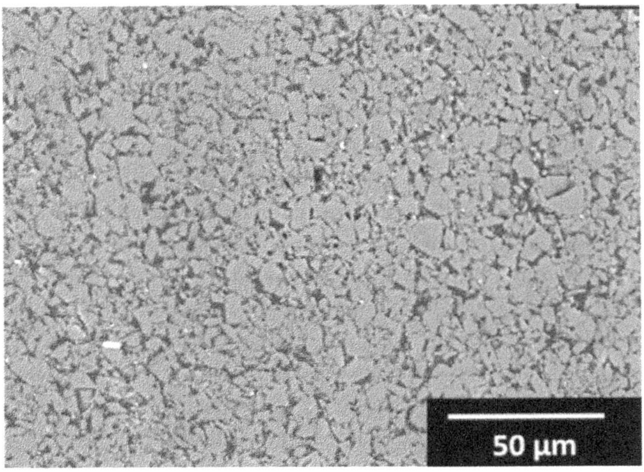

Figure 10.10 Polished microstructure of a polymer-infiltrated ceramic matrix (62) / with permission of Elsevier. Note the angularity of the particles without the necking seen in Figure 10.8a. The white spots are zirconia, and the dark interparticle area is the polymer; the medium gray is the glass.

Polymer-Veneered Metal Restorations

Another partial ceramic indirect restoration is composite veneering; this has been more popular outside the United States and can be more economical. Metal substructures were coated with polymers that were cured in a dental laboratory in layers; the coatings are subject to the requirements of ISO 10477/ADA 53 for polymer-based crown and bridge materials. These materials are included here because they are indirect restoratives, and the polymer coatings contain ceramic powders.

These veneering systems are modifications of composites used for direct restorations; heat and light curing are used, but the initiators have different wavelengths for activation. That is, UV light curing could be used because these devices are made extra-orally and then cemented intraorally. A thin opaque composite layer must be the first step, using a polymer that is more opaque (has more ceramic filler) than used in composite direct restorations, to mask the underlying metal. The anatomy is created by curing successive layers of polymers with ceramic powders, over the opaque layer, similarly to PFM restorations.

Several methods were developed to ensure adhesion of the polymer including retentive surface beads, mesh, and perforated metal. Surface treatment techniques for the metal were alumina sand-blasting, tin electroplating (to create a tin oxide surface), or etching. Composite veneering also required adhesives to bond the metal to the composite. The coatings included fluorinated alkyl methacrylate, SiO_x fume, or a silica/Cr solution, followed by a silane coating, and unidentified organic primer. Silane-coated alumina grains have also been used for sand-blasting the metal substructure (64, 65). After surface preparation, opaque composites were needed to cover the metals, which had more ceramic particles than conventional dental composites. Heat and light methods ensured curing of the opaque polymer layer, then more translucent esthetic polymers were similarly cured to create the anatomy. These polymer-veneered fixed prosthodontics are not as durable as PFM but have been a lower-cost alternative. Precious, non-precious, stainless steel, and even titanium substructures have been used for polymer veneering.

A unique use of composite veneering has been used to create esthetic crowns for primary teeth (Chapter 12). These pediatric crowns have a layered composite facial or buccal surface on stainless steel crowns as an esthetic alternative to plain stainless steel crowns and a lower-cost alternative to zirconia pediatric crowns. Unlike the customized crowns mentioned above, the manufacturer offers pre-made pediatric crows with an esthetic composite facing.

Tooth Preparation

Tooth structure, some dentin, enamel, and perhaps an older restoration, must be removed for fixed prosthodontics to be fitted. Dentists use instruments and abrasives to "prepare" the tooth/teeth (Chapter 17). Veneers only require removing about 0.4 mm of enamel on the facial side of the tooth because they are completely supported by the underlying tooth. Zirconia crowns require circumferential – 0.8 mm for crowns, and 1 mm for inlays and onlays, and extra if porcelain is to be applied over the zirconia. Lithium disilicate crowns require 1.0–1.5 mm tooth reduction, depending on the cement being used and the restoration. The shape of the margin for ceramic crowns should not be a knife edge, rough, or undercut, and the tooth preparation should not be "cylindrical," sharp, or grooved. Crown preparations for using ceramics should avoid point loading on the occlusal surface; that is, sharp cusps should be avoided because sharp edges create stress concentrations and possible fracture. If these contraindications are present, the risk of fracture is elevated. When a zirconia bridge is prescribed, the cross-sectional area between teeth should be more than 12 and 14 mm^2 for the anterior and posterior teeth, respectively; note that metal pontics need not be so large, which is a benefit of PFM bridges. The preparation guidelines vary among the possible indirect restorations, but every 0.1 mm removed of the tooth reduces the natural enamel and dentin protection of the pulp and roots. As mentioned before, while each dental intervention is performed to protect a tooth from further degradation, the risk for its ultimate demise and extraction also increases.

Impact of Ceramics on Indirect Restorations

Indirect, ceramic fixed prosthodontics have a long, important, and innovative history striving to meet the criteria in Table 10.5. Many ceramics have been tested, patented, and commercialized with the driving force to develop strong, durable, life-like restorations. The major ceramic systems for fixed prosthodontics have progressed from porcelain, glass-bonded alumina, alumina, magnesia, porcelain enamel on metal, glass-ceramics (especially lithium disilicate) to zirconia; the latter two are most commonly prescribed today.

Many systems of making ceramic copings have been used. Slip casting, glass casting, extrusion, powder pressing, and powder build-up techniques have been used before sintering. Tape-casting is not known to have been used, although tape-casting creates a flexible "green" ceramic that can be formed like 3D printing. The methods to make these restorations have often included the application of porcelain (glass/crystals) powders on metal or ceramic copings having formulas such as those listed in Table 10.3. The porcelain coatings for the stronger coping ceramics are silica-based (50–70% silica), often with boron oxide and always with other glass formers and modifiers (e.g., soda, potassia, lithia, alumina) to achieve compositions tailored in thermal expansion for the underlying coping.

Table 10.5 Characteristics Needed for Fixed Prosthetics.

Attribute	Desired trait
Esthetic	Tooth-like appearance, including color to match nearby teeth, with suitable translucency, opalescence, fluorescence
Biocompatible	Non-cytotoxic, non-irritating, and non-mutagenic (at a minimum)
Fracture resistance	Strong, with high fatigue strength, to avoid chipping or other fractures
Wear resistant	Resist erosion and abrasion from other teeth, other dental materials, and food, while not causing excessive wear of opposing dentition
Resistant to acids	Durable in common food acids such as vinegar
Adjustment of occlusion	Shape can be modified with dental abrasives, and polished as required in vivo
Marginal fit	Conforms to the tooth preparation (anatomy) within a few microns
Cementation	Easy to cement and preferably adhesive
Tooth reduction	Requires minimal tooth reduction (minimal thickness of restoration)
Easy to fabricate	Can be manufactured in dental laboratory, perhaps within a few hours for a one-appointment treatment
Cost	Affordable in 1st and 3rd world dental practices

Casting and ceramming of glass-ceramics, uniaxial hot-pressing of porcelains, and CAD-CAM milling of lithium disilicate and partially sintered tetragonal zirconia are more recent methods. The lithium disilicate base glasses vary in composition but always include more than 55% silica and at least 9% lithia and usually phosphorous pentoxide, zirconia and alumina and are composed of more than 50% crystals. Dental zirconia crowns are mostly 3 mol% yttria stabilized, although some materials contain slightly more yttria. The evolution of materials and methods is parallel to development of modern ceramics having higher strength; see Table 10.6 for comparisons of strength properties.

Table 10.6 Strengths and Toughness of Ceramic Crown Materials in approximate ascending strength.

Material or tradename	Approximate 3- or 4-point bending strength (MPa)	Fracture toughness ($MPa\text{-}m^{1/2}$)
Leucite porcelains	65–70, 80–100 (16)	
Higher leucite porcelains	90–120	
Dicor	45–101 (10), 150–180 (26)	0.94–2.1 (10)
Machinable Dicor	195–225 (26)	
Cerapearl	150–300 (28)	
Cerestore	170	1.4–1.94 (10)
Magnesia and forsterite, MagCor	125–140 (18)	
Glass-bonded alumina crowns	~380	
Empress II lithium disilicate	300–400	2.8–3.5 2.2–3.2 (66)
Other lithium disilicate materials (31)	210–420	1.4–2.5
Lithium disilicate, more crystallized	400–510 (33)	
In-ceram alumina	235–600	3.1–4.6
In-ceram zirconia	420–800	
Procera alumina	490–700	4.5–6.0
Zirconia (3Y-TZP)	900–1200	4–10

From Reference (19) / with permission of Elsevier, unless otherwise noted.

Metal substrates with porcelain enamel or composite coatings have also been used worldwide. Hybrid ceramic-polymer combinations are also available.

All-ceramic restorations require sufficient tooth removal for the required thickness of the crowns, bridges, and bridge connectors to resist fracture. Despite this need, yttria-stabilized zirconia has been the most successful ceramic for indirect restorations, including molar crowns and bridges, based on its strength, fracture toughness, and reasonable esthetics; lithium disilicate crowns are a close second. All-ceramic indirect restorations that mimic natural teeth can be realized today although improvements are certainly possible.

Ceramics in Chapter 10

The following ceramics and other inorganic materials were mentioned in this chapter. The ceramics for furnace construction, insulation, and heat treating feldspar are also mentioned generically:

- alumina
- alumina-zirconia
- aluminosilicates
  - of sodium, calcium, or potassium
- baria
- barium osumilite
- bismuth oxide
- boron oxide
- calcia
- calcium nitrate
- ceria
- cesium chloride, carbonate, sulfate, and phosphate salts
- chromium oxide
- cobalt oxide
- cordierite
- copper oxide
- feldspar
  - soda, calcia, or potassia based
  - nepheline syenite
  - sanidine
- fluoroapatite
- hafnia
- hydroxyapatite
- hydrofluoric acid

- iron oxide
- leucite
- lithia
- lithium disilicate
- lithium metasilicate
- lithium fluoride
- glass, Pyrex, Duran
- glass-ceramics
  - tetrasilicic fluoromica, Dicor & Macor
  - lithium disilicate
- iron oxide
- kaolin clay
- lanthana
- lithia
- lithium disilicate
- lithium metasilicate
- lithium phosphate
- leucite
- magnesia
- magnesia-alumina spinel
- magnesia with titania or zirconia
- magnesium fluoride
- magnesia silicate, forsterite
- manganese oxide
- mullite
- nickel oxide
- phosphorous pentoxide
- porcelain
  - with alumina crystals
  - with leucite crystals
- potassia
- potassium chloride, carbonate, nitrate, sulfate, and phosphate salts
- rubidium chloride, carbonate, sulfate, and phosphate salts
- silica: cristobalite, fumed amorphous silica, diatomaceous earth
- silica-alumina
- soda
- terbia
- tin oxide
- titania
- urania
- vanadia

- yttria
- zinc oxide
- zinc phosphate
- zirconia: tetragonal and partially stabilized (cubic and tetragonal)
  - magnesia and yttria-stabilized

References

1. Land, C.H. (1903). Porcelain dental art. *Dent Cosm* 45 (6): 437–444. and 615–20.
2. McLean, J.W., Hubbard, J.R., and Kedge, M.I. (1979). *The science and art of dental ceramics*, 344. Chicago: Quintessence Pub Co.
3. Burke, J.E. (2013). Lucalox alumina: the ceramic that revolutionized outdoor lighting. *MRS Bull* 21 (6): 61–68.
4. McLean, J.W. (2001). Evolution of dental ceramics in the twentieth century. *J Prosth Dent* 85 (1): 61–66.
5. Silva, N.R.F.A., Sailer, I., Zhang, Y. et al. (2010). Performance of zirconia for dental healthcare. *Materials* 3 (2): 863–896.
6. Al-Sanabani, F.A., Madfa, A.A., and Al-Qudaimi, N.H. (2014). Alumina ceramic for dental applications: a review article. *Am J Matl Res* 1 (1): 26–34.
7. Zheng, X., Sun, T., Zhou, J. et al. (2022). Modeling of polycrystalline material microstructure with 3D grain boundary based on laguerre-voronoi tessellation. *Materials (Basel)* 15 (6): 1–20.
8. Starling, L.B. (1985). Transfer molded “all ceramic crowns”: the cerestore system. *Ceram Eng Sci Proc* 41–56.
9. Drummond, J.L., Novickas, D., and Lenke, J.W. (1991). Physiological aging of an all-ceramic restorative material. *Dent Mater* 7 (2): 133–137.
10. Thompson, J.Y., Anusavice, K.J., Naman, A., and Morris, H.E. (1994). Fracture surface characterization of clinically failed all-ceramic crowns. *J Dent Res* 73 (12): 1824–1832.
11. Denry, I. and Holloway, J. (2010). Ceramics for dental applications: a review. *Materials* 3 (1): 351–368.
12. Seward, T.P. (1980). Coloration and optical anisotropy in silver-containing glasses. *J Non-Cryst Solids* 40 (1): 499–513.
13. Ruales-Carrera, E., Dal Bó, M., das Neves, W.F. et al. (2022). Chemical tempering of feldspathic porcelain for dentistry applications: a review. *Open Ceram* 9: 1–13.
14. Li, X.C., Lu, X.T., Bai, T. et al. (2024). Mechanical behavior and biological activity performance of Li+/Ca2+@Li+/K+ ion-exchanged lithium disilicate glass-ceramics. *Ceram Int* 50 (22): 47157–47171.
15. Haag, P. and Nilner, K. (2010). Bonding between titanium and dental porcelain: a systematic review. *Acta Odontol Scand* 68 (3): 154–164.

16 Naert, I. (2011). Materials in fixed prosthodontics for indirect dental restorations. In: *Comprehensive biomaterials* (ed. P. Ducheyne), 353–365. Oxford: Elsevier.

17 Shen, C., Rawls, H.R., and Esquivel-Upshaw, J.F. (2021). *Phillips' science of dental materials*, 13the, 448. Philadelphia: Elsevier, Inc.

18 O'Brien, W.J., Groh, C.L., Boenke, K.M. et al. (1993). The strengthening mechanism of a magnesia core ceramic. *Dent Mater* 9: 242–245.

19 Raigrodski, A.J. (2004). Contemporary materials and technologies for all-ceramic fixed partial dentures: a review of the literature. *J Prosthet Dent* 92 (6): 557–562.

20 Diego, A.A., Santos, C.D., Landim, K.T., and Elias, C.N. (2007). Characterization of ceramic powders used in the inCeram systems to fixed dental prosthesis. *Mater Res* 10 (1): 47–51.

21 Cesar, P.F., Miranda, R.B.P., Santos, K.F. et al. (2024). Recent advances in dental zirconia: 15 years of material and processing evolution. *Dent Mater* 40 (5): 824–836.

22 Adair, P.J. and Grossman, D.G. (1984). The castable ceramic crown. *Int J Period Restor Dent* 4 (2): 32–46.

23 Grossman, D.G. (1972). Machinable glass-ceramics based on tetrasilicic mica. *J Amer Cer Soc* 55 (9): 446–449.

24 Malament, K.A. and Grossman, D.G. (1987). The cast glass-ceramic restoration. *J Prosthet Dent* 57 (6): 674–683.

25 Grossman, D.G. (1988). The science of castable glass ceramics. In: *Proceedings of the fourth international symposium on ceramics perspectives in dental ceramics. Perspectives in dental ceramics* (ed. J.D. Preston), 117–133. Chicago, IL: Quintessence Publishing Co., Inc.

26 Fu, Q., Qin, F., Li, Y. et al. (2005). The study on strengthening of fluorophlogopite-based dental machinable ceramic. *Zhonghua Kou Qiang Yi Xue Za Zhi* 40 (1): 27–29.

27 Denry, I.L. and Rosenstiel, S.F. (1993). Flexural strength and fracture toughness of Dicor glass-ceramic after embedment modification. *J Dent Res* 72 (3): 572–576.

28 Nahara, Y., Sadamori, S., and Hamada, T. (1991). Clinical evaluation of castable apatite ceramic crowns. *J Prosthet Dent* 66 (6): 754–758.

29 Jiang, Y., Zhang, C., Xu, J. et al. (2024). An overview of dental glass–ceramics: from material design to the manufacturing process. *Int J Ceram Eng Sci* 6 (4): 1–19.

30 Al-Thobity, A.M. and Alsalman, A. (2021). Flexural properties of three lithium disilicate materials: an in vitro evaluation. *Saudi Dent J* 33 (7): 620–627.

31 Vallerini, B.F., Pinelli, L.A.P., Silva, L.D. et al. (2025). Assessment of the chemical solubility of experimental and commercial lithium silicate glass-ceramics. *Dent Mater* 41 (3): e8–e17.

32 Lohbauer, U., Fabris, D.C.N., Lubauer, J. et al. (2024). Glass science behind lithium silicate glass-ceramics. *Dent Mater* 40 (5): 842–857.

33 Kaur, K., Talibi, M., and Parmar, H. (2022). Do you know your ceramics? Part 3: lithium disilicate. *Br Dent J* 232 (3): 147–150.

34 Höland, W., Greenwood, G.W., Greer, A.L. et al. (1804). Control of nucleation in glass ceramics. *Philos Trans R Soc London, Ser A* 2003 (361): 575–589.

35 Abad-Coronel, C., Ordonez Balladares, A., Fajardo, J.I., and Martin Biedma, B.J. (2021). Resistance to fracture of lithium disilicate feldspathic restorations manufactured using a CAD/CAM system and crystallized with different thermal units and programs. *Materials (Basel)* 14 (12): 1–9.

36 Zarone, F., Di Mauro, M.I., Ausiello, P. et al. (2019). Current status on lithium disilicate and zirconia: a narrative review. *BMC Oral Health* 19 (1): 1–14.

37 Fu, L., Engqvist, H., and Xia, W. (2020). Glass-ceramics in dentistry: a review. *Materials (Basel)* 13 (5).

38 Su, G., Zhang, Y., Jin, C. et al. (2023). 3D printed zirconia used as dental materials: a critical review. *J Biol Eng* 17 (1): 1–19.

39 Zhang, F., Spies, B.C., Willems, E. et al. (2022). 3D printed zirconia dental implants with integrated directional surface pores combine mechanical strength with favorable osteoblast response. *Acta Biomater.*

40 Ebert, J., Ozkol, E., Zeichner, A. et al. (2009). Direct inkjet printing of dental prostheses made of zirconia. *J Dent Res* 88 (7): 673–676.

41 Marsico, C., Carpenter, I., Kutsch, J. et al. (2022). Additive manufacturing of lithium disilicate glass-ceramic by vat polymerization for dental appliances. *Dent Mater* 38 (12): 2030–2040.

42 Kim, Y.-S., Kim, Y.-R., Kang, J.-H. et al. (2023). Ceramic 3D printing using lithium silicate prepared by sol-gel method for customizing dental prosthesis with optimal translucency. *Ceram Int* 49 (24): 39788–39799.

43 Zhang, N.-Z., Wang, C., Ran, T.-F. et al. (2024). Intervertebral osteointegration and biomechanical performance of bioactive lithium disilicate glass-ceramic scaffold fabricated by digital light processing. *Ceram Int* 50 (24): 53674–53684.

44 Binobaid, A., De Lisi, M., Camilleri, J. et al. (2025). Zirconia-calcium silicate bioactive composites for dental applications using DLP additive manufacturing. *Bioprinting* 45.

45 Lawson, N.C., Frazier, K., Bedran-Russo, A.K. et al. (2021). Zirconia restorations: an american dental association clinical evaluators panel survey. *J Am Dent Assoc* 152 (1): 80–81. e2.

46 Ioannidis, A., Bomze, D., Hammerle, C.H.F. et al. (2020). Load-bearing capacity of CAD/CAM 3D-printed zirconia, CAD/CAM milled zirconia, and heat-pressed lithium disilicate ultra-thin occlusal veneers on molars. *Dent Mater* 36 (4): e109–e116.

47 Sundh, A. and Sjogren, G. (2006). Fracture resistance of all-ceramic zirconia bridges with differing phase stabilizers and quality of sintering. *Dent Mater* 22 (8): 778–784.

48 Denry, I. and Kelly, J.R. (2008). State of the art of zirconia for dental applications. *Dent Mater* 24 (3): 299–307.

49 Zhang, Y. and Lawn, B.R. (2019). Evaluating dental zirconia. *Dent Mater* 35 (1): 15–23.

50 Tabatabaian, F. (2019). Color aspect of monolithic zirconia restorations: a review of the literature. *J PORCN* 28 (3): 276–287.

51 Kocjan, A. and Shen, Z. (2013). Colloidal processing and partial sintering of high-performance porous zirconia nanoceramics with hierarchical heterogeneities. *J Eur Ceram Soc* 33 (15–16): 3165–3176.

52 De Aza, P.N., De Aza, A.H., and De Aza, S. (2005). Crystalline bioceramic materials. *Bol Soc Esp Ceram* 44 (3): 135–145.

53 Cho, M.H. and Seol, H.J. (2022). Optical properties, microstructure, and phase fraction of multi-layered monolithic zirconia with and without yttria-gradient. *Materials (Basel)* 16 (1): 41–54.

54 Swain, M.V. (2009). Unstable cracking (chipping) of veneering porcelain on all-ceramic dental crowns and fixed partial dentures. *Acta Biomater* 5 (5): 1668–1677.

55 Talibi, M., Kaur, K., and Parmar, H. (2022). Do you know your ceramics? Part 5: zirconia. *Br Dent J* 232 (5): 311–316.

56 Witz, G., Shklover, V., Steurer, W. et al. (2007). Phase evolution in yttria-stabilized zirconia thermal barrier coatings studied by rietveld refinement of X-ray powder diffraction patterns. *J Amer Ceram Soc* 90 (9): 2935–2940.

57 Spies, B.C., Zhang, F., Wesemann, C. et al. (2020). Reliability and aging behavior of three different zirconia grades used for monolithic four-unit fixed dental prostheses. *Dent Mater* 36 (11): e329–e339.

58 Zhang, Y., Wei, C., Fukui, T. et al. (2024). Ultrafast processing of zirconia ceramics by transient and selective laser absorption. *Ceram Int* 50 (14): 25273–25281.

59 Zhang, F., Vanmeensel, K., Inokoshi, M. et al. (2014). 3Y-TZP ceramics with improved hydrothermal degradation resistance and fracture toughness. *J Eur Ceram Soc* 34 (10): 2453–2463.

60 Brizuela-Velasco, A., Chento-Valiente, Y., Chavarri-Prado, D. et al. (2021). Zirconia and radioactivity: an in vitro study to establish the presence of radionuclides in dental zirconia. *J Prosthet Dent* 126 (1): 115–118.

61 Horvath, S.D. (2016). Key parameters of hybrid materials for CAD/CAM-based restorative dentistry. *Compendium* 37 (9): 1–6.

62 Della Bona, A., Corazza, P.H., and Zhang, Y. (2014). Characterization of a polymer-infiltrated ceramic-network material. *Dent Mater* 30 (5): 564–569.

63 Miura, S. and Fujisawa, M. (2020). Current status and perspective of CAD/CAM-produced resin composite crowns: a review of clinical effectiveness. *Jpn Dent Sci Rev* 56 (1): 184–189.

64 Al-Azar, I.C., Girish, M.S., Devraj, I.M. et al. (2024). An in-vitro evaluation of tooth discoloration and shear bond strength of glass ionomer cement bonded to tooth surface pretreated with silver diamine fluoride and glutathione biomolecule. *Niger J Clin Pract* 27 (11): 1322–1328.

65 Chou, Y.F., Maciel Pires, P., Alambiaga-Caravaca, A.M. et al. (2024). Remineralisation of mineral-deficient dentine induced by experimental ion-releasing materials in combination with a biomimetic dual-analogue primer. *J Dent* 152: 105468.

66 Kelly, J.R. (2016). *Ceramics in dentistry: principles and practice*, 117. Hanover Park, IL: Quintessence Publishing Co, Inc.

11

Cements and Adhesives

Dental cements and adhesives are interfacial "glues" for the dental practitioner to bond a material to teeth, whether it is polymeric, ceramic, or metal. Dental adhesives and cements are critical to the successful placement and retention of direct and indirect restoratives in modern dentistry to prevent secondary caries, with minimal tooth removal. The overall goal for dental adhesives and cements is to maximize bond strength and durability while minimizing postoperative sensitivity and pain for the patient.

The terms for attaching items in dentistry are confusing. Herein, these definitions are used.

- Bonding or Adhesion – joining a material or other device to a tooth
  - Luting is used to describe mechanical, nonchemical bonding/adhesion
- Cementing – using a material to bond one item or another or to a tooth
  - May be chemical or mechanical
  - Cements are the paste used to bond
  - Dental cements may have many compositions as described herein
  - Cement is also used to denote water-setting calcium silicate/aluminate powders
- Adhesive
  - Chemical bonding

Cementing techniques connect a device, such as a filling or a crown, to a tooth, which may be a single or multi-step procedure to create a mechanical or chemical bond or both. Mechanical adhesion has been denoted as "luting," a word derived from the Latin word for mud and was applied to the earlier cements where the roughness and friction of two interfaces were sufficient to retain a crown on a tooth. Chemical mechanisms create molecular bonds at the interface. Cements

Ceramics in Dentistry: Materials, Manufacturing, and Clinical Applications,
First Edition. Carolyn M. Primus.

that connect a device to a tooth, e.g. a crown or bridge, are usually present in a layer thinner than 25 μm.

Wax was a historical and ineffective cement for temporary attachment. Modern dental cements should be long-lasting; even orthodontic cements need to keep a bracket or band in place for months to years. To achieve long-term satisfaction, the cements must fulfill this list of attributes: be biocompatible, avoid tooth irritation, have dimensional stability with hot or cold food, remain adhesive under oral stresses, have low solubility in oral fluids (including food), a viscosity suitable to form a low enough film thickness, have easy application including removal of excess cement, wettability on the tooth (low contact angle), prevent bacterial infiltration to the underlying tooth, have high tensile, compressive, and fatigue strength, result in an esthetic appearance, resist discoloration over time – plus, have some chemical bonding to the tooth and restorative device. Antimicrobial activity is also desirable. The selection of a suitable cement for a case is based on understanding these features of cement.

This chapter describes the zinc oxide, glass ionomer, and resin cements/adhesives. Ceramic powders have been necessary for all of these cements. The ISO 9917-1/ADA 96 and ISO 3107/ADA 30 standards have requirements for the glass ionomer and zinc oxide cements, which are shown in Table 11.1. The zinc oxide-based cements and the glass ionomer cements have similar requirements for film thickness (<25 μm), setting time (1.5–10 minutes), and low acid erosion and include freedom from arsenic or lead. The latter requirements for metallic purity seem to be a historical reference from the early 20th century zinc oxides or chlorides that were considered to be of questionable purity (1), perhaps containing lead or arsenic. The requirements for compressive strength are low (>5 MPa).

Table 11.1 ISO 9917-1 and ISO 3107 requirements for cements for indirect restorations.

Cement type	Max. film thickness (μm)	Min. setting time (min.)	Max. setting time (min.)	Min. compressive strength (MPa)	Max. acid erosion (mm)	Max. acid-soluble as content (ppm)	Max. acid-soluble Pb content (ppm)
ZnO phosphate	25	2.5	8	8	50	2	100
ZnO polycarboxylate	25	2.5	8	8	50	2	100
ZnO-eugenol	25	1.5	10	5, <35	NR	2	NR
Glass ionomer	25	1.0	8	8	50	2	100

NR = no requirement.

No separate standards exist for the resin-based cements apart from ISO 4049 discussed in Chapter 9.

Testing bonding/adhesion or strength is always a cement topic, as discussed in ISO 11405 and ADA 111 documents. The stress on the bond may be tensile, shear, or a combination of the two. No laboratory or clinical tests are valid for all the various clinical applications of cements; however, the relative performance of materials is often compared in the dental literature. While laboratory bond test results may not predict clinical behavior, tensile and shear bond tests have been used to compare adhesive materials.

Zinc Oxide Cements

Four formulas of dental cement have been based on zinc oxide (ZnO) powder; each has played a significant role in dentistry: zinc oxide-eugenol (ZOE) (>1858), zinc oxide-oxychloride (>1860), zinc oxide-phosphate (>1879) (2), and zinc oxide-polycarboxylate (>1968). These cements were very significant advancements in their time, by mixing fine white zinc oxide powder with a liquid – eugenol, zinc chloride, phosphoric acid, or carboxylate solutions, respectively. Zinc oxychloride cement (Eq. (5.11)) was used as a temporary filling material but was found to have high solubility, making it less successful. ZOE cement remains popular for its broad uses in temporary restorations or as a temporary cement, and as a root canal sealing material (Chapter 8). The phosphate and carboxylate ZnO cements were popular in the 20th century and merit description although these two cements are now passé but remain available and inexpensive compared to resin cements.

Zinc phosphate cement was the standard in the early 20th century for cementing metal crowns on teeth because of its fast setting and good strength. The zinc oxide powder was mixed with a potent phosphoric acid (39–59%) solution, which formed hopeite (hydrated zinc phosphate, $Zn_3[PO_4]_2.4H_2O$, refer to Eq. (5.13)) as a matrix with embedded unreacted ZnO particles. The reaction is fast and exothermic. Manufacturers sintered zinc oxide with magnesia and then ground them into a powder (3) for blending with radiopaque powders. Some products contained 2–3% aluminum phosphate, which slows the reaction by creating an amorphous aluminum phosphate ($AlPO_4.nH_2O$) on the zinc oxide particles, with concomitant formation of some zinc aluminophosphate ($Zn_{0.06}Al_{0.94}PO_4$) (4), for a harder cement. Other fillers have included anhydrous silicic acid, hydrous silicic acid, aluminum oxide, titanium oxide, calcia zirconia, magnesia, aluminum hydroxide, calcium hydroxide, magnesium hydroxide, aluminum silicates (Al_2SiO_5-type clays), calcium silicate (wollastonite), zirconium silicate, magnesium silicate, and barium sulfate (US Pat. 4,773,933). "Red copper" cements were based on zinc oxide with about 24% copper oxide (cuprous oxide, Cu_2O) in the powder (5). Silver salts were also used in some products in the unsubstantiated hope that the Zn-phosphate cement would be antimicrobial.

Zinc phosphate cement is nonadhesive but was widely used to cement (affix) inlays, crowns, and bridges, and as a base under deep cavities by providing thermal insulation to protect the pulp. Its exothermic setting reaction could damage the pulp; therefore, clinical experience and training for the dentist and assistant were needed to mix the cement and control the reaction temperature and rate (3, 6). Mixing small portions helps control the heat of the cement, as does using a cool glass slab, which needs to be kept above the ambient dew point to prevent condensation moisture from diluting the phosphoric acid concentration. A prosthesis should be seated quickly before the zinc phosphate cement's matrix forms, and should be held under pressure, keeping the area (field) as dry as possible until the cement initially sets; then excess cement can be removed. A lower powder-to-liquid ratio (more liquid) is useful when a longer working time is needed because it creates a slightly thinner mix for cementing a bridge; however, the lower powder-to-liquid ratio is more acidic and a hazard. A layer of varnish or other nonpermeable coating applied at the margin helps prevent dissolution of the cement in oral fluids before the complete setting. Land (7) devised a method of coating zinc oxychloride and orthophosphate on the intaglio of porcelain restorations before cementing with zinc phosphate to enhance adhesion with zinc phosphate cements. Such practical approaches are important to clinical success. Resin cements have superseded the use of zinc phosphate cement for crowns and bridges.

Zinc oxide-carboxylate (polycarboxylate) cements are an alternative cement to zinc phosphate for fixed prosthodontics and have a chemical bond to teeth. Polycarboxylate cements are also powder–liquid products where zinc oxide is mixed by the dentist with a water-based liquid solution of 32–42 weight percent of acrylic acids, such as polyacrylic acid or itaconic acid, with molecular weights from 30,000 to 50,000. The zinc oxide powder is often blended with magnesia, tin oxide, and bismuth oxide (MgO, SnO_2, Bi_2O_3). Stannous fluoride (Tin[II] fluoride, SnF_2) is present in some cement brands to slow the setting time, raise the strength, and enhance the manipulative properties. This cement is more viscous than zinc phosphate cement, but vibration after mixing can be used to ensure the film thickness is less than 25 μm, as required in ISO 9917-1. Thinner (less powder) mixtures reduce the cement's compressive strength, which is slightly less than that of zinc phosphate cement. See Table 11.2 for comparisons of cement properties.

The setting reaction of the zinc polycarboxylate is similar to that of zinc phosphate cement, beginning with the dissolution of the ZnO powder particles. The powder releases zinc, magnesium, and tin ions that bind and crosslink the acrylic acid carboxyl groups, forming an amorphous polycarboxylate matrix phase and encapsulating the unreacted portion of the particles. The working time for

Table 11.2 Comparisons of cements for fixed prosthodontics.

Cement type	Compressive strength (MPa)	Elastic modulus (GPa)	Solubility	Pulp irritation	Microleakage	Esthetics
ZnO phosphate	48–133	20	High	Medium	High	Low
ZnO polycarboxylate	57–99	16–19	High	Low	High	Low
Zinc oxide eugenol	8 (8)	7.6	Medium	High	Medium	Medium
Glass ionomer	93–226	3.5–10 (9), 11	Low	Medium	Low	Low
RMGIC	85–126	1.6	Very low	Medium high	Very low	Medium
Resin	52–224	12–16	Very low	Medium high	Very low	High

Source: (10) / MDPI / CC BY 4.0.

polycarboxylate cement is much shorter than that for zinc phosphate cement, approximately 2.5 versus 5 min. A cool slab for mixing lengthens the working time for zinc carboxylate cement but thickens the polyacrylic acid, which hinders mixing; the slab should not be colder than the dew point, thus avoiding water condensation. Refrigerating the powder is helpful because it retards the setting reaction without raising the viscosity of the liquid. Rapid spatulation reduces the viscosity of the polycarboxylate cement so that a suitably thin cement film can be created, as needed, to affix a crown or bridge. During setting, the polycarboxylate cement passes through a rubbery stage. Excess cement should not be removed while the cement is rubbery because some of the cement may be pulled out from beneath the margins, leaving a void; excess cement can be removed when the prosthesis is fully seated or when the cement becomes hard.

The polycarboxylate cements are known to have excellent biocompatibility and lack of postoperative sensitivity. They are mainly used for crowns, or for long-term, but temporary cementation. The outstanding characteristics of polycarboxylate cements are their chemical bond (chelation) of the polyacrylic acid and calcium ions on the surface of enamel or dentin, minimal pulp irritation, and reduced penetration of the irritating acid into the dentinal tubules due to the larger size of the polyacrylic acid molecules compared with phosphoric acid. Its adhesive qualities are beneficial in thermal cycling the polycarboxylate cements, unlike the zinc phosphate cements, that lose their retentiveness. However, early washout (dissolution of the ZnO-carboxylate cement) has caused loss of retention, from either too thick or improperly mixed cement. The ZnO-carboxylate cements and the silicate restoratives were the foundation for glass-ionomer developments as can be discerned by the formula similarities.

Despite the adhesion of the cement to tooth structure, polycarboxylate cements are not superior to zinc phosphate cement in the retention of metal prosthetics. Polycarboxylate cements fail at the cement–metal interface; zinc phosphate cements fail at the cement/tooth interface. Polycarboxylate cement failure may be related to its higher shrinkage versus zinc phosphate cements. Neither zinc polycarboxylate nor zinc phosphate cement is used for restorative purposes because the cements are opaque. Furthermore, zinc oxide cements with phosphoric acid or carboxylic solutions are subject to long-term acid dissolution in the oral cavity, unlike the resin cements described later in this chapter.

ZOE cements are multi-purpose because of their neutral pH; it has been used as a temporary filling, impression material, a periodontal dressing, and a low-cost root canal sealer. Here, its use is discussed for a crown cement. ZOE hardens when the zinc oxide powder and eugenol liquid are mixed; the setting reaction starts when water in the eugenol solution begins hydrolyzing the zinc oxide to form zinc hydroxide, which chelates with eugenol to harden. The setting reaction is slower than zinc phosphate, but zinc acetate dihydrate ($Zn(CH_3COO)_2(H_2O)_2$) in the powder accelerates the setting reaction; the acetate is more soluble than zinc oxide or hydroxide. Acetic acid (CH_3COOH) in the eugenol solution also accelerates the dissolution of the zinc oxide particles. Other powder additives may be wax, kaolin, talc, diatomaceous earth, or zinc stearate ($Al_2O_3.2SiO_2.2H_2O$, $Mg_3Si_4O_{10}[OH]_2$, SiO_2, or $C_{36}H_{70}O_4Zn$). Canada balsam resin was part of some liquid formulas to increase flow and improve mixing properties.

The versatility of ZOE cement is reflected in the ADA 30/ISO 3107 standards, which list two types of ZOE cement by clinical application: temporary cementation, and for base or temporary restorations. ZOE cement requirements are presented in Table 11.1. The ZOE luting cements for fixed prosthetics have high film thicknesses and excess cement removal is difficult. ZOE cements have a lower compressive strength than other zinc oxide cements. Although not listed in ISO 3107, the ZOE cements have also been used as impression materials, as noted in Chapter 14.

Resin-bonded composites or resin restoratives are not placed over a ZOE base because residual, unreacted eugenol is believed to interfere with the proper setting of polymeric materials. To avoid this incompatibility, other carboxylic acids have been used instead of eugenol to produce a similar material, known as zinc oxide non-eugenol cements. Zinc oxide's antimicrobial attribute is a benefit in all these ZnO-based cements compared to glass-ionomer cements or resin composites.

Glass Ionomer Cements

The Type I glass ionomer cement (GIC) cements to attach a device to a tooth are mixed with a lower powder-to-liquid ratio (more liquid) than the glass ionomer restoratives (GIs) of Chapter 9. GICs are weaker but have better handling properties for cementing, than GI restoratives. For instance, one product line of GIC changes the powder-to-liquid ratio changes from 3.6 to 1.2 for restoratives for cementing of crowns, bridges, inlays, or onlays. Other low-viscosity mixtures of glass ionomers are placed on the occlusal surface of primary and immature permanent teeth as pit and fissure sealants to cover the anatomical crevices where caries often start. The GICs are also used for cementing orthodontic devices, such as bands or brackets to teeth. Their removal is facilitated by drying, as noted before. The fluoride release of glass ionomer cements is beneficial for preventing caries around the orthodontic devices or crowns.

Resin-modified glass ionomer materials have also been formulated for cementing crowns. The resin-containing GICs may require an adhesive "conditioner" to bond to the tooth surface before their placement. One GIC cement combines calcium aluminate cement with a glass ionomer to attach crowns and has been used with success (11).

Adhesively Bonding Direct Resin Composite Restoratives and Fixed Prosthodontics

The 1950s ushered in the modern era of dentistry with acid etching and acrylic resin restoratives initiated by Buonocore and Hagger (12). The goal for the new resin restorative materials was to perform like dentin and enamel, distributing stresses to avoid breakage and loss of adhesion of crowns. Resins reduced the need for creating retentive features – dovetails, grooves, undercuts, and sharp internal angles – during the preparation of teeth and started the "conservative dentistry" movement focused on less tooth removal. Unlike glass ionomers, resin composites are non-adherent to the tooth structure; therefore, a bonding system was needed to intimately attach direct resin restorations to dentin and enamel. Bonding systems for the direct resin composites spawned the resin cements designed for fixed prosthodontics, including ceramic crowns.

Current adhesive resin monomers include organophosphates such as MDP (10-methacryloyloxydecyl dihydrogen phosphate), organo-phosphonates, hydroxyethyl methacrylate (HEMA), and/or 4-methacryloxyethyl trimellitate anhydride (4-META). Polymerization of resin cement with these monomers may be initiated by light curing, chemical curing, or dual curing (both light and chemical initiators). Light-cured cements are suitable for bonding veneers, and dual-cure cements are useful for dark-shade and opaque restorations.

Adhesives Systems for Direct Resin Composites

Direct resin composites are bonded to etched enamel which has a rough surface. The first successful adhesive system for composite resins required three liquids applied in three steps, denoted as the "total etch" technique. The first step was to etch enamel with 33–37% phosphoric acid for a few seconds. Etching dissolves surface debris and the tips of enamel crystals, creating a rough surface that can be wet by acrylic resins. Phosphoric acid etchants are formulated as gels for intraoral use to ensure local application of the acid on the teeth and not the tender mucosa. Adhesion to etched dentin is more complicated because phosphoric acid dissolves the hydroxyapatite, leaving exposed collagen fibrils and open dentinal tubules. The second total-etch step is to apply a "primer" resin monomer (2-hydroxyethyl-methacrylate) dissolved in a solvent (water, acetone, or alcohol) to interlock with the enamel. On dentin, this primer diffuses and wets the collagen fibrils, creating the "hybrid layer" up to 10-μm deep for good bonding. Primer is gently dried with the clinician's air gun to evaporate the solvent but not displace the resin. The third step is the application of an "adhesive." The adhesive contains methacrylate resin, light-sensitive initiators, and 20–50% ceramic filler (usually fumed silica); it requires light-curing. After curing, the direct composite is applied and cured. The adhesive is bonded to the primer and to the direct resin composite. Descriptions of the adhesive monomers are clarified in reference (13).

Later bonding systems used an etchant and a primer/adhesive; the latter contains less ceramic filler, 3–10%. Later, an etchant was combined with a primer, and a separate adhesive was created the latter containing 20–50% filler. Recently, single-component, self-etching adhesives have been introduced that contain less than10% ceramic filler. Self-etching adhesives contain an acid, replacing phophoric, and with its other monomeric components, as a single step bond.

The dental bonding systems can be classified as "etch & rinse" (total etch) and "self-etch." Recent self-etch adhesives have been called "universal" adhesives with broader applicability and usage indications; these products include mild organic acids that do not completely expose collagen or dentinal tubules but are similar to the other self-etch adhesives. Universal adhesives rely on the ionic bonding of acidic monomers and the calcium in the hydroxyapatite of teeth; they adhere to zirconia, metals, ceramics, and polymers because they contain phosphate monomers and silane molecules. The universal adhesives can be used to add/augment composite to indirect restorations such as ceramic crowns, porcelain-fused-to-metal crowns, or amalgam; there indications are in addition to bonding composite resin direct restoratives to the tooth.

Resin Cements for Indirect Restorations

Resin cements for indirect restorations are divided into "adhesive cements" – a resin cement that requires a separate adhesive – and "self-adhesive cements" that do not need an additional component (10). Resin cements of either type are mixtures of monomers with hydrophilic groups (to wet a tooth's hydroxyapatite) and hydrophobic groups for polymerization with the restorative material. The adhesive cements contain curing initiators, inhibitors, or stabilizers, and in some products, inorganic fillers. Self-adhesive resin cements also contain acidic monomers to improve the bond strength to the tooth structure. Like resin composite restoratives, the monomers of these cements are never completely converted to polymers. The components of the adhesive resin cements are discussed in ISO technical specification 16,506, which contains bonding strength test methods for adhesive polymer-based materials for bonding to dentine. Resin cements may be mechanically, hand, or auto-tip mixed for self-curing or light curing to affix inlays, onlays, veneers, posts, crowns, and bridges.

The low solubility; higher compressive, flexural, and fatigue strengths; lower thermal expansion; higher hardness; and better wear resistance, especially the adhesive cements, are superior to the zinc oxide and GIC cements discussed above. Importantly, the resin cements have a lower elastic modulus than earlier cements; the absorption of stress is key to avoiding fracture of all-ceramic restorations such as Dicor, Cerestore and ceramic veneers (Chapter 10). The benefits of these properties are more secure retention of fixed prosthodontics and fewer cases of marginal degradation. Resin cements are suitable for affixing restorations of metal or porcelain-fused-to-metal ceramics, including veneers, indirect composites, implant-supported crowns and bridges, and endodontic posts placed in a root. Shades of cement are needed for cementing translucent veneers for the facial side of anterior teeth for esthetic results. Low-viscosity resin cements are also used as pit and fissure sealants placed on the occlusal surface of primary and immature permanent teeth, like the glass ionomer cements, to cover crevices where caries begin. The polymeric pit and fissure sealant materials are standardized under ISO 6874/ADA39 documents for self-curing and light-curable materials.

Ceramic Fillers in Resin Adhesives and Resin Cements

Resin bonding cements contain less ceramic (inorganic) filler powder than composite restoratives; cement require a low film thickness. The lower filler contents are concomitant with lower viscosity and strength compared to resin composite restorative materials. Ceramic fillers in bonding systems have included colloidal or fumed silica (SiO_2), baria-alumino-borosilicate glass, barium alumino-silicate

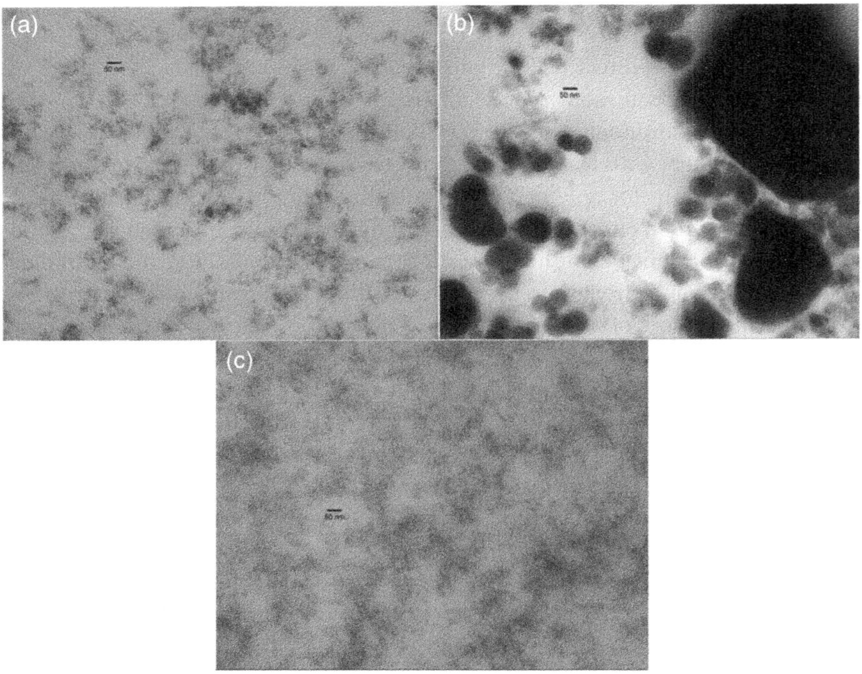

Figure 11.1 TEM images of adhesives containing (a) fumed silica; (b) microhybrid particles and (c) nanoparticle filler particles. *Source:* Courtesy of Solventum Company.

glass, fluoroalumino-silicate glass, and sodium fluorosilicate (Na_2SiF_6) (13), which are preferably nano-sized (<0.1 μm) and silanated. Hybrid metal oxides, fumed silica, and nanoparticle fillers have improved the bond strengths. The hybrid oxides may include alumina, titania, zirconia, and hydroxyapatite. Radiopaque ceramic fillers (baria or strontia containing glass, or zirconia) have been included to enable the dental practitioner to distinguish between a thick "pooled" adhesive, a gap, or a carious lesion in an X-ray. Fumed silica is used to increase the viscosity of the bonding liquids to facilitate their local application on a tooth using a tiny brush. See Figure 11.1 for TEM micrographs of fumed silica, microhybrid glass particles, and nanoparticles. The nanoparticle bonding materials have been known to penetrate up to 10 μm deep into the dentin tubules to perhaps assist with adhesion. Problems with adhesives have included aggregation and settling of the filler particles in the bottle although nanoparticles do not settle out of solution. Brownian motion, rather than gravitational forces, governs the motion of nanoparticles, which keeps them in suspension.

Summary of Adhesives and Cements

A dentist's armamentarium for bonding must be stocked with multiple cementing systems because one adhesive or cement product can be used for every case. The resin composite bonding systems, the resin cements, glass ionomer cements, and a temporary cement are necessary so that a suitable choice can be made based on the needs of a case. Earlier cements were based on zinc oxide powders but were not as elastic as resin cements, hindering the longevity of stiff, all-ceramic restorations.

Before cementation of indirect restorations, a clinician must follow the manufacturer's surface treatment protocol for the substrate and the restoration. The manufacturer's instructions are important to follow for creating the thin cement layer thickness to ensure the long-term success of a restoration. The type, shade, and thickness of cements contribute to a final restoration's esthetics. Many similarities exist between the direct resins composites and the resin bonding systems, including the ceramic fillers and they both rely on chemical adhesion. Ceramic powders and modern monomers have evolved together to create successful, durable, esthetic cements. Ceramic powders have been important for every type of dental cement from zinc oxide-based to glass ionomers, and resins.

Ceramics in Chapter 11

The following ceramics or inorganic materials were mentioned in this chapter:

- alumina
- aluminum phosphate
- bismuth oxide
- hydroxyapatite
- kaolin clay
- magnesia
- phosphoric acid
- silica
  - diatomaceous earth
  - fumed
- baria-alumino-borosilicate glass
- fluoroalumino-silicate glass
- stannous fluoride
- talc
- tin oxide

- titania
- zinc chloride
- zinc oxide
- zinc stearate
- zirconia

References

1 AlRughaib, M.B., Marafi, A.A., and Gutmann, J.L. (2024). Historical perspectives and comparisons on the use plastic-based cements in endodontics and prosthodontics: part 2 – oxyphosphates. *J. Hist. Dent.* 72 (2): 139–146.

2 Mahant, R., Agrawal, S., Kapoor, S., and Agrawal, I. (2017). Milestones of dental history. *CHRISMED J Health Res.* 4 (4): 229–234.

3 Shen, C., Rawls, H.R., and Esquivel-Upshaw, J.F. (2021). *Phillips' Science of Dental Materials*, 13the, 448. Philadelphia: Elsevier, Inc.

4 Jabri, M., Mejdoubi, E., El Gadi, M., and Hammouti, B. (2012). Optimisation of hardness and setting time of dental zinc phosphate cement using a design of experiments. *Arab. J. Chem.* 5 (3): 347–351.

5 American Dental Association (1974). *Guide to dental materials and devices*, 7the, 297. Chicago: American Dental Association.

6 O'Brien, W.J. (2008). *Dental materials and their selection*, 4the, 425. Hanover Park, IL: Quintessence Pub. Co.

7 Land, C.H. (1903). Porcelain dental art. *Dent Cosm.* 45 (6): 437–444. and 615–20.

8 Hamdy, T.M. (2024). Evaluation of compressive strength, microhardness and solubility of zinc-oxide eugenol cement reinforced with E-glass fibers. *BMC Oral Health.* 24 (1): 1–8.

9 He, L.-H., Purton, D.G., and Swain, M.V. (2010). A suitable base material for composite resin restorations: zinc oxide eugenol. *J. Dent.* 38: 290–295.

10 Heboyan, A., Vardanyan, A., Karobari, M.I. et al. (2023). Dental luting cements: an updated comprehensive review. *Molecules* 28 (4): 1–16.

11 Jefferies, S.R., Pameijer, C.H., Appleby, D.C. et al. (2012). Prospective observation of a new bioactive luting cement: 2-year follow-up. *J. Prosthodont.* 21 (1): 33–41.

12 Van Meerbeek, B., Yoshihara, K., Van Landuyt, K. et al. (2020). From Buonocore's pioneering acid-etch technique to self-adhering restoratives. A status perspective of rapidly advancing dental adhesive technology. *J. Adhes. Dent.* 22 (1): 7–34.

13 Van Landuyt, K.L., Snauwaert, J., De Munck, J. et al. (2007). Systematic review of the chemical composition of contemporary dental adhesives. *Biomaterials* 28 (26): 3757–3785.

12

Temporary Devices and Posts

Temporary devices are needed in dentistry, with their use required for a few weeks to several years. Impression materials and many solutions are used temporarily during a treatment but are discussed in other chapters. The materials for primary tooth crowns, orthodontic brackets, temporary cements/restoratives, and posts are described in this chapter.

Pediatric Crowns

Humans have evolved, like other mammals, to have two sets of teeth. We have 20 primary teeth (baby, deciduous) and 32 permanent teeth (adult). The primary teeth are smaller, thinner, more fragile and prone to decay and sometimes need long-term temporary crowns until they are exfoliated. Caries arresting treatments may suffice for primary teeth, as described in Chapter 8, but children and adolescents need extra dental treatment when they have rampant caries or molar incisor hypomineralization (MIH, insufficient hydroxyapatite in the enamel or permanent teeth). The treatments in terms of increasing intervention by the dentists are direct restorations of the enamel, and the pulp treatments in Chapter 8. Pulpotomies may be differentiated as partial or full, but both involve the removal of coronal pulp tissue. Root canal therapy, pulpectomies, of primary teeth may be required in severe cases where a tooth needs to be retained (for jawbone growth) or to treat young permanent teeth.

Large composite resin restorations (Chapter 9) can be placed on decayed primary teeth via the strip crown technique using thin, flexible transparent polycarbonate crown forms. The crown form is trimmed to fit the tooth, then filled with chemical or light-curable composite resin material and hardened on the primary tooth. Next, the outer polycarbonate is removed, and the composite resin

Ceramics in Dentistry: Materials, Manufacturing, and Clinical Applications,
First Edition. Carolyn M. Primus.

restorative is contoured to its final shape. This technique is faster than the direct composite resins placed in adults but less precise; speed is crucial for treating pediatric patients.

As mentioned in Chapter 2, early childhood caries occurring on multiple teeth may be so significant that full coverage pediatric crowns may be prescribed to protect the primary tooth, alleviate pain and enable speaking and mastication. The crowns for primary teeth are preformed, unlike the custom crowns used on adults' permanent teeth, where a precise fit is imperative to ensure decades long-term protection of the tooth. The pediatric dentist customarily prepares (grinds off enamel) the tooth to fit the preformed crown rather than fitting the crown to the tooth preparation.

Stainless steel crowns for primary teeth have been the standard restorative option beginning in 1947 but for esthetic reasons, these metal crowns are usually reserved for posterior teeth. Esthetic alternative crown materials include composite-veneered stainless steel, fiberglass, polymer, or zirconia crowns. These esthetic options are available in preformed shapes for every primary tooth, in various sizes, and some color (shade) variations. The "pre-veneered" stainless steel crowns mentioned in Chapter 10 have a composite coating on the anterior or occlusal surfaces, making these preformed crowns more esthetic than the unadorned stainless steel. See Figure 12.1. The pioneering company for this technology was NuSmile Ltd., which manufactures stainless steel crowns with composite polymers as a low-cost esthetic crown. Aluminum has been used instead of stainless steel as a substrate for a tooth-colored epoxy coating, containing ceramic

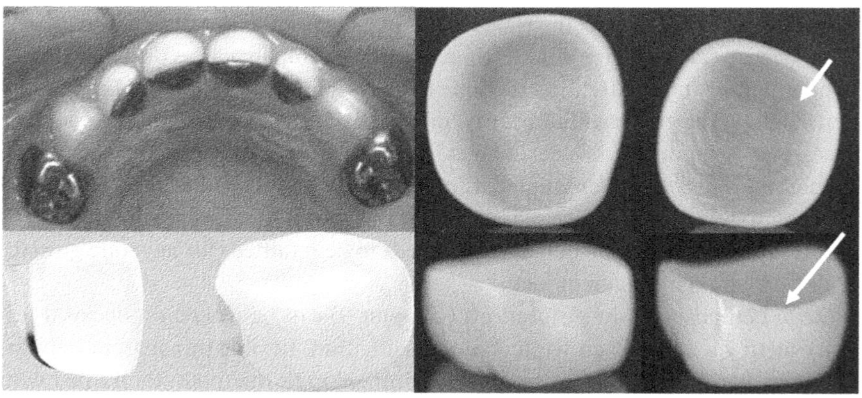

Figure 12.1 Crowns for primary teeth. On the left are composite-coated stainless steel crowns in situ (top) and two side views of individual crowns. On the right are machined/milled crowns. These zirconia crowns have distinct machining marks and flaws in the margin (arrows). *Source:* Courtesy of NuSmile Ltd.

pigments; these crowns can be easily cut and crimped but are softer and less durable (1) than stainless steel.

Flexible materials are useful as crowns for primary teeth, where they can stretch over the bulges on the molars' facial and lingual surfaces near the margin; the bulges help retain the crowns and creating a "snap fit." Preformed fiberglass pediatric crowns, composed of ceramic fibers and polymers have such flexibility. These crowns contain a mesh of quartz or E-glass fibers and may include barium borosilicate glass powder, as disclosed in the US Pat. Application 2017/0333158 Al. E-glass is a well-known glass fiber composition used industrially, whose formula is in Table 12.1 and was mentioned in Chapter 9. The glass fibers are embedded in epoxy resin or other dental resins, with pigments such as titania. Carbon, aramid, or quartz fibers are alternatives to the E-glass. These crowns are flexible, tooth-colored, and low-cost but are less durable than metal or zirconia.

Table 12.1 Glass-ceramics for brackets and fiber posts.

	Glass-ceramic orthodontic brackets**				
Oxide	**4,789,649**	**5,032,081, 5,261,814**	**Glass for dental post***	**E-glass**	**AR glass**
SiO_2	43–50	56–63	40–60	52–56	55–75
Al_2O_3	26–30	17–22	3–4	12–16	0–5
CaO	0.1–3		5–6	16–25	1–10
MgO	11–15		4–7	0–5	
BaO			5–10		
SrO			9–16		
ZnO		10–14	2–5		
Na_2O, K_2O, & Li_2O	7–10.5	1.5–5, 0.1–1, 4–6	1.5–2.0	0–2	11–21, 1.5 Li_2O
TiO_2			5–10	0–0.8	0–12
B_2O_3				5–10	0–8
ZrO_2					1–18
P_2O_5					
F/Cl	3.3–4.8, 0.01–0.6				
Sb_2O_3		0.5–2			

* Preferred composition ranges are from US 2011/0045440 Al.
** Preferred composition ranges from US Patents.

Polymer crowns for pediatric use have also been used, including polycarbonate (1); other polymers in US Pat. Application 2010/0297587 Al: polyacetal, polyacrylate, polymethylmethacrylate (PMMA), polyamide, polyaryletherketone (PAEK), polyetherketone (PEK), polyether-ether-ketone (PEEK), polyetherimide (PEI), polyethersulfone (PES), polysulfone (PSU), and mixtures thereof. Fillers, ceramic or organic, may be included for pigmentation. Injection molding is a common manufacturing technique for these preformed polymer pediatric crowns. Hybrid ceramic-polymer crowns are available, which may be similar to the Ceramir lithium disilicate-resin CAD-CAM materials of Chapter 10; such crowns may advantageously be repaired with composite, which is problematic for zirconia crowns described below.

Zirconia pediatric crowns are indisputably stronger, more durable, and more attractive than stainless steel or composite-faced stainless-steel crowns. However, zirconia lacks the elasticity of the other crown materials, and it cannot be crimped at the gingival margin for fitting, unlike stainless steel crowns. Careful tooth preparations and the use of fluoride-containing cement are needed for using of zirconia crowns. Yttria (Y_2O_3)-stabilized (<6% by weight) zirconia (2) is used, indicating the preference for the strong tetragonal zirconia. The zirconia pediatric crowns have been manufactured by milling or injection molding zirconia. The milled zirconia crowns are shaped using partially sintered zirconia, then sintered to a final shape; these zirconia crowns tend to have interior machining tracks and may have defective margins compared to injection molded crowns. See Figure 12.1. Manufacturers smooth the exterior surfaces of zirconia crowns by "tumbling," polishing with diamond, or applying an external glaze. The axial thickness of these crowns is about 0.4 mm, less than the thickness required for zirconia crowns on permanent teeth. However, compared to stainless steel crowns, more tooth reduction is required for zirconia pediatric crowns: about 2 mm on the occlusal surface. Colorants include titania and iron oxide to tint the zirconia, but shades are limited for these temporary crowns.

Zirconia pediatric and custom crowns are "tried in" for their fit before final cementing. Salivary proteins adhere to the zirconia and contaminate the intaglio such that bonding is poor; therefore, thorough cleaning is needed before final cementation. Common cleaners are sodium hydroxide solutions applied to the crown extraorally. Zirconia particles smaller than 100 nm may be dispersed in the alkaline solution to attract the proteins off the surface (US Pat. 10,995,306). Lanthanum chloride solutions for cleaning are also effective at attracting the phosphates off the zirconia surface, an idea borrowed from fish tank maintenance. One manufacturer makes pink-tinted zirconia crowns for "try-in" to avoid cleaning the final crown before seating.

Glass ionomer and resin-modified glass ionomers (Chapters 9 and 11) cements are popular for cementing pediatric crowns because they release fluoride to reduce subsequent decay; this is beneficial for children who have already had caries that destroyed the underlying tooth. The cements can be used to partially restore the anatomy before the crown is seated, such as when a pulpotomy or pulpectomy is performed. The shade of these cements can influence the esthetics of these thin zirconia crowns.

Pediatric Endodontics

Some primary teeth present with massive decay and bacterial invasion, so a pulpectomy is required. These teeth are treated similarly to permanent teeth with removal of the pulp, some shaping, and irrigation. If a primary tooth does not have a permanent successor, the root canal is filled with gutta-percha and sealer, the same as for permanent teeth. If a permanent tooth is forming underneath, the primary tooth is obturated with materials that are uniquely designed to be temporary; the filling material should undergo resorption at the same speed as the primary tooth is being resorbed by the body, until the tooth exfoliates (is replaced by its successor, permanent tooth).

Debates have occurred about obturation materials for primary tooth pulpectomies. Several materials are available based on zinc oxide-eugenol, zinc oxide with iodoform, and calcium hydroxide with eugenol and zinc acetate, calcium hydroxide and iodoform (CHI_3) in water, or iodoform with calcium hydroxide in silicone oil (3). All such products are antimicrobial but differ in their speed of resorption, but the silicone oil-containing products are known to resorb faster than the primary teeth (4–6); the other obturation products resorb more slowly and incompletely. Products with low calcium silicate cement, derived from the "bioactive cement" endodontic sealers (Chapter 8) are being tested to create an endodontic filler with a resorption rate that is "just right" for soon to be exfoliated primary teeth that are; the cement offers antimicrobial and bioactivity benefits.

Orthodontics

The permanent teeth form in the jawbone and force the primary teeth to exfoliate. The permanent teeth may not be in perfect alignment develop and erupt, creating malocclusion. Beginning in the early 20th century with Edward Hartley Angle, dentists began orthodontic treatments of malocclusion (7). Orthodontic brackets long term (present for more than 30 days) devices, but are used temporarily in a lifetime.

Orthodontic treatment of children and adults is performed to include esthetic benefits such as closing diastemas (gaps between teeth) or aligning "crooked" teeth. Other benefits include improved speaking or chewing ability, avoiding biting one's lips or cheeks, mitigating gum disease, and preventing long-term excessive wear or trauma of the teeth against one another. Headgear, arch (jaw-bone) expanders, temporary implants, polymer aligners, and brackets (braces) may be implemented to achieve changes in the tooth positions. Brackets are common and require connections (ligation) using archwires and elastomers, such as rubber bands or polymer chains, to exert the forces of alignment. The popular polymer aligners and retainers are entirely polymeric; no ceramic or metal is included.

Brackets must be made of a non-corroding, chemically and biologically inert material, having enough strength to withstand archwire ligation forces (the forces causing tooth movement) and mastication (eating) force for a few months to as long as three years. The brackets are bonded individually to each tooth and then attached to one another with a wire to effectuate the desired permanent tooth movement. The shape of the orthodontic brackets is complex; they have a base for adhesion, a face with a groove for the archwire, and tie wing features to manage complex movements of the teeth during treatment, as depicted in Figure 12.2. Orthodontic brackets are designed for each tooth, maxillary and mandibular, right and left – centrals, laterals, cuspids, 1st and 2nd bicuspids, and molars. Originally, brackets were only made of stainless steels such as 304L, 316L, 17-4 PH, or super-austenitic stainless steel SR-50A (9). Stainless steels are successful only because they spontaneously form a thin, coherent, chromia (ceramic) coating. Brackets are standardized under ISO 27020/ADA 100.

Ceramic orthodontic brackets have been used since 1986, especially for adult orthodontic patients who require more esthetics. The first ceramic brackets

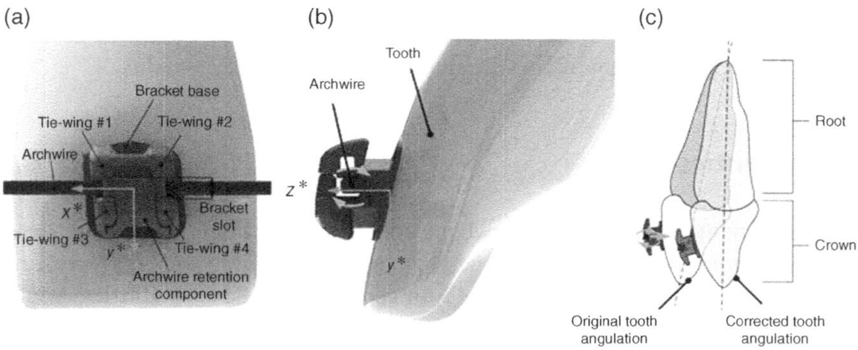

Figure 12.2 Self-ligating orthodontic bracket components. (a) Facial view of bracket showing tie wings, archwire, and bracket base. (b) Side view of the bracket showing the bracket slot (the prescription). (c) Control of tooth angulation using an archwire. *Source:* (8)/Springer Nature.

were made of sapphire, single-crystal, alpha alumina (Al_2O_3), a transparent and hard material. These sapphire brackets were larger than the metal brackets but were significantly less apparent. Sapphire brackets were manufactured by slowly "drawing" a crystal from a pool of molten alumina (>2072 °C) using the Czochralski or the edge-defined, film-fed growth (refer to US Pat. 4,639,218) methods depicted in Figure 7.5. With either method, a seed crystal of sapphire was inserted into molten alumina, and a long sapphire crystal was drawn from the crucible. Using the edge-defined method, the molten alumina was pulled through a die into the approximate desired bracket shape. Forming such crystals by the edge-defined method is difficult because the metal dies used for the edge-defined method must operate at high temperatures (>2000 °C) and the metal die can color the sapphire crystals or be a sourced of bubble (defect) formation. The preferred crystal orientation was the c-axis perpendicular to the direction of drawing the crystal, but the preferred orientation of the archwire groove in the crystal has been debated (US Pat. 4,932,865). The flexural strength of sapphire has been claimed to be at least 240 MPa and as high as 670 MPa, which is at least as high as the stainless steel used in brackets but sapphire has lower fracture toughness.

After the sapphire crystals are drawn, they must be cut and machined with diamonds into the bracket shapes. Many designs are required for the various teeth, but all have a 0.5 mm deep groove for the archwire. Machining is followed by a stress-relieving heat treatment at 1850 °C for four to six hours, where slow heating and cooling are needed because alumina is sensitive to thermal shock. The brackets are polished after annealing to smooth the contours and reduce the depth of any surface cracks. Polishing ensures transparency and low friction of the sapphire bracket with the metal archwire. Mechanical diamond polishing and flux polishing have been used. For instance, sapphire brackets can be immersed in a molten flux of lithium meta- and tetraborate, alumina and lithium fluoride ($LiBO_2$, $Li_2B_4O_7$, Al_2O_3, and LiF) at 850–900 °C for about 4–30 minutes, then immersed in hydrofluoric acid to remove any residual flux, resulting in a smoother surface (US Pat. 4,932,865).

Three problems were inherent with sapphire brackets: high hardness of alumina compared to tooth enamel, low fracture toughness, and high cost relative to metal brackets. The high hardness can wear or damage opposing tooth enamel and has limited its orthodontic use. The low toughness has led to breakage of the tie wings during fabrication or use, particularly on the anterior brackets. Elastomeric modules (polymer ligatures, not metal) and coated low-friction ligature wires were recommended to prevent fracture. When the sapphire brackets failed during treatment, usually torsion was too high, which is influenced by the ligature wire's composition, shape, thickness, and the bracket's slot size, depth, and vertical position.

The expense of ceramic brackets was reduced by the development of the polycrystalline alumina brackets. Polycrystalline brackets have higher friction than sapphire but about equal to metal brackets. The polycrystalline alumina ceramic brackets are made by injection molding, a technique described in Chapter 7. The composition of the polycrystalline alumina brackets in US Pat. 4,219,617 was 93.5% Al_2O_3, with the remainder being magnesium–calcium–silicate interstitial glass phase; this is not as strong or translucent as the high-purity Lucalox material mentioned in Chapter 10. US Pat. 4,954,080 discloses a 99.5% pure alumina, translucent bracket having grains preferably larger than 10 µm; alternative materials were also claimed – spinel, zirconia, zircon, and yttrium aluminum garnet. Three brands of single-crystal alumina brackets were found to be stronger than three brands of polycrystalline alumina brackets (10). Alumina brackets have been marketed with various surface treatments for low friction of the wires, base designs and coatings for adhesion, and metal or polymeric clips in the raceway for the wire.

A glass-ceramic orthodontic bracket was patented (US Pat.4,789,649) that contained mica and cordierite crystals $(K,Na,Ca)_2(Al,Mg,Fe)_{4-6}(Si,Al)_8O_{20}(OH,F)_4$ and $(Mg,Fe)_2Al_4Si_5O_{18}$. This glass-ceramic consisted of large flat mica crystals (<200 µm) and finer cordierite crystals (<5 µm), having a compressive strength of 450 MPa and fracture toughness of about 2 MPa-m$^{-1/2}$. Another patented glass-ceramic bracket (US Pat. 5,032,081, 5,261,814) had large crystals on the interior and an outer layer of smaller crystals that created a compressive stress for higher strength. See Table 12.1 for the compositions of these glasses before crystallization. Transparent spinel ($MgO.Al_2O_3$) has also been investigated for orthodontic brackets (11).

Cubic, not tetragonal, zirconia brackets have been manufactured (12). Their pale, yellowish tint and opacity were less esthetic than alumina. No reduction in friction has been reported of zirconia compared to alumina brackets (13), and these are no longer manufactured.

Orthodontic brackets are bonded to enamel, not dentin; the enamel facial surface is etched using phosphoric acid. Erbium-doped yttrium aluminum garnet and erbium-chromium-doped yttrium aluminum gadolinium garnet (Er: YAG and Er, Cr:YSGG) lasers have also been used to etch teeth prior to bracket bonding. Ceramic brackets presented unique challenges for bonding to the tooth because the ceramics were unlike metal brackets that have a metal mesh on the tooth-facing side for embedding the cement. Originally, the chemical retention method of bonding was used for ceramic brackets; manufacturers applied a thin glass coating on a smooth, concave ceramic bracket base by cathode sputtering, plasma deposition, or electron beam evaporation. The glass coating was coated with silane (<1-µm thick), which strongly adhered to the glass coating on the bracket base and to the adhesive. Alternatively, the sapphire brackets were heated to remove adsorbed water and treated with a dilute solution of 2–2.5% silane solution in toluene/propylene glycol monomethyl ether – the same process used to adhere ceramic fillers to resin in direct composites. However, the bond of the silane to the bracket was so strong that the tooth enamel was damaged during the removal of the brackets. The tooth's enamel was weaker than the cement-silane-bracket adhesive bond, leaving minor fractures and roughness on the tooth surface after "debonding." Protecting tooth enamel integrity is crucial during debonding and avoiding aspiration or ingestion of brackets or fragments. This chemical adhesion method is obsolete for ceramic brackets and has been superseded by using slightly weaker cements.

Current ceramic bracket bases have undercuts and a patterned undersurface to mechanically engage an adhesive. The patterned base can also serve as a slot to insert pliers for the purpose of adjusting the position during adhesion or later removal. Resin cements are now commonly used to adhere ceramic brackets to teeth. These cements are based on formulas for the weaker, flowable direct composite resin restoratives discussed in Chapters 9 and 11. Several techniques have been used to debond (remove) the ceramic brackets without damage: mechanical, ultrasonic, electrothermal, and lasers. Laser heating can weaken/soften the resin cement so that lesser forces are needed for debonding, reducing the risk of enamel damage. However, the heat produced by some lasers can damage the tooth pulp (14); thus, caution is needed.

After brackets are bonded to teeth, the patient needs to keep the brackets free of biofilm. Cleanliness minimizes friction, protects the teeth from decay, and produces the quickest alignment. Ceramic brackets may be better than metal for minimizing plaque accumulation, but professional cleaning (Chapter 13) during orthodontic treatment is essential.

Ceramic coatings have been applied by chemical vapor deposition to disguise metal orthodontic brackets or wires made of titanium, stainless steel or nickel-titanium. Zirconium nitride and tungsten disulfide (ZrN, WS_2) have been applied to stainless steel and NiTi orthodontic wires to hide the reflective metallic appearance. Some stainless steel brackets products boast a zirconia or zirconium nitride coating to create a light gold color. Orthodontic wires of various metals, sizes, and shapes are covered under ISO 15841/ADA 32 standards.

An interesting advantage of ceramic brackets is that they do not need to be removed for an MRI scan. Stainless steel or ceramic brackets with metal components, such as a metal wire guide, must be removed to avoid MRI artifacts when the anatomy under examination is near the brackets.

Polymer orthodontic brackets (15) formed of polycarbonate, polyurethane, polyethylene, polyester polyamides, or polymethyl methacrylate have been available since the 1970s. These polymers have a much lower elastic modulus than metals or ceramics, making distortion of the slot more likely and tooth alignment more difficult; adding a metal slot liner helped their usefulness. Plus, polymer brackets tend to discolor during treatment time. As with food packaging, concerns have arisen about the release of Bisphenol-A (BPA), potentially from polycarbonate brackets or adhesive monomers and polycarbonate degradation. Adhesives are evolving to avoid BPA, particularly because orthodontics is primarily for adolescents. A few polymer brackets have about 30% of an undisclosed ceramic filler.

Temporary implants may be needed for the process of aligning teeth; these protrude through the mucosa and are attached to ligating wires. Orthodontic anchor screws provide temporary intraoral skeletal anchorage and are removed at the end of the orthodontic treatment. Similar to endosseous dental implants (Chapter 16), they are inserted into the maxillofacial bone structures. These implants have been composed of titanium, like endosseous implants for crowns; titanium is successful because of it forms a tenacious surficial ceramicit forms a tenacious surficial ceramic oxide. Newer products include aligned carbon fibers embedded in PEEK thermoplastic polymer. ISO 19023/ADA 178 for orthodontic anchor screws have methods to compare physical and mechanical properties of these screws.

Temporary Restoratives and Treatments

Temporary restoratives and cements are between appointments, while a permanent (fixed prosthodontic) restoration is being made in a dental laboratory, or when longer term root-canal disinfection is required. Between appointments, a temporary restorative material is needed to cover the opening to the interior of the tooth. This interval between appointments may be used to see if the pulp will heal, for a crown to be made, or for root canal disinfection. In the late 1800s, zinc oxychloride and zinc phosphate cements were used as short-term (days to a few weeks) or long-term (months) temporary filling materials. Sometimes, zinc oxide and the silicate glass powder of a silicate cement restorative (Chapter 9) were combined before mixing with phosphoric acid solution as a temporary material.

Another early temporary material included copper oxide, hydroxide, or carbonate powder that was mixed with phosphoric acid to form copper (II) phosphate, $Cu_3(PO_4)_2$ (16). The so-called black copper phosphate cements contained about 90% copper oxide (CuO), with the remainder being cobalt oxide (Co_3O_4) (17). As mentioned in Chapter 11, zinc oxide eugenol cement products are still in use as a temporary medicament or restorative.

A popular temporary restorative has been Cavit™ material, which contains zinc oxide (30–50%) but no eugenol and sets with water reacting with the other components: calcium sulfate, (<30%) barium sulfate (<20%), talc (<20%), zinc sulfate (5–10%), glycol acetate, polyvinyl acetate (1–5%), and triethylene glycol diacetate. This rather high viscosity material is useful as a base because it has some setting expansion to help seal the margins (18). Variations of the

Cavit-type formula from other manufacturers contain different resins (e.g. ethyl-vinyl acetate), but the setting occurs by reaction of calcium sulfate and zinc oxide with water, creating zinc sulfate as the set material. Zinc sulfate, diatomaceous earth, and sodium fluoride may also be included. An alternative temporary material includes light-curing dimethacrylate monomers, polyester, and silica (systemp.inlay or onlay).

Zinc oxide-eugenol (ZOE) cement is used as a temporary pulp medicament in indirect contact with the pulp because it is known to have a sedative effect on an irritated pulp; however, the ZOE cements should not be used directly on a pulp because excess eugenol is cytotoxic and may cause pulp necrosis. ZOE products have been modified to raise the strength and abrasion resistance by adding alumina to the powder and substituting orthoethoxybenzoic acid ($C_9H_{10}O_3$) for part of the eugenol liquid; these are denoted as Super-EBA cements, having good durability as a temporary material, such as before a crown or bridge is completed. Another modified ZOE product (IRM) has a powder containing 20–40% of fine powdered polymethacrylate powder, zinc oxide and zinc acetate that can be mixed with a eugenol/acetic acid liquid to create this popular long-term temporary material. Silane-coated, E-glass fibers (1.6 μm in diameter, 110 μm in length) have also been mixed in ZOE (18), to increase the compressive strength and lower the solubility for use as temporary material; its commercialization is not known. A putty-like restorative consistency should be mixed with a high powder-to-liquid ratio. A cool glass mixing slab slows the setting, but like the other ZnO cements, the slab should not be colder than the dew point to prevent water from condensing and accelerating the setting.

Two-paste, rather than powder-liquid, ZOE products are available. The zinc oxide base paste is suspended in a non-reactive organic liquid, which may include a rosin; the other paste contains eugenol and additives such as zinc acetate ($Zn[CH_3CO_2]_2.2H_2O$), magnesium chloride ($MgCl_2$), talc or kaolin for easy mixing and fast setting. A putty-like restorative consistency should be mixed with a high powder-to-liquid ratio. A cool glass mixing slab slows the setting, but like the carboxylate cements, the slab should not be colder than the dew point to prevent water from condensing and accelerating the setting.

Self-cure and light-curable temporary materials have been developed for temporary fillings that contain glycols, methacrylates, and these ceramics: calcium sulfate, zinc oxide, barium sulfate, silica, or sodium fluoride. Chopped glass fibers in a flowable composite have been used in a temporary material, which is also indicated for a "core build-up."

Temporary – provisional – restorations (crowns) protect teeth that have been prepared for a crown until the final crown is manufactured and cemented to obviate chemical and thermal trauma to the dentin. Most temporary crowns are made from weaker polymeric materials, such as the methacrylate resins, with little or no ceramic filler. Temporary materials may be formed by hand or 3D printed in a dental laboratory, often within the dental office so the patient can have the teeth prepared for a crown or bridge but leave the office with a "crown" that will enable them to enjoy food, and disguise missing tooth anatomy.

Preformed, temporary polycarbonate crowns are available but require an inventory of shades and sizes for many teeth shapes and adjustment intraorally. Provisional crowns also require temporary (provisional) cements that ensure the temporary crown can be easily removed for the final crown's placement. Zinc oxide-eugenol, polycarboxylate, and non-eugenol zinc oxide cements are used for this purpose but have modifications in these temporary cement products to avoid strong adhesion. Dycal®, a calcium hydroxide pulp medicament has also both been used for the temporary cementation of crowns.

Temporary, antimicrobial medicaments are used for root canal therapy, which contain a non-setting paste of about 40% calcium hydroxide. Clinicians may mix their own pastes with water, but paste products are available, usually including polyethylene glycol, a radiopaque powder (e.g. barium sulfate), and perhaps some cellulose, dispersed in water. Such medication is applied after the pulp extirpation, canal preparation (shaping with instruments), and irrigation before obturation (Chapter 8). The high pH of calcium hydroxide reduces residual infection, particularly if the infection had progressed into the alveolar bone. During its residence, the calcium hydroxide particles gradually form calcium carbonate, changing to the neutral pH of calcium carbonate. At the second endodontic appointment, usually 1 week, the unset paste is flushed from the root canal system before the obturation phase of root canal therapy.

Temporary denture liners are used to improve the comfort of mastication, particularly for new denture wearers. For patients with insufficient ridge height or dry, thin tissues, soft liners may be the only way that a denture can be worn. Soft denture liners are used temporarily (<30 days) until a denture reline is performed or a new denture is made. Titania and fumed silica are ceramic powders in these reline materials. The short-term soft liners, tissue conditioners, are applied to the denture by the dentists without having to send the denture to a dental laboratory but are not intended for long-term use. Powdered polymers are mixed with ethyl alcohol and other dissolved polymers, which avoid tissue irritation. Water gradually replaces the alcohol, and the substance hardens and loses its cushioning function.

Denture-bearing, hard (bone) tissue resorbs as the wearer ages, causing the alveolar ridge to thin and flatten; this change interferes with denture fit and stability. Longer-term, soft denture liners are either silicone elastomers or acrylic resins, containing ethyl alcohol and/or ethyl acetate to preserve the softness. The silicones last longer but are harder than the short-term liners. Cold-cure acrylic (polymethacrylate powder and monomer liquid) or heat-cured acrylic is used when a harder lining material is selected for dentures. Hard liners may provide more stability but must have a precise fit to avoid tissue irritation and pain. Such materials are the subject of ISO 10139-1 (short term) and 10139-1 (longer term) (ADA 75 and 160) standards. Hard denture liner requirements are in ISO 23401.

Posts

Dental crowns for permanent teeth are designed to fit over the remaining coronal tooth anatomy like a closely fitting helmet. Unfortunately, some teeth become so fractured or so decayed that little of the coronal tooth anatomy remains. For such cases, a clinician must recreate the basic shape of a tooth for the crown to be placed via a post and core build-up. Posts are placed in such teeth after a root canal treatment and become the foundation for a coronal buildup – recreation of the core anatomy for placement of a crown.

Originally, such posts were preformed metal posts or a custom-made (laboratory made) metal post and core. Fiberglass post-and-core build-up is now a popular alternative – see Figure 12.3; the posts are cemented within the root using a self-curing, resin cement (Chapter 11). The posts contain bundled glass fibers, formed into a tapered shape and bound with less than 25 weight percent resin. The advantage of such posts is that their elastic modulus (13–15 GPa) is similar to that of dentin (11–28 GPa), unlike the lower elasticity (stiffer) stainless steel posts. A similar elastic modulus of dentin and post material is preferred, which minimizes the risk of root fracture from mastication forces. After the cementation of a post, the core-build-up composite material is cured over the post. The core recreates enough anatomy that a crown can be affixed to the tooth.

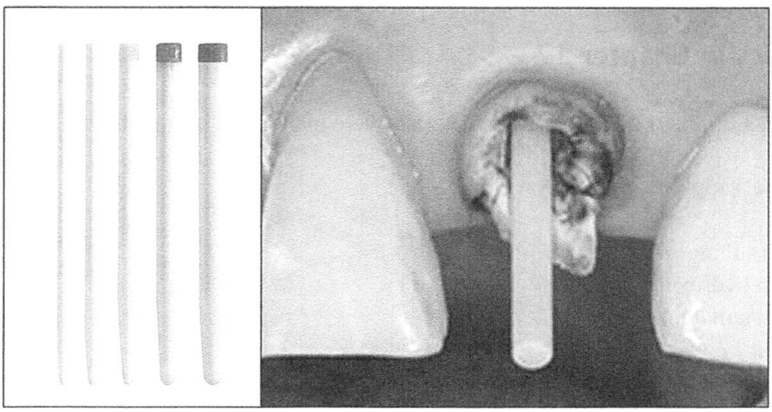

Figure 12.3 Various sizes of fiberglass posts for dentistry (left) and a post after being cemented in a tooth (right), which is ready for application of core build-up material to recreate coronal anatomy as the foundation for a crown to be fabricated.

The first fiberglass posts contained conventional E-glass fibers, which were augmented with radiopaque particles. However, the particles weakened the posts compared to posts without particles. Alkaline-resistant glass fibers (AR-glass fibers) for concrete have been used, which contain zirconia in the glass, imparting modest radiopacity but less strength. More radiopaque glass fibers have been submitted for patenting, which have the attributes of insolubility, enough strength for use in a post, and do not devitrify (crystallize) during fiber manufacture (drawing from molten glass). See Table 12.1 for three glass fiber formulas; all are silicate glasses with some alumina and calcia. Minor oxides may be present in the US Pat. Application 2011/0045440 Al glass composition, including iron oxide and fluoride. Current glass posts have radiopacity up to four times that of dentin (~4 mm Al) for visibility on an X-ray; the baria (BaO) and strontia (SrO) in the glass fibers distinguish the glass.

Summary Regarding Temporary Devices and Posts

Dental treatments may require long-term but temporary devices. For instance, "stock" zirconia or fiberglass pediatric crowns are used on primary teeth. Similar glass fiber posts are used for crown build-up but remain permanently. Sapphire and polycrystalline alumina orthodontic brackets are also long-term temporary ceramic devices as are the special oxide coatings on ligation wires. Many composite formulas are modified to create products suited for temporary cements or temporary crowns; these usually are have lower strength for their easy replacement with a permanent material. Calcium hydroxide pastes are temporarily placed to enhance root canal therapy. Ceramics as fillers, fibers or pediatric crowns are essential for these temporary uses.

Ceramics in Chapter 12

The following ceramics or inorganic materials were mentioned in this chapter:

- alumina, sapphire, or polycrystalline
- baria
- barium sulfate
- calcium hydroxide
- calcium sulfate
- chromia
- copper oxide, carbonate, and hydroxide
- copper phosphate
- cordierites

- diamond
- hydrofluoric acid
- iron oxide
- kaolin clay
- lanthanum chloride
- lithium borates
- lithium fluoride
- magnesium chloride
- mica
- phosphoric acid
- silica, E-glass, AR-glass, fluoride containing glass
- sodium fluoride
- strontia
- talc
- titania
- titanium nitride
- tungsten sulfide
- yttria
- yttrium aluminum garnet
- yttrium aluminum gadolinium garnet
- zinc oxide
- zinc oxychloride
- zinc sulfate
- zirconia
- zirconium nitride

References

1 Mittal, G.K., Verma, A., Pahuja, H. et al. (2016). Esthetic crowns in pediatric dentistry: a review. *Intl J Contemp Med Res.* 3 (5): 1280–1282.

2 Sztyler, K., Wiglusz, R.J., and Dobrzynski, M. (2022). Review on preformed crowns in pediatric dentistry – the composition and application. *Materials.* 15 (6): 2081–2100.

3 Navit, S., Jaiswal, N., Khan, S.A. et al. (2016). Antimicrobial efficacy of contemporary obturating materials used in primary teeth – an in-vitro study. *J. Clin. Diagn. Res.* 10 (9): ZC09–ZC12.

4 Rewal, N., Thakur, A.S., Sachdev, V., and Mahajan, N. (2014). Comparison of endoflas and zinc oxide eugenol as root canal filling materials in primary dentition. *J Indian Soc Pedod Prev Dent.* 32 (4): 317–321.

5 Hu, X., Liang, Z., Wang, Q., and Liu, L. (2023). A retrospective study of iRoot BP Plus pulpotomy compared with vitapex pulpectomy for irreversible pulpitis of primary molars with the presence of coronal pulp tissue. *Int. J. Paediatr. Dent.* / the British Paedodontic Society [and] the International Association of Dentistry for Children 33 (2): 216–226.
6 Pandranki, J., Vanga, N.R., and Chandrabhatla, S.K. (2018). Zinc oxide eugenol and Endoflas pulpectomy in primary molars: 24-month clinical and radiographic evaluation. *J Indian Soc Pedod Prev Dent.* 36 (2): 173–180.
7 Mundhada, V.V., Jadhav, V.V., and Reche, A. (2023). A review on orthodontic brackets and their application in clinical orthodontics. *Cureus.* 15 (10): 1–10.
8 Melenka, G.W., Nobes, D.S., Major, P.W., and Carey, J.P. (2013). Design of an orthodontic torque simulator for measurement of bracket deformation. *Sens. Imaging.*: An International Journal 14 (3–4): 57–80.
9 Oh, K.T., Choo, S.U., Kim, K.M., and Kim, K.N. (2005). A stainless steel bracket for orthodontic application. *Eur. J. Orthod.* 27 (3): 237–244.
10 Kieling, T.C.B., Correr-Sobrinho, L., Godoi, A.P.T. et al. (2019). Fracture strength of monocrystalline and polycrystalline ceramic brackets during archwire torque. *Rev Odon da UNESP.* 48: 1–7.
11 Krishnan, M., Tiwari, B., Seema, S. et al. (2014). Transparent magnesium aluminate spinel: a prospective biomaterial for esthetic orthodontic brackets. *J. Mater. Sci. Mater. Med.* 25 (11): 2591–2599.
12 Srinidhi, R., Dilip, S., Gopinath, A. et al. (2023). Orthodontic bracket materials – an up-to-date review. *Intl J Chem and Biochem Sci.* 24 (6): 45–54.
13 Elekdag-Türk, S. and Yilmaz, H. (2019). Ceramic brackets revisited. In: *Current approaches in orthodontics*, 5–22. Intechopen.
14 Azzeh, E. and Feldon, P.J. (2003). Laser debonding of ceramic brackets: a comprehensive review. *Am. J. Orthod. Dentofacial Orthop.* 123 (1): 79–83.
15 Hassan, R., Aslam Khan, M.U., Abdullah, A.M., and Abd Razak, S.I. (2021). A review on current trends of polymers in orthodontics: BPA-free and smart materials. *Polymers (Basel).* 13 (9): 1409–1421.
16 AlRughaib, M.B., Marafi, A.A., and Gutmann, J.L. (2024). Historical perspectives and comparisons on the use plastic-based cements in endodontics and prosthodontics: Part 2 – oxyphosphates. *J. Hist. Dent.* 72 (2): 139–146.
17 American Dental Association (1974). *Guide to dental materials and devices*, 7the, 297. Chicago: American Dental Association.
18 Hamdy, T.M. (2024). Evaluation of compressive strength, microhardness and solubility of zinc-oxide eugenol cement reinforced with E-glass fibers. *BMC Oral Health.* 24 (1): 1–8.

13

Teeth Maintenance

Earlier chapters described how to "fix" damaged teeth. This chapter describes how people and dentists maintain teeth before and after restorative treatment, including maintenance for partial and full dentures.

Dental enamel is protected by a pellicle, a layer created by salivary glycoproteins. This layer is vulnerable to staining, but it shields the tooth from food acids and bacteria. The ever-present bacteria in our mouths accumulate over the pellicle and form plaque, a soft sticky coating. Plaque can "mature" by calcification – hardening – facilitated by the calcium and phosphate ions in our saliva forming calculus (tartar), which may be above or below the gingival (supra- or subgingival calculus). Plaque is detrimental because it is a home to microbes: biofilms resistant to destruction.

As a practical matter, microbes cannot be eliminated, but home care and professional teeth cleaning with treatments with fluoride ions (F^-) help preserve healthy teeth and minimize the growth of these films and microbial-related diseases. Cleaning the teeth, performed personally or by professionals, helps remove the biofilms and obviate bacterial attack on teeth. Cleanliness is particularly important around implants and at the interface where dental restorations meet the tooth structure. Abrasive ceramic powders with detergents are used to remove the microbial layers and prevent their acidic, cariogenic buildup. Fluoride treatments, home care, professional maintenance, and bleaching, internal and external, are described in more detail next.

Fluoride in Dentistry

Only a century ago, dentists recognized the benefits and hazards of fluoride with modern analytical chemistry.[i] Fluoride ions are valuable for tooth maintenance because the ions can become incorporated into our tooth mineral,

i https://www.nidcr.nih.gov/health-info/fluoride/the-story-of-fluoridation

Ceramics in Dentistry: Materials, Manufacturing, and Clinical Applications,
First Edition. Carolyn M. Primus.

hydroxyapatite. Even though dental enamel is the most acid-resistant substance in the human body, it is constantly subjected to acidic cariogenic plaque and fermentable carbohydrates (food). Fluoride ions can substitute, via ion exchange at room or body temperature, with some of the hydroxide ions in the enamel's hydroxyapatite ($Ca_{10}(PO_4)_6(OH)_2$) crystals, forming surficial fluorapatite crystals ($Ca_{10}(PO_4)_6F_2$) or a solid solution (combination) of hydroxyapatite and fluorapatite ($Ca_{10}(PO_4)_6(OHF)$). Fluoride makes the mineral more resistant to acids created by caries attack compared to pure hydroxyapatite. "Hardening" of enamel by fluoride ions has proven very effective in preventing dental caries, particularly in children (1). Fluoride is present in some of the restorative materials products described in earlier chapters: silicate restoratives, glass ionomer cements, and the resin-hybrids containing fluoride glasses or salts. As noted in Chapter 5, fluoride presence in teeth is indicative of fewer caries (2). Based on evidence, fluoride-containing toothpaste and silver diammine fluoride are on the list of "Essential Medicines" issued by the World Health Organization (3) even though fluoride is not considered an essential dietary mineral. Fluoride is recognized by the ADA as a safe and effective agent that can be used to prevent and control dental caries in children and adults when used as directed or within the context of community water fluoridation programs.

A daily supply of fluoride ions is needed to retain some fluorapatite in the enamel, which may be meted out systemically or topically. Systemic fluoride provides topical protection because fluoride will be present in saliva, which continually bathes the teeth. Small quantities of fluoride are absorbed systemically from a few plants and animals (e.g. peanuts, tea, and fish). Water is another systemic source of fluorine. All natural water sources contain traces of the ionic form of fluorine, having been leached from soil and rocks into groundwater. Systemic fluoride is beneficial for developing teeth in children; only systemic fluoridation provides lifelong resistance to acid by becoming incorporated into developing enamel.

Fluoride is supplemented in some public water systems in 25 countries. Community water fluoridation processes adjust the fluoride content of water to the recommended level for optimal dental health, 0.7 parts fluoride per million (0.7 mg/L) (4) by the addition of sodium fluoride (NaF), fluorosilicic acid (H_2SiF_6), or sodium fluorosilicate (Na_2SiF_6). Community-wide alternatives to drinking fluoridated water have included fluoride supplementation of table salt (5, 6), milk (7), and chewing gum (8). In 1985, France authorized fluoridated salt (250 ppm of potassium fluoride [KF] in food). Fluoride supplements can be prescribed for children ages six months to 16 years who are considered at high risk for tooth decay and whose primary drinking water has a low fluoride concentration. Reverse osmosis and distillation systems reduce the fluoride levels, decreasing the decay-preventive effects of optimally fluoridated water, although carbon/charcoal filtration systems do not remove fluoride. Many bottled waters do not contain optimal levels of fluoride.

Arguments have presented against water fluoridation that are unsubstantiated or specious (5, 9, 10). Water fluoridation has been maligned as a health hazard for children causing neurodevelopment. A recent review of the recommended community fluoride levels concluded that this fluoride exposure does not affect children's (age 0–5 years) IQ (11). Another study confirms that fluoride has not diminished neurodevelopment (11). A meta-analysis of fluoride and children's IQ concluded that at concentrations below 1.5 mg/L in water, any correlation with ill effects was uncertain; a concentration of 1.5 mg/L is twice as high as used in community fluoridation.

The story of fluoride exemplifies the statement of the German philosopher, Paracelsus, who in the 15th century said, "Sola dosis facit venenum" (Solely the dose determines that a thing is not a poison). Some water sources around the world do contain more fluoride than recommended by the WHO or EPA (12). Too much fluoride in water can lead to children developing permanently mottled enamel, a problem recognized in the early 20th century (9) called fluorosis (13). The affected teeth vary in appearance, from having opaque, white striations to stained, pitted enamel (14), as depicted in Figure 13.1. Fluorosis occurs when an excess quantity of fluoride is ingested for a sufficient period during the growth of the permanent teeth. The level of fluoride intake between the ages of about 15 and 30 months is thought to be most critical for the potential of fluorosis occurring in the maxillary central incisors. The mechanisms by which fluoride modifies tooth development are not fully understood but may result from alterations in protein metabolism that disrupt the crystal organization in the developing tooth. Excessive fluoride exposure is minimized by reducing the fluoride in public water sources having naturally occurring high

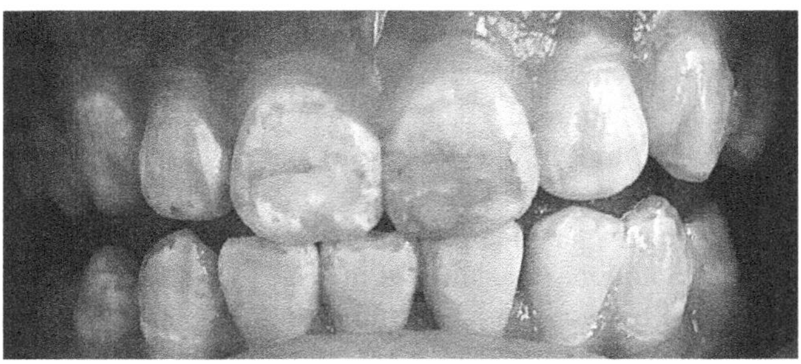

Figure 13.1 Examples of fluorosis from high-fluoride water sources. *Source:* Wang et al., (2020) / SAGE Publications / CC BY-NC 4.0.

levels of fluoride, ranging from 3 to 17 mg/L (15). Also, children should be prevented from ingesting fluoride-containing toothpaste to avoid fluorosis. Fluoride concentration in enamel is not permanent but cyclic, with the availability of fluoride absorbed systemically or topically. The exception is the retention of high fluoride doses in children's developing permanent teeth.

Fluorosis differs from tetracycline staining, which is also a problem for developing teeth. When immature teeth are exposed to tetracycline, in utero or through oral administration up to the age of 8 years, it will bind to calcium ions (calcium orthophosphate) in the teeth. If this happens before the eruption of the teeth, the tetracycline bound to calcium orthophosphate will initially be fluorescent yellow, changing to non-fluorescent brown discoloration, after eruption.

Professionally Applied Topical Fluoride

The benefits of a modest dose of fluoride ions in reducing caries have led to topical fluoride treatments that are applied or prescribed by clinicians. Dental hygienists and pediatric dentists frequently use fluoride varnishes (ISO 17730/ADA 117), rinses (ISO 16408/ADA 116), foams, gel-like topical treatments, and sealants (ISO 6874/ADA 19) with fluoride. Varnishes are effective for children and high-risk adults, such as the elderly with impaired brushing skills, those having little or poor dental care, or those suffering from xerostomia. Fluoride varnishes have a thin consistency and are composed of a resin or natural gum and a solvent for sodium fluoride (NaF), fluorapatite ($Ca_{10}(PO_4)_6F_2$), or calcium fluoride (CaF_2) (8, 16) although nano-silver fluoride (AgF) has also been tested (17). Several layers of very low viscosity fluoride varnish are brushed onto the occlusal tooth surfaces to provide fluoride for the enamel; varnish is more substantive than toothpaste in providing fluoride but also temporary. Two or more applications per year are typical. Casein phosphopeptide-amorphous calcium phosphate (CPP-ACP) and tricalcium phosphate ($Ca_3(PO_4)_2$) are additives used to augment the benefits of fluoride in varnishes. CPP is a milk-derived phosphopeptide that binds calcium and ACP ($Ca_3(PO_4)_2.3H_2O$), a precursor in hydroxyapatite formation. Tricalcium phosphate is sometimes added to augment the benefits of fluoride in varnishes. Other products contain 0.2% sodium fluoride (900 ppm) and include zinc oxide, the latter for antimicrobial benefit.

Acidulated fluoride rinses may be applied professionally although diluted formulas may be used at home. Solutions of acidulated fluoride (1.23% APF) have a low pH (~3.5) for professional use containing sodium fluoride (1–3% NaF) and orthophosphoric acid (1–5% H_3PO_4) equivalent to 12,300 ppm F. Oral rinses are required to have a pH value between 3.0 and 10.5; if below 5.5, the rinse needs to pass a demineralization test or erosion test; erosion screening tests are in ISO 28888 and ADA 151. Precautions are necessary for its use because the acid may etch any porcelain restorations present in a patient's mouth. Gel-like rinses containing 5000 ppm sodium fluoride, phosphoric acid, and sodium phosphate monobasic (NaH_2PO_4) are also available by prescription for topical fluoride treatment. The rinses cover more tooth surfaces than the varnish to help prevent interproximal caries. Fluoride released from these materials gradually diminishes over time.

Silver diammine fluoride (SDF) solution – 12–38% – is a topical treatment gaining US popularity to arrest early childhood caries (noticeably slow the carious destruction of a tooth). SDF solutions have been incorrectly referred to as silver diamine fluoride, but SDF contains an "ammine" (NH_3) group and not an "amine" (NH_2). SDF solutions are also known as silver fluoride and silver ammonium fluoride; the 38% SDF solution contains 25% silver, 8% ammonia, 5% fluoride, and 62% water. Its use arose from earlier dental treatments with silver nitrate ($AgNO_3$) and sodium fluoride (NaF) to slow carious destruction, as noted in Chapter 8. The product has 4.5% F, approximately twice that of sodium fluoride varnish (2.2% F). SDF liquid is swabbed on teeth to kill the caries and the fluoride ions form fluorapatite, and the silver ions form a layer of silver phosphate (Ag_3PO_4) (18). Its significant disadvantage is that the solution will darken the caries, same as silver nitrate treatment; the caries are arrested, but the decay is apparent. However, evidence indicates that nano-sized silver particles in a fluoride solution (1%) will not discolor enamel (19). Potassium iodide (KI), an inorganic salt, is used after the SDF solution is applied to counteract the silver discoloration (20, 21) by creating silver iodide with any free silver. SDF is a low-cost, less-invasive alternative to a direct restorative due to its strong ability to stop caries, including secondary caries near restorations, and its ease of application is suitable for primary teeth and people "in care".

SDF was designated by the FDA in 2016 as a "breakthrough therapy" to arrest – stop the progression – of tooth decay in children and adults. Before 2016, the FDA had only approved SDF for treating sensitivity in the permanent teeth although, notably, SDF was used in other countries for 80 years before the FDA designation (Argentina, Australia, Brazil, China, and Japan). The World Health Organization has designated SDF – along with fluoride toothpaste and glass ionomers (Chapter 9) – as essential medications.

Titanium tetrafluoride (TiF_4) is also known to slow the progression of caries. The compound can replace calcium in hydroxyapatite, enhancing acid resistance. However, the solution is very acidic (pH ~1). Recently, polymeric dendrimer solutions of TiF_4 at 0.5% have been created to mitigate the acidity and provide benefits without demineralizing surrounding dentin (22). The titanium and fluoride ions penetrated 100 μm in dentin and were an improvement over the earlier acidic solution. Another future alternative without discoloration may be a copper tetraamine fluoride solution combining copper fluoride (CuF, CuF_2) ammonia (NH_3) solutions (23).

As mentioned in Chapters 9 and 11, sealants are applied to children's teeth to cover the occlusal surface's pits and fissures, which are decay sites because these narrow and deep crevices for cleaning. Sealants may be based on glass-ionomer, resin, or hybrid formulas to cover the teeth with a low-viscosity material, similar to those materials described in Chapter 9, 10, or 11. The sealants may wear away over time. Although varnishes, topical fluorides, and sealants are present temporarily after application, they are not usually distinguished as a temporary material because they are not intentionally removed. As with the silicate and glass ionomer restoratives discussed in Chapter 10, they release localized fluoride that diminishes over time. Fluorides have also been added to amalgam and zinc oxide cements with the hope of providing localized fluoride benefits. Please note that sealants refer to a covering on the occlusal surface; "sealers" refer to materials used endodontically, within the root, a topic discussed in Chapter 8.

Home Care

Humans have always had to manage the effects of food residue in one's mouth, including stains, plaque, and calculus. In antiquity, people used their fingers, plant material, animal bristles, or feathers to apply powders of chalk or eggshells (fine calcium carbonate, $CaCO_3$), salt (NaCl), pumice (SiO_2), magnesia (MgO), or ash (containing residual silica) to clean their teeth and freshen their breath. Hydrogen peroxide and sodium bicarbonate were popular and remain in use today. Some disastrous attempts were made to dissolve plaque and calculus with inorganic acids (HCl and H_2SO_4); unfortunately, the acids also dissolved the teeth (24).

As early as 1800, dentists recommended chalk (calcium carbonate) for daily use to clean teeth (25). Dentifrices – usually paste but also powders, tablets, and liquids – have been used by people to remove food residues, abrade plaque, reduce tooth stains, eliminate or mask halitosis, and deliver active agents into the oral cavity to fluoridate and reduce plaque formation. Tooth powders, either home-made or manufactured, have been supplanted by toothpaste (pastes, including gel forms) and came into general use by the mid-20th century with higher awareness of the appearance of teeth and dental treatments. Many designs of nylon-tufted toothbrushes (ISO 22254/ADA119) for toothpaste application have been used and patented although no one design is known to be the best.

Modern toothpastes have nine components: abrasive, detergent, liquid, humectant, thickeners, flavor, color, anti-corrosive substance to control the pH, and active ingredients (for fluoridation or anti-plaque formation) (24). Abrasive ceramic powders have provided a wonderful armamentarium for home care both for stain removal and to disrupt the biofilm. Silica gel nanoparticles or precipitated silicate are commonly included in toothpastes. Other ceramic powders that have been or are used in dentifrices for plaque abrasion are silica, calcium carbonate, zircon, wollastonite, aluminum hydroxide, alumina, titania, and montmorillonite (magnesium aluminosilicate); plastic resin particles have also been added (US Pat. 4,980,153). Some abrasive particles are coarse but easily crushable to less than 10 μm. Titanium dioxide (titania) thickens and whitens toothpaste.

Anionic and amphoteric detergents are used in toothpastes to create a foam, reducing the surface tension to loosen films or debris and imparting antibacterial and plaque inhibition properties. The detergent compound most often used in toothpastes is the anionic sodium lauryl sulfate (SLS); other anionic detergents are sodium lauryl sarcosinate, sodium C14–16 olefin sulfanate, and cocamidopropyl betaine. Toothpaste detergents are controversial (26) because of cytotoxicity, oral epithelial destruction, ulceration, and inflammation by denaturing glycoproteins of the mucin layer formed on the teeth from glycoproteins.

The common humectants and liquids in toothpaste are 10–30% sorbitol, glycerol, polyethylene glycols, and water. The humectants do not solidify under normal conditions, and they dry (evaporate) slowly because they have a low vapor pressure. Organic thickeners, such as sodium carboxymethyl cellulose and xanthan gum, may be included to achieve a suitable viscosity and reduce separation of the liquid and powder; fumed silica also serves that function. Pleasant flavors – essential oils, aromas, or sweeteners – and pigments in toothpaste formulas encourage their use. Toothpaste-related standards (ISO 11609/ADA 130) require dentifrices to have a pH of less than 10.5 – hence buffering agents (anti-corrosives) are needed. One manufacturer adds sodium bicarbonate to neutralize the acidity in plaque. Preservatives are also needed in toothpaste for shelf life.

Active agents are present in some dentifrices for properties such as desensitizing, anti-bacterial, anti-caries, anti-plaque, anti-gingivitis, and anti-calculus. For instance, fluoride compounds for anti-caries are sodium fluoride, sodium mono-fluorophosphate, and stannous fluoride (NaF, Na_2PO_3F, and SnF_2) although potassium fluoride (KF) and organic amine fluoride have been used in the past. Stannous fluoride and sodium fluoride are also known to reduce gingivitis (gum inflammation). The FDA's monograph on over-the-counter oral products states that dental products with 1500 ppm fluoride or less are generally safe and effective. A method (ISO 11948/ADA 171) exists to determine the fluoride content of dentifrices – or other fluoride-containing dental products – using a fluoride ion–selective electrode in aqueous samples derived from dental products. Fluoride-containing toothpastes, mouthwashes, or similar products help recharge (ion exchange with the enamel) the fluoride in surficial hydroxyapatite via ion exchange.

Phosphate ceramic compounds are active ingredients in dentifrices, including dicalcium phosphate, calcium pyrophosphate, and tetrasodium pyrophosphate ($Na_4P_2O_7.10H_2O$), to inhibit supragingival calculus formation; the latter is often accompanied by zinc citrate ($C_{12}H_{10}O_{14}Zn_3$) in concentrations of 3.3–5%. Calcium sodium phosphosilicate (a bioactive glass, nominally formulated as $CaNaPSiO_6$) and tricalcium phosphate ($Ca_3(PO_4)_2$) are used to decrease sensitization and potentially re-mineralize enamel. New ideas for re-mineralization of enamel surfaces include using nano-sized hydroxyapatite particles dispersed in toothpastes at about 10%; the nano-apatite toothpaste may be augmented with fluoride to hopefully form fluoroapatite for greater hardness and acid resistance of the tooth enamel. Potassium and strontium salts (potassium chloride, citrate, and nitrate [KCl, $K_3C_6H_5O_7$, and KNO_3]; strontium chloride and acetate [$SrCl_2$ and $Sr(C_2H_4O_2)_2$]; sodium monoflurophosphate (Na_2PFO_3); and stannous fluoride [SnF_2]) also reduce sensitivity. The desensitizers may temporarily block the orifices of exposed dentin tubules so that oral fluids do not move in and out, eliminating the pain stimulated by their motion.

Toothpaste tablets are available as a toothpaste alternative; they may contain fluoride compounds for strengthening, nano-hydroxyapatite for re-mineralizing, xylitol to help prevent cavities, and other dry ingredients usually used in paste dentifrices. Chewing the tablets creates a foaming paste with one's saliva. Tablets reduce packaging for ecological benefits and convenience but are without whitening ingredients.

Carbon powder (charcoal) has been added to some toothpastes. Social media sites have advocated charcoal for whitening teeth (extrinsic stain removal). Historically, carbon powder has been used on teeth, but the modern formulas of carbon-containing dentifrice contain finer powder forms of activated charcoal. Unlike peroxides, charcoal toothpastes do not provide a whitening benefit (27). Charcoal particles can lodge in the margins of restorations, which can locally discolor the teeth.

Toothpastes and mouthwashes (oral rinses) have been formulated with zinc oxide or zinc salts to inhibit plaque and tartar formation with antimicrobial action. Zinc compounds (e.g., $ZnCl_2$ at more than 0.2%) inhibit tartar formation, are antimicrobial, and reduce the volatile sulfur compounds that cause halitosis (bad breath) (28).

Scoring methods exist to quantify plaque/tartar removal (29), but no consensus exists on how abrasive a toothpaste must be. Toothpaste abrasion plays a very small role in tooth erosion compared to other dietary microbial and salivary factors. The abrasive characteristics of ceramic powders are more complex than comparisons of hardness. Abrasion is influenced by the shape, porosity, particle size distribution, percent by volume, and a particle's tendency to fracture during application to a surface. These considerations apply to toothpastes, hygienist's professional products, dental laboratories polishing restorations, and abrasive instruments used to finish the shaping of a restoration by a dentist. The Relative Dentin Abrasion – Profilometry Equivalent (RDA) test method in ISO 11609 has been developed for testing dentifrices. Precisely flat samples, a profilometer, human teeth, and a brushing machine are required. After the test's brushing protocol is completed, the mean depth of abrasion is measured using profilometry versus the unbrushed control area on the dentin or enamel surface. Any toothpaste with an RDA of less than 250, the recognized threshold for safety, is considered safe for lifetime use. An alternative method using irradiation with 1 mCi of ^{32}P ß-radiation has also been used (30).

A particular concern for abrasion is the thinner layer of enamel present in the cervical region, where, if enamel crystals are lost, it will create a divot. This area is vulnerable to acids and abrasion, especially vigorous brushing or the presence of gum recession, exposing dentin. Abfraction is a controversial topic related to the cervical region where cyclic loading and bending (chewing, clenching) is believed to cause the gradual loss of enamel crystals, creating defects shown in Figure 6.7; abrasion may be a contributing factor to abfraction. Tooth-colored flowable resin-based composites are popularly used for covering cervical enamel loss. Pink-pigmented composite materials (Chapter 9) are also effective for masking unesthetic gingival recession characterized by abfraction, replacing the lost enamel, and protecting the dentin near the gingiva. Such cervical resin-based composites contain more ceramic powder pigments to match the many shades of the gingiva in the world.

Dental floss filaments are made of nylon, silk, polytetrafluoroethylene, or polyester that may be unwaxed or waxed. Waxed floss has a coating of microcrystalline wax, candelilla wax, beeswax, carnauba, castor oil, or rice bran wax but no ceramic powder. Flavorings with essential oils, aromas, or sweeteners are common. Only one floss brand and some "floss picks" are known to contain ceramic powders – silica – probably embedded in the wax or gum coatings on the floss fibers, which may be useful in removing biofilm.

Brushing one's teeth with toothpaste is an essential and effective part of personal hygiene, but teeth cleaning by a dental professional is superior. Hygienists have better access to the teeth and can use special equipment, instruments, and materials to remove biofilm clinging to the enamel and dentin as described in the next section. Diagnosis of potential problems is another benefit of professional prophylaxis.

Professional Cleaning

Periodic, professional teeth cleaning (prophylaxis, prophy) is now customary. Dental hygienists apply their skills with specialized materials and equipment that are more aggressive than those used at home, while avoiding harm to the soft tissue surrounding teeth. Prophylactic abrasive pastes and slurries of powder are applied using rotating brushes or rubber cups on the end of slow-speed dental handpieces rotating at less than 3000 rpm or with an airjet. At the height of the 2020 COVID-19 pandemic, rubber cups were popular again to reduce the dispersion of aerosols into the operatory rather than brushes or airjets. Air abrasion to clean teeth is more common and faster, reducing the hygienist's hand fatigue. The air abrasion nozzle projects a slurry of powder onto the tooth, possibly occluding some exposed dentinal tubules with the powder to reduce sensitivity. This process may be called "polishing" in a patient's vernacular. Air abrasion reaches tooth surfaces that are less accessible with a rubber cup or brush for removing biofilms.

The prophy pastes or slurries contain ceramic powders of low-to-medium hardness to abrade or dislodge plaque. The size of powders in prophylactic pastes may be classified as coarse, medium, or fine; however, no standard exists for defining these particle size categories. Relatively large particle sizes, greater than 70 μm, impart momentum and dislodge the layer without becoming embedded in the biofilm. Glycerin, preservatives, and flavors are combined with the ceramic powders to make professional cleaning more pleasant for the patient.

The hardness of these powders must be considered because cleaning should not abrade the enamel, gingiva, exposed dentin, cementum (the root sheath), dental cement, or resin-based composite restorations. See Table 13.1 for hardness comparisons among the prophy powders, tooth surfaces, and common restorative materials. The hardness of enamel exceeds that of dentin and most resin-based composite filling materials, but the prophylactic powders are harder; they must be administered with care to avoid harm to teeth or other tissues. Exposed dental cement at the margins of restorations is vulnerable to abrasion. Loss of cement at the margin of a restoration is detrimental to the longevity of the restoration because of the increase in the potential for bacterial re-infiltration (secondary caries). This highlights the skills needed by hygienists. The all-ceramic restorations (discussed in Chapter 10) are much harder than enamel and will not be harmed by prophylactic pastes or abrasive sprays. As mentioned for toothpastes, abrasion is influenced by the shape, porosity, particle size distribution, percent by volume, impact velocity, and a particle's tendency to fracture during impact on a surface.

Silica has been prominently used for prophylaxis, usually a pumice powder or perlite. Other abrasive ceramic particles used in commercial prophylaxis polishing pastes include aluminum hydroxide ($Al(OH)_3$) and sodium bicarbonate ($NaHCO_3$), calcium carbonate ($CaCO_3$), aluminum oxide (alumina, Al_2O_3), aluminum silicate, garnet ($(Ca,Mg)_3(Al,Fe,Cr)_2(SiO_4)_3$), feldspar $(K/Na/Ca)AlSi_3O_8$), zirconium oxide (ZrO_2), and silicon carbide (SiC). Sodium bicarbonate is recognizable by patients for its grittiness, salty taste, and the fine deposits of overspray on their face. Aluminum hydroxide particles are a little harder than sodium bicarbonate; therefore, the hydroxide can abrade cement margins or create scratches on resin-based composite materials having a lower fill percentage of glass.

Table 13.1 Knoop hardnesses.

Tooth structure	Knoop hardness number
Cementum	40
Dentin	68
Enamel	355–461
Restorative materials	
Porcelain	14
Metal reinforced glass ionomer	14–24
Glass ionomer	18–30
Anterior resin-based composites	46–48
Micro-filled resin-based composites	19–58
Posterior resin-based composites	45–64
Hybrid resin-based composites	51–65
Gold, gold alloys	20–90, 120–170
Abrasives used in prophylaxis pastes and dentifrices	
Sodium bicarbonate Na_2CO_3	120
Calcium carbonate $CaCO_3$	135–170
Aluminum hydroxide $Al(OH)_3$	330
Pumice	590
Bioactive glass	840
Feldspar (various compositions)	840–930
Garnet ($[Mg,Fe,Mn]_3Al_2(SiO_4)_3$)	930–1220
Alumina (Al_2O_3)	2100
Silicon carbide (SiC)	2780

Source: (31) / Wolters Kluwer Health, Inc.

Calcium carbonate (chalk, $CaCO_3$) is less abrasive (lower hardness) than pumice and aluminum hydroxide. Alumina, garnet, feldspar, and zirconia are more abrasive and only used as minor components. Silicon carbide powder has been used as part of a slurry for specialized prophylaxis within periodontal pockets, a challenging area for prophylaxis; however, this powder is gray.

Serious stains can require the dentist to intervene to improve the appearance of the dentition. The more aggressive pastes – more aggressive prophylactic pastes – require careful application to avoid damaging anatomy. ADA 62 has requirements for in-office abrasive pastes for removing stains and other exogenous materials from natural tooth structures and prostheses.

Ultrasonic Cleaning

Ultrasonic teeth cleaning is used to remove recalcitrant biofilm, particularly below the gum line, in periodontal pockets and exposed furcations, considerable more thoroughly than can be achieved by hand scaling. A metal tipped scaler, vibrating at about 25,000–50,000 cycles per second, is used with water irrigation. The ultrasonic vibration and water cause cavitation and violent bubble motion that contribute to plaque removal while irrigating and flushing debris from periodontal pockets without an abrasive powder. The efficacy of ultrasonic scaling is undisputed, as shown in Figure 13.2, for an in vitro display of the results of hand and ultrasonic scalers used to remove biofilm.

Two kinds of ultrasonic scalers are used: piezoelectric and magnetostrictive. The ceramics that make ultrasonic instruments vibrate are discussed in Chapter 18. Piezoelectric scaling may be preferred over the original magnetostrictive scalers because piezoelectric motion is a more precise linear scaling motion; magnetostrictive vibration provides a wider but imprecise elliptical motion. The linear

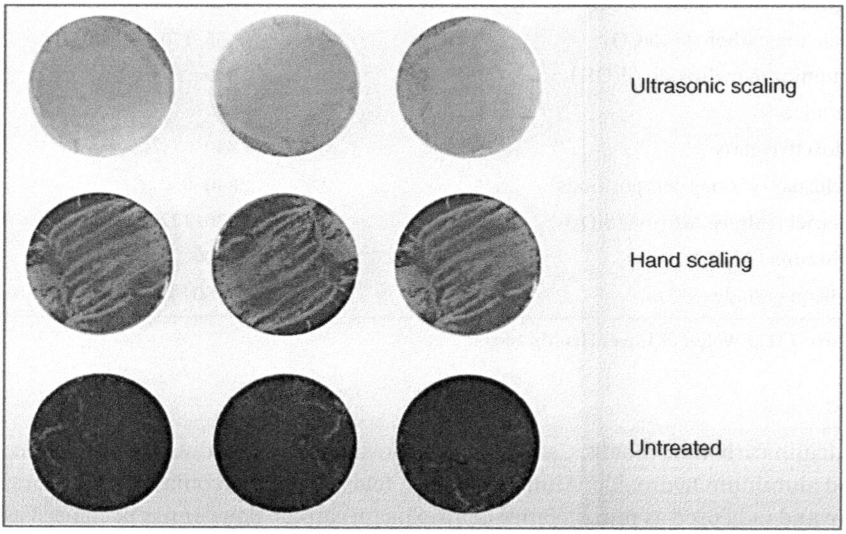

Figure 13.2 Ultrasonic scaling results (top) in a petri dish showing very little biofilm remaining. Hand Scaling (middle row) shows streaks removed by hand scaling. The control biofilm (bottom) shows untreated biofilm. *Source:* Dentsply Sirona USA / https://www.youtube.com/watch?v=VKpthcW1llU/last accessed on April 28, 2025.

motion of piezoelectrics also reduces the hygienist's exposure to the bioburden in aerosols generated by scaling and allows the hygienist to use lower power settings. The amount of ultrasonic energy is crucial to control because too much power can destroy cells on the root surface or within the pulp or damage tooth enamel. Polymers are used for ultrasonic tips to clean dental implants; they prevent damage to the implant. Training is necessary to achieve the correct instrument angulation against the tooth surfaces and avoid damage to the more delicate root dentin or restorations. The requirements and test methods for air or electrical piezoelectric, ferrostrictive, and magnetostrictive ultrasonic scalers and tips are in ISO 18394/ADA 157.

Lasers for Cleaning

One laser has been FDA-cleared for reducing bacteria in the periodontal regions surrounding teeth. This laser equipment is based on the InGaAs semiconductor diode operating at 980 nm with a power of less than 10 W in continuous or pulsed modes. The laser light can "reduce inflammation and reduce bacteria" while simultaneously inducing hemostasis.

Bleaching Teeth – Outside and Inside

Professional prophylaxis can remove the majority of extrinsic discoloration, but stain removal can be augmented by bleaching techniques and products for in-office bleaching, dentist-prescribed at-home bleaching, and over-the-counter bleaching products. Most bleaching products use hydrogen peroxide (H_2O_2) as the active agent, applied to the facial tooth surface to achieve a lighter, whiter color. Hydrogen peroxide can diffuse through the interprismatic spaces of the enamel; the reactive oxygen species (ROS) generated by the decomposition of hydrogen peroxide will break down chromophores (stains) to lighten the enamel.

Hydrogen peroxide bleaching can cause mild-to-severe dentin hypersensitivity. Adverse effects have occurred with higher hydrogen peroxide concentrations and longer treatment times on soft tissues, hard tissues, and restorative materials – oral mucosa irritation, pulpal sensitivity, pulpitis, or alteration of the enamel surface (32). Bleaching with hydrogen peroxide is a relatively safe procedure; the European Scientific Committee on Consumer Products[ii] (SCCP) rates tooth whitening products containing 0.1–6.0% hydrogen peroxide or equivalent to hydrogen peroxide–releasing substances are safe, but a consultation with a dentist is recommended.

ii https://www.ncbi.nlm.nih.gov/pmc/articles/PMC5804394/st

Carbamide peroxide ($CH_6N_2O_3$, $CH_4N_2O.H_2O_2$) is an organic oxidizer created by reacting urea with hydrogen peroxide. A product with 30% carbamide peroxide contains around 10% hydrogen peroxide and is a common component of bleaching products for longer shelf life and a prolonged effect for home products. ISO 28399/ADA 136 documents have test methods and requirements for external bleaching agents, not including abrasives, for home or office application. Erosion is to be avoided!

Bright white or violet-colored LED light is sometimes used to enhance the effectiveness of external bleaches (33, 34). The effectiveness of light activation of bleaching materials is controversial. Using a light may dry the teeth during treatment, giving an initial perception of greater whiteness.

Some testing has shown antimicrobial and enhanced bleaching with titania (TiO_2) nanoparticles that were co-doped with nitrogen, fluorine, or silver to accelerate the hydrogen peroxide decomposition. More bleaching efficacy with the nanoparticles may lead to lower hydrogen peroxide concentrations and less post-treatment sensitivity.

Endodontic treatments with antibiotics have caused internal discoloration which can be treated by internal bleaching. The first documented intracoronal (internal) tooth bleaching was in the 1800s and included calcium chloride, $CaCl_2$, hydrogen peroxide, H_2O_2, sodium perborate (NaH_2BO_4, $Na_2H_4B_2O_8$, $[Na]_2[B_2O_4(OH)_4]$), sodium peroxide of various hydration formulas ($Na_2O_2.2H_2O_2.4H_2O$, $Na_2O_2.2H_2O$, $Na_2O_2.2H_2O_2$, and $Na_2O_2.8H_2O$), and pyrozone (25% hydrogen peroxide/75% ether). In the mid-1900s, the walking bleach technique was developed in which sodium perborate was mixed with water and placed in the pulp chamber of the tooth that had previously had an endodontic treatment. Sodium perborate reacts with water, producing hydrogen peroxide; it can be left for several days in the pulp chamber and may be repeated (35, 36). Although more complicated than extra coronal bleaching, intracoronal bleaching is viewed as a minimally invasive procedure to improve dental esthetics at a relatively low cost that conserves tooth structure as opposed to placing a crown to disguise a badly discolored tooth. This bleach does not correct tetracycline or SDF discolorations.

Denture and Night-Guard Cleaners

Removable appliances – full or partial dentures, nightguards, or the like – need cleaning and disinfection, which is easily performed with sodium hypochlorite (NaOCl) solutions. The antimicrobial action of sodium hypochlorite is attributed to the hydroxyl and chloride ions (OH^-, Cl^-) dissociation in water, which dissolves microbial cell walls and mucins, degrades lipids and fatty acids, and inactivates enzymes. The common concentrations are 1.5 to 2% and may include sodium hydroxide (1.7% w/o). A solution with 0.5% hypochlorite for three minutes has antimicrobial activity against *Streptococcus mutans* and *Candida albicans* without affecting denture color, surface smoothness, or strength. Inorganic acid-based cleansers, typically containing weak solutions of hydrochloric or phosphoric acids, chemically dissolve calcified biofilm deposits and the cell membrane of microorganisms in biofilms. It is notable that some denture cleaners will discolor exposed metal of partial dentures.

Effervescent denture cleaner tablets contain inorganic oxidants, such as sodium bicarbonate, sodium percarbonate, and sodium persulfate ($NaHCO_3$, $Na_2H_3CO_6$, $Na_2S_2O_8$), which release carbon dioxide bubbles and oxygen when they dissociate in water to attack surface films. Sodium sulfite and sodium triphosphate (Na_2SO_3, $Na_5P_3O_{10}$) are also used, which are common in laundry detergents. Sodium lauryl sulfate detergent in tablets also can disrupt the biofilm and improve cleaning efficacy. Effervescent-type denture cleaners are used for cleaning metallic dentures, but they are less antimicrobial than the sodium hypochlorite cleaners; also they may disrupt the adhesion and softness of "relined" dentures. Enzyme-based cleaners are similar to effervescent-type cleaners but contain lipases, amylases, and proteases. The enzymes are formulated to degrade fats, glycoproteins, and other proteinaceous organic matter, creating antimicrobial effects. These are primarily used with dentures having soft reline materials present.

Summary of Ceramics and Tooth Maintenance

Maintenance of teeth is essential and should be performed at home and by dental professionals. Systemic and topical fluoride compounds used in home and professional care have significantly reduced the incidence of dental caries by slightly hardening the enamel through forming fluoroapatite; repeated fluoride application is required to maintain this protection. The scientific consensus adopted by the World Health Organization lists three fluoride-eluting material as essential medications – silver diammine fluoride, fluoride toothpaste, and glass ionomers.

The keys to successful tooth maintenance are mechanical removal of biofilms and use of fluoride compounds, especially in toothpaste and water systems. Abrasive ceramic powder acid and base have been essential for cleaning teeth and removable prosthodontics for home and professional uses. Internal and external bleaching is achieved with hydrogen peroxide and sodium perborate, respectively.

Ceramics in Chapter 13

The following ceramics and other inorganic materials were mentioned in this chapter:

- acidulated fluoride
- alumina

- aluminum hydroxide
- calcium carbonate
- calcium chloride
- calcium fluoride
- charcoal
- feldspar
- fluoroapatite
- fluorosilicic acid
- garnet
- hydrochloric acid
- hydrogen peroxide
- hydroxyapatite
- indium-gallium-arsenic
- magnesia
- montmorillonite clay
- phosphoric acid
- potassium chloride
- potassium fluoride
- potassium iodide
- potassium nitrate
- silica
  - gel
  - fumed
  - pumice, perlite
  - calcium sodium phosphosilicate glass
- silicon carbide
- silver diammine fluoride
- silver fluoride
- silver phosphate
- sodium bicarbonate
- sodium fluoride
- sodium fluorosilicate
- sodium hypochlorite
- sodium hydroxide
- sodium mono-fluorophosphate
- sodium perborate
- sodium percarbonate
- sodium persulfate
- sodium peroxide
- sodium phosphate monobasic
- stannous fluoride

- sulfuric acid
- tetrasodium pyrophosphate
- titania
- tricalcium phosphate
- wollastonite
- zinc oxide
- zircon
- zirconia

References

1 Yu, O.Y., Zhao, I.S., Mei, M.L. et al. (2018). Caries-arresting effects of silver diamine fluoride and sodium fluoride on dentine caries lesions. *J Dent* 78: 65–71.

2 Mitrut, I., Scorei, I.R., Manolea, H.O. et al. (2022). Boron-containing compounds in dentistry: a narrative review. *Romanian J Morphol Embryol* 63 (3): 477–483.

3 Benzian, H. (2022). Dental public health breakthrough. *Br Dent J* 232 (7): 421.

4 Gooch BF. U.S. Public Health Service Recommendation for Fluoride Concentration in Drinking Water for the Prevention of Dental Caries. Public Health Reports; 2015.

5 Bergmann, K.E. and Bergmann, R.L. (1995). Salt fluoridation and general health. *Adv Dent Res* 9 (2): 138–143.

6 Hescot, P., Roland, E., and Desfontaine, J. (1995). Fluoridated salt in France. *Adv Dent Res* 9 (2): 144–145.

7 Ivanova, K., Pakhomov, G.N., Moeller, I.J., and Vrabcheva, M. (1995). Caries reduction by milk fluoridation in Bulgaria. *Adv Dent Res* 9 (2): 120–121.

8 Shen, C., Rawls, H.R., and Esquivel-Upshaw, J.F. (2021). *Phillips' science of dental materials*, 13the, 448. Philadelphia: Elsevier, Inc.

9 Unde, M.P., Patil, R.U., and Dastoor, P.P. (2018). The untold story of fluoridation: revisiting the changing perspectives. *Indian J Occup Environ Med* 22 (3): 121–127.

10 Samaranayake, L., Porntaveetus, T., Tsoi, J., and Tuygunov, N. (2025). Facts and fallacies of the fluoride controversy: a contemporary perspective. *Int Dent J* 75 (4): 1–12.

11 Do, L.G., Sawyer, A., John Spencer, A. et al. (2025). Early childhood exposures to fluorides and cognitive neurodevelopment: a population-based longitudinal study. *J Dent Res* 104 (3): 243–250.

12 McMahon, P.B., Brown, C.J., Johnson, T.D. et al. (2020). Fluoride occurrence in United States groundwater. *Sci Total Environ* 732: 1–15.

13 DenBesten, P. and Li, W. (2011). Chronic fluoride toxicity: dental fluorosis. *Monogr Oral Sci* 22: 81–96.

14 Wang, Q., Meng, Q., and Meng, J. (2020). Minimally invasive esthetic management of dental fluorosis: a case report. *J Int Med Res* 48 (10): 1–7.

15 Edmunds, W.M. and Smedley, P.L. (2013). Fluoride in natural waters. In: *Essential of medical geology*, 2nde (ed. O. Selinus, B. Alloway, J. Centeno, et al.), 311–336. Springer.

16 Cochrane, N.J., Shen, P., Yuan, Y., and Reynolds, E.C. (2014). Ion release from calcium and fluoride containing dental varnishes. *Aust Dent J* 59 (1): 100–105.

17 Nozari, A., Ajami, S., Rafiei, A., and Niazi, E. (2017). Impact of nano hydroxyapatite, nano silver fluoride and sodium fluoride varnish on primary teeth enamel remineralization: an in vitro study. *J Clin Diagn Res* 11 (9): ZC97–ZC100.

18 Alhothali, M., Exterkate, R., Lagerweij, M. et al. (2021). The effect of equal fluoride concentrations in silver diamine fluoride and potassium fluoride on demineralized dentin during pH-cycling: chemical data. *Eur J Oral Sci* 129 (4): 1–8.

19 Ammar, N., El-Tekeya, M.M., Essa, S. et al. (2022). Antibacterial effect and impact on caries activity of nanosilver fluoride and silver diamine fluoride in dentin caries of primary teeth: a randomized controlled clinical trial. *BMC Oral Health* 22 (1): 657–668.

20 Nguyen, V.N.C., Felsenfeld, J., and Primus, C.M. (2017). Potassium Iodide. The Solution to Silver Diamine Fluoride Discoloration? *Adv Dent Oral Health* 5 (1): 1–6.

21 Freire, P.L., Stamford, T.C., Albuquerque, A.J. et al. (2015). Action of silver nanoparticles towards biological systems: cytotoxicity evaluation using hen's egg test and inhibition of *Streptococcus mutans* biofilm formation. *Int J Antimicrob Agents* 45 (2): 183–187.

22 Estedlal, T., Omrani, L.R., Abdi, K. et al. (2024). Development of TiF4-dendrimer complex gel as an anti-demineralization agent for dentin: an in vitro study. *Dent Mater* 1–10.

23 Xu, V.W., Yin, I.X., Niu, J.Y. et al. (2024). The anti-caries effects of copper tetraamine fluoride on enamel: an in vitro study. *J Dent* 151: 1–7.

24 Breuer, M. (1978). *Cosmetic science*, 355. Academic Press.

25 Spielman, A., Koshki, J., Lepor, A., and A S. (2024). John Greenwood's sidenotes on a 1778 John Hunter text at the New York Academy of Medicine. *J Hist Dent* 71 (3): 158–171.

26 Birant, S., Duran, Y., Gokalp, M. et al. (2021). Effects of different detergent-containing children's toothpastes on the viability, osteogenic and chondrogenic differentiation of human dental periodontal ligament stem cells and gingival stem cells in vitro. *Tissue Cell* 72: 1–12.

27 Franco, M.C., Uehara, J., Meroni, B.M. et al. (2020). The effect of a charcoal-based powder for enamel dental bleaching. *Oper Dent* 45 (6): 618–623.

28 Ziyati, O., Abou-Obeida, S., Mtalai, N., and Boussiri, K.E. (2024). Zinc and oral health: literature review. *OALib* 11 (07): 1–23.

29 Lee, J.B., Choi, D.H., Mah, Y.J., and Pang, E.K. (2018). Validity assessment of quantitative light-induced fluorescence-digital (QLF-D) for the dental plaque scoring system: a cross-sectional study. *BMC Oral Health* 18 (1): 1–11.

30 Hefferren, J.J. (1976). A laboratory method for assessment of dentrifrice abrasivity. *J Dent Res* 55 (4): 563–573.

31 Sawai, M.A., Bhardwaj, A., Jafri, Z. et al. (2015). Tooth polishing: the current status. *J Indian Soc Periodontol* 19 (4): 375–380.

32 Bizhang, M., Domin, J., Danesh, G., and Zimmer, S. (2017). Effectiveness of a new non-hydrogen peroxide bleaching agent after single use – a double-blind placebo-controlled short-term study. *J Appl Oral Sci* 25 (5): 575–584.

33 Kury, M., de Oliveira Ribeiro, R.A., de Souza Costa, C.A. et al. (2024). Co-doped titanium dioxide nanoparticles decrease the cytotoxicity of experimental hydrogen peroxide gels for in-office tooth bleaching. *Clin Oral Investig* 28 (10): 1–11.

34 Kury, M., Hiers, R.D., Zhao, Y.D. et al. (2022). Novel experimental in-office bleaching gels containing co-doped titanium dioxide nanoparticles. *Nanomaterials (Basel)* 12 (17): 1–23.

35 Amer, M. (2023). Intracoronal tooth bleaching – a review and treatment guidelines. *Aust Dent J* 68 (Suppl 1): S141–S152.

36 Barakah, R. and Alwakeel, R. (2019). Non-vital endo treated tooth bleaching with sodium perborate. *Curr Health Sci J* 45 (3): 329–332.

14

Modeling Teeth for Treatments

In the 18th century, dentists were improving fixed prosthodontics and needed to improve and customize the fit thereof. Dentists sketched the dentition to help them make restorative devices, but impression materials were needed to make models of teeth for better fitting indirect restorations. Impression materials are molded in the mouth, usually with a tray, to fit over the teeth and gums; when removed, the impression is an intaglio – a negative likeness – of the tooth anatomy. Impressions may cover several teeth, a whole arch, or create a record of the occlusion (bite registration) between the maxillary and mandibular arches. Impression materials are also needed for making maxillofacial prostheses, such as obturators (maxillectomy, cleft lip, and palate prostheses), ear prostheses, and prostheses of the eyes. A modeling material is cast in the impression to replicate the teeth and create a positive – a three-dimensional replica – of the dental anatomy that can be examined without the patient.

For fixed prosthodontics (Chapter 10), the dentist removes some tooth structure (prepares the tooth) so that the dental laboratory can make an appropriate indirect restoration for attachment (cementing). Then the dentist has to communicate (prescribe) the precise shape of the prepared tooth to the dental laboratory via an impression of the prepared tooth. Traditionally, impression material was molded over the prepared tooth and adjacent teeth, allowed to set, and then removed from the mouth, and these are described in this chapter. However, digital impressions now constitute about 35% of dental prescriptions; digital impressions do not need a tray of material to be inserted in the mouth to capture the tooth shape; optical scanning equipment is used to record the teeth and their positions, including the occlusal relations of the surrounding teeth.

Impression materials – or the intraoral optical scanners discussed later in this chapter – should accurately capture anatomical detail. Like most dental materials, the desirable characteristics for impression materials include biocompatibility

Ceramics in Dentistry: Materials, Manufacturing, and Clinical Applications,
First Edition. Carolyn M. Primus.

and non-toxicity; they should be non-irritating to oral tissues as well as odorless, tasteless, immune to oral fluids, and easy to prepare and use. Impressions must withstand disinfection, which is required after removal from the mouth, without losing shape or detail. Finally, impression materials should have short enough working and setting times for patients' and dental professionals' patience. A "good" shelf life and a reasonable cost make any dental material ideal. Compatibility with gypsum (hydrated calcium sulfate) is useful because gypsum is ordinarily used to create the positive model of the dentition from the impression.

Historic impression materials have been wide-ranging, beginning with warmed beeswax in the 18th century (1). Waxes are frequently mentioned in duplicating the anatomy and for crafting dental restoratives for both fixed prosthodontics (Chapter 10) and dentures (Chapter 15). Metal trays were developed to ease the insertion and removal of the wax with as little distortion as possible; porcelain trays for holding wax or other materials were used but were fragile and less common.

Wax is also an auxiliary impression material used for bite registration, but other formulas have had multiple uses in a dental laboratory based on easy melting and conform ability. Soft and hard waxes have been used to make a prototype of a restoration – metal or ceramic – and for various denture pattern creations (baseplate wax). In addition, waxes are a frequent (minor) component in dental materials from gutta-percha to the impression materials described herein. Ceramic fillers can be a minor part of a wax formula to control flow, e.g., mica, talc, and alumina. Dental waxes are standardized in ISO 15854 and ADA 122 documents.

The so-called "modeling compounds" or impression compounds were developed in the mid-1800s (2); they contained gutta-percha (transpolyisoprene rubber), waxes of various types, resins, and ceramic powders. The fillers constituted about 50% of the material, usually talc ($Mg_3Si_4O_{10}[OH]_2$, magnesium silicate), calcium carbonate ($CaCO_3$), and iron oxide (Fe_3O_4) although white lead (hydrocerussite, trilead dihydroxide dicarbonate, $2PbCO_3.Pb[OH]_2$) was used in some formulas. This thermoplastic material, available as sheet or rope, was warmed to soften the gutta-percha in an impression tray before insertion in the mouth; gutta-percha softens) at about 40 °C (its glass transition point) and melts at about 64 °C. The elasticity from the gutta-percha was an improvement over wax. The "set" modeling compounds had high enough viscosity and rigidity, that they were unsuitable for impressions with undercuts and unable to record fine details of the dentition. Therefore, modeling compounds were best for denture fabrication; however, modeling compound was used for the archaic use of copper tubes (3) and single-tooth impressions.

In the same era, plaster of Paris (calcium sulfate hemihydrate, $CaSO_4.1/2H_2O$) began being used for impression taking. Plaster impressions had less distortion than wax but had to be removed in pieces. Shellac was painted on plaster impressions after removal from the mouth and functioned as a separator so that gypsum could be poured into the plaster impression to create models. Wax and plaster were sometimes combined for impressions, with the wax against the teeth. Metal foil was also used in the early 20th century for making impressions. The metal foil would become part of the earliest ceramic crowns by Land (4) as described in Chapter 10.

Zinc oxide-eugenol (ZOE) impression materials were developed in the 20th century and became well-known for making impressions for fixed prosthodontics. The ZOE impression materials contained about 87% ZnO powder dispersed in an oil to make a paste. Just before use, this paste was combined with another paste containing eugenol (12–15%), and organic resins (~50%), such as balsam resin, and pigments. Silica was present in both pastes to equalize the viscosities, which made apportioning and mixing easier. See Table 14.1 for a typical composition, which includes zinc acetate dihydrate $Zn(CH_3CO_2)_2.2H_2O$ and an alkaline earth chloride ($Mg/CaCl_2$). ZOE impression material becomes rigid as it absorbs water and sets, which makes removal difficult and unsuitable for impressions with undercut

Table 14.1 Typical ZOE, agar, and alginate compositions (*wt.%*) (ceramic components listed first)

Component	ZOE	Agar–agar	Alginate
Zinc oxide (reactor)	42.5		
Zinc oxide (filler)			4
Borate		0.2–0.5	
Calcium sulfate		1–2	16
Silica, as diatomaceous earth (filler)			60
Magnesium or calcium chloride	2.5		
Potassium titanium fluoride (accelerator)			3
Sodium phosphate (retarder)			2
Other unidentified ceramic fillers	10		
Zinc acetate (accelerator)	1		
Oil & eugenol & rosin	44		
Agar		13–17	
Wax		0.5–1.0	
Potassium alginate			15
Water		75–80%	1:1 with powder above

areas; its strength is lower than the elastomeric materials discussed later in this chapter, and the eugenol can be irritating to the soft tissue. Higher heat and humidity accelerate setting, as does adding a drop of water when the powder and liquid are mixed. On the positive side, ZOE impression material has dimensional stability for 24 hours, is of lower viscosity than modeling compound, and is suitable for casting gypsum models for dentures and interocclusal records (bite registration).

Hydrocolloids

Hydrocolloids were the first elastic impression materials; they form a gelatin-like biocompatible solid, easy to mix and use on wet tissues, and flexible enough to be removed as an accurate rendition of the teeth. Two types have been used, agar–agar and alginate, which are flexible carbohydrates based on seaweed. Agar–agar became the first elastic impression material in the 1930s; it's a mixture of agarose and agaropectin in a 70/30 proportion. When mixed with water, it forms a gel at body temperature but melts at about 85 °C. The agar impression material contains ceramic powders of borax, silica (diatomaceous earth), clay, and potassium sulfate (K_2SO_4). See Table 14.1 for a typical composition. This material is boiled in water to melt, then incubated at 45 °C to create a gel for making impressions; it needs to be swiftly placed to avoid cooling. Agar is used for denture impressions, duplicating models, and sometimes for crown preparation with a subgingival margin because it is hydrophilic. When removed, a model should be made within an hour; otherwise, the impression will undergo imbibition or syneresis (absorb or expel water) and become inaccurate. Agar differed from earlier materials because it was elastic, non-toxic, and affordable, but it is not easily disinfected without distortion. The need for equipment to melt then incubate the agar in a gel state, and its sensitivity in making models makes it unpopular now. It is the only reversible impression material.

Sodium alginate impression material was developed in the United States during World War II when agar–agar from Japan was in short supply. Alginate ($[C_6H_8O_6]_n$, alginic acid) is an insoluble polysaccharide extracted from some brown algae species. Alginic acid is converted to sodium or potassium alginate ($[Na/K]C_6H_7O_6$), which is soluble in water. Alginate impression powder typically contains about 15% sodium or potassium alginate, 16% calcium sulfate, 60% diatomaceous earth, with minor amounts of zinc oxide, potassium titanium fluoride (K_2TiF_6), trisodium phosphate (Na_3PO_4), and optional pigments, flavors, and glycol. Minor components may be magnesium oxide, sodium ethylene diamine tetraacetic acid, and fluorides of sodium, lithium, zinc, or barium (US Pat. 4,515,913A). A typical powder composition is found in Table 14.1 (5).

A dental assistant mixes the alginate powder with water and loads it in an impression tray where the powder to set quickly and irreversibly. The alginate compounds readily dissolve in water and react with Ca ions from $CaSO_4$ forming insoluble calcium alginate. Trisodium phosphate modulates the reaction rate because the calcium ions preferentially react with the phosphate ions from sodium phosphate to form tricalcium phosphate ($Ca_3[PO_4]_2$). Eventually there are more calcium ions in the mixture than phosphate ions. At this point, the extra calcium ions rapidly bind to the dissolved alginate. This accelerated setting phenomenon is also known as "snap-set"; that is, a slow setting followed by a rapid setting event. Calcium phosphate in the set material may sparingly dissolve, which contributes to the alginate's dimensional instability after setting; alginate must be swiftly used for making a model – within an hour, like agar–agar. Potassium titanium fluoride (K_2TiF_6) (3%) is included to create a harder gypsum surface when calcium sulfate is poured into the impression; otherwise, the alginate can inhibit setting of the calcium sulfate in dental stone. The inexpensive alginate impression material is easy to use but has low tear strength versus the polymeric materials described below. Alginates are popular impression materials because they have low viscosity, do not compress tissue, and set quickly.

These two hydrocolloids are classified in ISO 21563 and ADA 128 into three types – heavy, medium, and light body formulas – for various impression uses.

Polymeric Impression Materials

Three popular, polymeric impression materials were developed in the mid-20th century: polysulfide, polyether, and polyvinyl siloxane. These two-part, monomer materials, consisting of base and catalyst/accelerator pastes, chemically react when mixed to quickly form an elastic polymer. The elasticity, stability, and tear strength of the polymers are much higher than earlier materials, a great advantage for recording undercuts and details. The overall composition and ceramic components are discussed below. A wide range of ceramic filler powders have been mentioned for use in polymeric impression materials (US Pats. 9,549,881, 8,921,475); among the fillers are silica (glass powder or fibers, quartz powder, cristobalite, diatomaceous earth), calcium silicate (wollastonite), carbon powder, iron oxide, zinc oxide, calcium carbonate, calcium sulfate, magnesium carbonate, talc, zircon, montmorillonite, bentonite, zeolite, sodium aluminum silicate, feldspar, nepheline syenite, alumina, titania, and barium sulfate.

Polysulfide rubber, introduced in the mid-1950s, was the first polymeric (elastomeric) impression material. The base paste contains rubber-based monomers with thiol groups and ceramic fillers – silica, titania, and lithopone (zinc sulfide and barium sulfate, ZnS and $BaSO_4$) – to increase the viscosity and elastic modulus. The second paste contains 60–68% of brown-colored lead dioxide (PbO_2) in an inert carrier oil. When the two pastes are mixed, the lead dioxide reacts with the hydrogen of the thiol (organosulfur [R – SH]) groups, forming lead oxide (PbO), oxygen, and water while polymerizing the polysulfide rubber. About 0.5% sulfur is included to ensure lead sulfide (PbS) is formed rather than the metal Pb. Higher temperature and humidity accelerate the reactions. The lead (Pb) compounds pose no patient hazard because the lead is encapsulated and immobilized in the monomer and is used for less than 10 minutes. The polysulfide rubber is hydrophilic, strong and flexible, having good flow (low viscosity), a longer working time than the other elastomers, and better biocompatibility than the other elastomeric impression materials – surprising given the PbO_2/PbO content! However, polysulfide impression materials are messy and have a sulfurous odor. Impressions for dentures are often made with polysulfide rubber impression material, but the polysulfide materials' indications are versatile.

Polyether rubber was introduced as an impression material in the 1960s; it is used for preparing impressions for indirect restorations, implants, and denture borders. The base and catalyst pastes react to form imine-terminated polyether rubber, cross-linked by an aromatic sulfonate. Silica, titania, zeolites, zinc oxide, and pigments, such as cobalt aluminate (cobalt blue $Co[AlO_2]_2$), are known to be fillers in polyether impression material.

Polyether impression material is also hydrophilic, has good tear strength, has no odor or taste, is tidier than the polysufides, and is compatible with gypsum. However, polyether rubber is the stiffest, least elastic, of the polymeric impression materials. Its disinfection time should be limited because it is hydrophilic – prolonged soaking can cause distortion – but it is suitable for fixed prosthodontics, implants, inlay, and onlay impressions.

Polyvinyl siloxanes became popular elastomeric polymers for taking tooth impressions in the 1980s, either "condensation" or "addition-reaction" types. Silicon, a ceramic, is a component of the monomers, but the silicone monomers are organic, having methyl groups (C-H bonds).

The condensation silicone impression materials contain hydroxy-terminated poly-dimethylsiloxane and fillers in the base paste. The accelerator paste contains tetraethyl silicate (tetraethyl orthosilicate, tetraethoxysilane, TEOS, $SiC_8H_{20}O_4$) with stannous octoate ($C_{16}H_{30}O_4Sn$) as the catalyst. The tin catalyst hydrolyzes with trace water and forms tin hydroxide ($Sn(OH)_2$ or $Sn(OH)_4$); when the pastes are combined, the tin hydroxide causes the silicone monomers to polymerize, set, and release ethanol, which gradually evaporates. The condensation silicones are accurate and pleasant for the patient but prone to shrinkage because of the ethanol released; they require immediate pouring of a model. The fillers include amorphous and crystalline silica, with pigments including titania and iron oxide.

The addition silicone impression materials are the most popular elastomeric material for impressions (6). Their base paste contains hydroxy-terminated polysiloxane polymer and fillers. The accelerator/catalyst paste contains divinylpolysiloxane prepolymers, palladium powder (Pd), and inorganic chloroplatinic acid (H_2Cl_6Pt), or platinum-divinyltetramethyldisiloxane ($C_{24}H_{54}O_3Pt_2Si_6$). When the addition silicone pastes are mixed, the base paste's hydrosilane-terminated molecules react with the catalyst's siloxane oligomer's vinyl groups and polymerize. A relatively dry mouth is needed to overcome the hydrophobic nature of these polymers; surfactants are included in the formulas to enable intimate contact with the dental tissues. A secondary reaction produces hydrogen gas by the reaction of water with the hydride of the base polymer. Unlike other impression materials that require a gypsum model material to be poured immediately, the addition silicones require a waiting period of at least 30 minutes to allow the hydrogen gas to dissipate. Advantages of the addition silicone impression materials are their excellent accuracy, short setting time, good tear resistance, and compatibility with gypsum. Because of the polymers' stability, multiple models can be cast from the same impression. Fillers for the polyvinyl siloxanes include the usual inert and common ceramic powders: cristobalite, fumed amorphous silica, diatomaceous earth, titania, zeolites, and calcium carbonate and cobalt oxide pigment. A fun fact is that addition silicone was used to make the astronauts' boots for the first moon landing, and created the first human impression in lunar dust.

The polymeric impression materials are available in more than one viscosity to accommodate different case needs. Impression materials of several consistencies are commonly combined in an impression tray to balance high fidelity around the prepared teeth and high tear strength for removal. The ability of an impression material to record fine details depends on its consistency and ability to "wet" the tissues, ideally by being hydrophilic; wettability implies close contact can be made with tissues to capture fine details. The viscosity, or more loosely, the consistency, of the monomeric impression materials is codified in the ISO 4823 – elastomeric impression materials standard (ADA 19), which lists four types of consistency from thick to thin (0–3) This standard includes a test method and requirements for consistency (spread). The consistency test is used rather than a viscosity measurement because viscosity values depend on the method, and the consistency test is considered easy and practical. An impression is expected to reproduce 20–70 µm and 100–150 µm for fixed and removable prosthodontics, respectively. High dimensional stability – low linear dimensional change – is also needed, as well as a lack of distortion (high elastic recovery) and low strain after compression. See Table 14.2 for the standards' requirements for consistency, detail reproduction and overall requirements.

Table 14.2 ISO 4823/ADA 19 requirements for elastomeric impression materials.

<table>
<tr><th>Type</th><th>Description of consistency</th><th colspan="2">Diameter of disc in consistency test (mm)</th><th>Detail reproduction (μm)</th><th>Linear dimensional change (%)</th><th>Elastic recovery (%)</th><th>Strain in compression (%)</th></tr>
<tr><td>0</td><td>Putty</td><td>—</td><td>75</td><td>75</td><td rowspan="4"><1.5</td><td rowspan="4">>96.5</td><td rowspan="2">0.8–20</td></tr>
<tr><td>1</td><td>Heavy bodied</td><td>—</td><td>50</td><td>50</td></tr>
<tr><td>2</td><td>Medium bodied</td><td>31</td><td>20</td><td>20</td><td rowspan="2">2.0–20</td></tr>
<tr><td>3</td><td>Light bodied</td><td>36</td><td>20</td><td>20</td></tr>
</table>

Table 14.3 Typical working & setting times and elongation for elastomeric impression materials.

Elastomer	Mean working time (min.)	Mean setting time (min.)	Elongation at break (%)
Polysulfide	4:20	12:30	500
Polyether	2:20	8:20	300
Condensation silicone	2:30	9:00	350
Addition silicone	1:50	6:00	150

The typical working and setting times of the elastomeric materials are presented in Table 14.3. Note that the working time to get the impression material mixed and placed over the teeth may be as brief as 2.3 minutes. All the elastomers set in less than 15 minutes, which is usually tolerable except for children. Some impression materials have been modified for faster setting in pediatric dentistry. The elastomeric impression materials may be stretched at least 150% before tearing, a convenient attribute for removing an impression from the mouth.

Bite registration impressions are needed to confirm how the maxillary and mandibular teeth occlude, a crucial aspect of designing restorative devices. Bite registration impressions are usually performed after other impressions are made; elastomers and zinc oxide-eugenol materials are common.

Polyether urethane dimethacrylate material was developed in the late 20th century as a light-curable impression material. The impression material contained fumed silica, titanium dioxide, zinc sulfide, and iron oxide; it had excellent mechanical qualities, long working time, short setting time when initiated, dimensional stability, accuracy, high tear strength, good wettability, and biocompatibility. Plus, it was suitable for cold disinfection and compatible with gypsum. However, light curing in a large portion of the dental arch is problematic, requiring time and access to the posterior teeth, so its popularity was never realized. A combination of materials of vinyl polysiloxane and polyether has recently been promoted for its hydrophilic behavior and dimensional stability achieved by the monomer combination (7).

Impression Materials' Adjuncts

A dentist's preparation of a tooth for a crown always includes a finishing line very close to the mucosa (gingival tissue), and this margin is very important to replicate; therefore, the mucosa may need to be temporarily displaced to get a precise impression. This is sulcus expansion, formerly known as retraction of the gingival tissue, and it is needed for high-fidelity impressions for implant restoration or crowns with subgingival margins. Astringent, inorganic salts are impregnated into a retraction cord (thin, knitted, cotton string) or are added to high-viscosity polymeric materials to shrink the soft tissue, avoid bleeding, and prevent interference with recording the margin (edge of the tooth's preparation) in an impression material or digitally. The retracting agents are aluminum sulfate (alum), aluminum chloride, aluminum potassium sulfate, or ferric sulfate ($Al_2(SO_4)_3$, $AlCl_3$, $KAl(SO_4)_2.12H_2O$, or $Fe_2(SO_4)_3$). Other hemostatic agents used in cords are ferric subsulfate, ferric chloride, aluminum ammonium sulfate, aluminum acetate, potassium permanganate, silver nitrate, and hydrogen peroxide ($Fe_4H_2O_{22}S_5$, $FeCl_3$, $(NH_4)Al(SO_4)_2{\cdot}12H_2O$, $C_6H_9AlO_6$, $KMnO_4$, $AgNO_3$, and H_2O_2) per US Pat. 8,382,476. Aluminum chloride gel solutions (25%) are also used for hemostasis before an optical or physical impression is made. Certain kaolin clays are expansive and hemostatic with water; both are benefits to use in sulcus expansion materials. Addition-silicones, without a platinum "getter", are present in some products because they emit hydrogen gas to create an expanded sulcus.

Materials for Models

After an impression is taken, a model is made – a positive replica that imitates the dental arch. To make a physical model, plaster (calcium sulfate) is mixed with water and placed in (poured into) disinfected impressions. When the plaster hardens, a gypsum (hydrated plaster) model has been formed that is removed from the impression. The calcium sulfate powders are manufactured via different processes to create the distinct types, but all are mixed with water to use the reversible reaction of Eq. (14.1), the reverse of Eq. 5.3:

$$\begin{array}{c}(CaSO_4)_2.H_2O + 3H_2O \Leftrightarrow 2(CaSO_4.H_2O)\\ \text{Plaster (hemihydrate)} + \text{water} \Leftrightarrow \text{gypsum (dihydrate)}\end{array} \tag{14.1}$$

The chemical reaction proceeds as the plaster dissolves in the water, achieves saturation of calcium ions, and precipitates as the dihydrate. As the dihydrate is precipitated, more plaster powder can dissolve into the water. Potassium sulfate (K_2PO_4) increases the solubility of the plaster, which accelerates the setting. Borax (sodium borate, $Na_2B_4O_7.10H_2O$) retards setting by an unclear mechanism. This setting reaction is exothermic, and large models feel warm during setting. As with other setting reactions described for cements, the reaction never goes to completion, but 90% conversion is possible. Minor amounts of gypsum in the hemihydrate powder act as nuclei to speed the precipitation and hardening. The gypsum products are somewhat fragile compared to restorative materials but can reproduce detail as fine as 20 μm. Since the plaster powders of hemihydrate appear identical except under a microscope, dyes have been allowed to signal to the user what calcium sulfate product they are using. Dental plaster is white, dental stone is tan, and other shades are at the manufacturer's discretion.

Five types of gypsum materials are identified according to their use in ISO 6873 and for Dental Duplicating Material and ADA 25 – Gypsum Products: (1) impressions; (2) models for mounting in an articulator and diagnostic models; (3) models for fixed and removable prosthodontics (stronger than Type 2); (4) stronger, for low expansion dies, model base, and dies for CAD/CAM cases; and (5) high-expansion dies. The standards have requirements for expansion and compressive strength for each type as listed in Table 14.4. The die materials must be more robust than models because they are used with other materials to make a restorative device. The Type 1 gypsum for impressions needs less compressive strength but must be faster setting (less than five minutes) and more fluid than the other types although plaster intraoral impressions are now uncommon. Starch powder has been added to plaster impression materials so that a plaster model can be cast into the impression, soaked in water, and the impression material disintegrates.

The gypsum products are made from mined gypsum mineral, which is heat-treated to drive off water. The manufacture of the hemihydrate powder is critical to controlling the strength and setting speed of the plaster. Heating gypsum at about 120 °C produces irregular, porous particles of the hemihydrate suitable for dental (or medical orthopedic) plaster. When gypsum is heated above 120 °C under steam pressure, a less porous hemihydrate powder is made. These forms

Table 14.4 Requirements for gypsum products per ISO 6873.

Type	Class	Maximum linear setting expansion (%) @ 2 h	Compressive strength (MPa)	Uses	Color	Approximate water to powder ratio
1	—	0.15	4–8	Impressions	White	0.5–0.75
2	1	0.05	>9	Models for articulators and diagnostics. Class 2 may be fast setting.		0.5
2	2	0.30	>9			
3	—	0.20	>20	Models for full or partial dentures, and dies for fixed prosthodontics, CAD/CAM cases. Stronger than Type 2.	Blue or yellow	0.3
4	—	0.15	>35	Dental stone for models bases CAD/CAM dies	Tan	0.25
5	—	0.30	>35	Dental stone for high strength & high expansion dies, to compensate for shrinkage of the dental restoration.	No requirement	0.2

of plaster are referred to as alpha and beta (α and ß), respectively, but these are not different crystal forms as α and ß usually designate. The α and ß designations describe the crystal morphology; α is the less porous form. The morphology of α and ß plaster powders is shown in Figure 14.1a. Very dense hemihydrate particles are manufactured by boiling gypsum powder in a chloride ($CaCl_2$) salt solution and sold as dental stone. Dental stone is stronger than the other gypsum powders and requires less water to set because it has fewer pores.

Key factors for mixing and reacting calcium hemihydrate to dihydrate include

- Water to plaster ratio: more water means that more of the plaster has to dissolve to achieve saturation, which delays crystallization (setting) but causes less expansion.

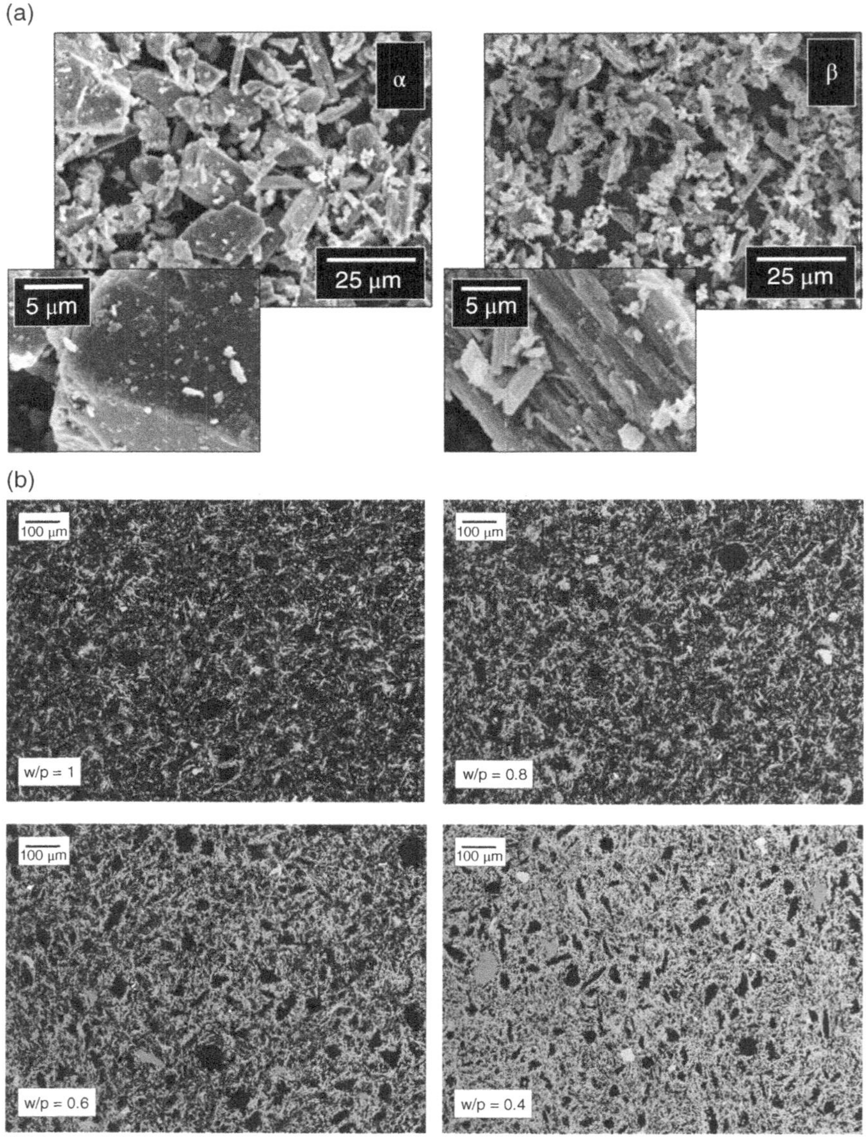

Figure 14.1 (a) SEM photomicrographs of the α and ß forms of calcium sulfate hemihydrate powder. (b) SEM photomicrographs of polished sections of hardened gypsum, prepared with decreasing water-to-plaster weight ratios (w/p). White areas are gypsum crystals and black areas are voids. *Source:* (8) / American Chemical Society.

- Spatulation (vigorous mixing) increases the number of nuclei by dispersion of the particles and has a shorter setting time.
- Hot water increases the rate of plaster dissolution but slows crystallization/precipitation for a net effect of slower setting.
- Vibrating a model removes bubbles and increases its strength.

The typical water to powder ratios are in Table 14.4; naturally, less water makes the stronger products, which can be surmised from Figure 14.1b showing the increasing density of gypsum with increasing powder. The water is apportioned by volume, and the powder is weighed; mixing is commonly performed in a rubber bowl to facilitate spatulation for homogeneity. A working model for the dental technician may be made to include some individual teeth (dies) that can be removed from the rest of the arch. Dies are hard gypsum models of an individual tooth, which can be separated from the rest of the model for the convenience of a dental technician who uses them for building a restoration. Copper has been electroplated on dies for durability.

Other materials are used for models: epoxy, polyurethane, and heavy body silicone materials for 3D printing, or better durability as a die for repeated duplication. The silicone materials are stable in their dimension as they set; the epoxy resin materials vary widely but have the dimensional fidelity similar to gypsum, with a "bit" of shrinkage. The amount of shrinkage upon polymerization is quantitatively about equal to the expansion with gypsum. These alternative models and die materials have ceramic fillers for viscosity control and pigmentation, including silica, titania, glass fibers, and undisclosed pigments. The fillers absorb some of the heat of setting.

Duplicating Materials

Several models may be needed for different aspects of creating a restorative dental device. For instance, a study model of the dental arch may be mounted on an articulator to study occlusion from viewpoints that are impossible intraorally, allowing the dentist or dental technician to meticulously visualize the teeth and their interaction. Duplication of models is also necessary when a refractory die is required for firing a ceramic restoration, such as a veneer. When multiple models are required, a duplicate impression of the first model is required. Duplicating materials used for the refractory die manufacture are required to be flexible and to have the same elastic recovery requirements as elastomeric impression materials, per ISO 14356/ADA 141. The refractory model materials are discussed in Chapter 15.

Optical/Digital Impressions

Digital dentistry advances in the 21st century are making impression materials outdated. Optical sensors for recording images of the dentition give better patient comfort because a small interoral camera is used rather than a full arch tray with impression material that must be retained for several minutes on the teeth. Patient comfort was also improved when scanners no longer needed spray-on coatings containing titania propelled by ethanol and pentane, to record the teeth positions. Like toothpaste, such sprays contained pigments and flavors.

Many advantages of intraoral scanning have been noted: the material and armamentarium used in analog impressions are avoided (e.g. impression trays, impression material, gypsum); the communication between the clinician and laboratory technician is improved since both parties can view and image on a screen, a "soft" copy can be stored without distortion concerns, and infection control is eliminated due to absence of contact, except for the scanner.

Currently, the resolution of detail is about 20–40 μm, depending on the scanner. However, the depth of field, accuracy, resolution, speed, and field of view are ever-improving with new equipment. Critical aspects of a scanner design are autoclavability, lightweight construction, ability to access the molars, depth of field of the optics, ease of use, and real-time imaging speed. Equally important is the accuracy of the scanners for capturing the anatomy for models, restoration design and manufacture. ISO 20896-1 and ADA 132 – Scanning Accuracy of Dental Chairside and Laboratory CAD/CAM Systems – were created for this topic. Notably, the scanners require an investment of $10,000–$70,000.

Optical created impressions fit into a digital workflow of dental devices creation. Electronic models are created as images from the impressions that can be virtually rotated for viewing and diagnosis. The virtual model images are used to design indirect restoratives, such as all-ceramic crowns. These electronically generated crown designs are sent to a CAD machine for subtractive or additive methods of creating the indirect restorative or other dental device.

Digital impressions have disadvantages: the expense of the equipment, less accuracy of entirely edentulous arches, interference of blood and saliva obscuring subgingival finish lines, and incomplete occlusal information for full arch prosthodontic treatments. For single units or a bridge (not a full arch), the intraoral scanners are accurate.

Summary of Impression, Model, and Duplicating Materials

Impression, model, and duplication materials have been essential to the precise practice of dentistry and making custom indirect restoratives that fit. A summary of the various impression materials and their features is in Table 14.5, and their

Table 14.5 Summary of impression materials.

Material	Elastic?	Hydrophilic?	Best use?	Muco-compressive?
Wax	No	Yes	Dentures	
Calcium sulfate (plaster)	No	Yes	Dentures	No
Modeling compound	No	No	Dentures	No
Zinc oxide-eugenol	No	Yes	Fixed prosthodontics	No
Agar	Yes	Yes	Dentures	
Alginate	Yes	Yes	Dentures	No
Polysulfide	Yes	Yes	Putty for dentures; light body for fixed prosthodontics including implants	No for light body; yes for putty
Polyether	Yes	Yes		
Condensation silicone	Yes	No		
Addition silicone	Yes	Yes and no		

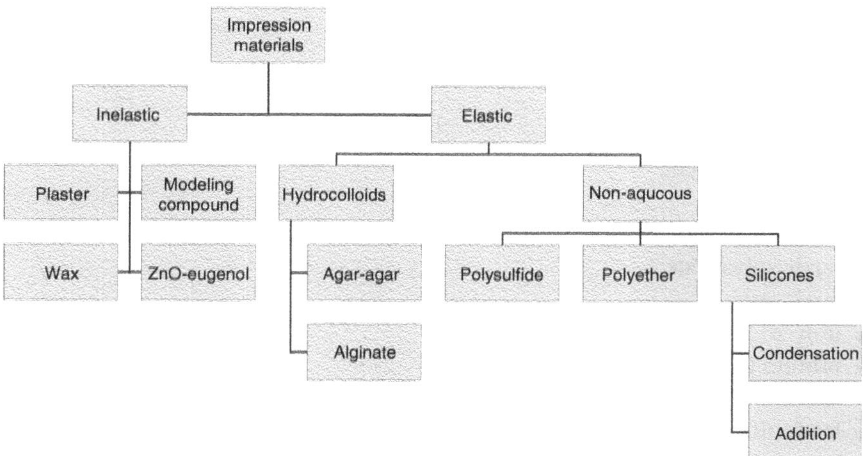

Figure 14.2 Classification of impression materials.

classification is in Figure 14.2. The choice of materials has been influenced by the tissue to be copied and the level of detail reproduction necessary. The materials used for primary impressions for removable complete dentures were alginate, impression compound, and elastomers in putty consistency. Alginate and elastomers are used to impress the oral tissues for constructing partial removable and fixed dentures. Addition-silicones and polyethers are commonly used impression materials in implant prosthodontics. The materials have been diverse but often included inorganic salts or ceramic powders, especially calcium sulfate. Gypsum is needed for models made from impressions. Duplicating materials to copy the models are similar to the impression materials and also require accuracy. Optical scanning will make these dental materials obsolete in developed countries.

Ceramics in Chapter 14

The following ceramics and other inorganic materials were mentioned in this chapter:

- alumina
- aluminum chloride
- aluminum potassium sulfate
- aluminum sulfate, alum
- barium fluoride
- barium sulfate
- bentonite
- borax
- calcium carbonate
- calcium chloride
- calcium sulfate and its hydrates
- carbon
- chloroplatinic acid
- cobalt aluminate
- feldspar
- ferric chloride
- ferric subsulfate
- ferric sulfate
- iron oxide
- lithium fluoride
- lead oxide
- lead sulfide
- magnesia
- magnesium carbonate
- magnesium chloride
- mica
- montmorillonite clay
- porcelain
- potassium permanganate
- potassium sulfate and its hydrate

- potassium titanium fluoride
- silica
- barium-alumino fluroroborosilicate glass
- diatomaceous earth
- glass fibers
- quartz, cristobalite
- sodium fluoride
- sodium phosphate
- talc
- titania
- tricalcium phosphate
- trisodium phosphate
- white lead
- wollastonite
- zeolites
- zinc fluoride
- zinc oxide
- zinc sulfide
- zinc sulfide

References

1 Papadiochos, I., Papadiochou, S., and Emmanouil, I. (2017). The historical evolution of dental impression materials. *J Hist Dent* 65 (2): 79–89.

2 Gupta, R. and Brizuela, M. (2024). *Dental impression materials*. StatPearls. Treasure Island (FL): StatPearls Publishing.

3 Singer, L. (1976). Simplified copper tube impressions for full crown coverage. *J Prosth Dent* 36 (5): 588–592.

4 Land, C.H. (1903). Porcelain dental art. *Dent Cosm* 45 (6): 437–444. and 615–20.

5 Shen, C., Rawls, H.R., and Esquivel-Upshaw, J.F. (2021). *Phillips' science of dental materials*, 13the, 448. Philadelphia: Elsevier, Inc.

6 Harcourt, J.K. (1978). A review of modern impression materials. *Aust Dent J* 23 (2): 178–186.

7 Craig, R.G. and Hare, P.H. (1990). Properties of a new polyether urethane dimethacrylate photoinitiated elastomeric impression material. *J Prosthet Dent* 63 (1): 16–20.

8 Jaffel, H., Korb, J.-P., Ndobo-Epoy, J.-P. et al. (2006). Probing microstructure evolution during the hardening of gypsum by proton NMR relaxometry. *J Phys Chem B* 110 (14): 7385–7391.see Table 14.2

15

Artificial (Denture) Teeth

In antiquity, a few missing teeth were replaced using natural substances for missing teeth – wood (common in Japan), ox, horse, or cadaver teeth, hippopotamus teeth and bone, and sea cow ivory tusks. The devices were affixed to remaining abutment teeth with wire, sinew, or thread. However, a vital need existed for those with few or no teeth: they needed larger sets of replacement teeth, dentures. Full or partial dentures are crucial to enunciation, mastication, and appearance for people who are partially or entirely edentulous. Early dentures had frameworks/bases carved from bone or ivory, or fashioned from gold, to fit the bony alveolar ridges. The replacement teeth were often from cadavers – sometimes called Waterloo teeth – which had been severed from their roots. Tools were used to remove the pulp and replace it with lead, which could be easily melted and poured into the pulp chamber. These dentures were never that satisfactory because the natural materials inevitably discolored and the organic components decomposed, emitting a foul odor.

Modern artificial teeth – denture teeth – are affixed to a framework/base and are removable by the wearer for cleaning. Porcelain, and then polymeric, artificial teeth were invented to make denture-wearing tolerable and affordable, which were long-lasting improvements to the quality of life for the edentulous. Polymeric and ceramic teeth standards are ISO 22112/ADA 15 Artificial Teeth for Dental Prostheses.

Porcelain Artificial Teeth

In the late 1700s, people had access to refined sugars, so caries and tooth loss were prevalent even though tooth "powders" were also available for cleaning. Dr. Pierre Fauchard is credited with suggesting the use of porcelain (1) for dentures.

Ceramics in Dentistry: Materials, Manufacturing, and Clinical Applications,
First Edition. Carolyn M. Primus.

Fauchard made porcelain dentures with a gold base, but he may have used enamel (glass coatings) to create the gum and tooth colors. Alexis Duchateau, a pharmacist, used porcelain to make a denture in 1774, an invention sparked by his own ill-fitting, odoriferous ivory denture (2); he denoted his dentures as mineral paste teeth. His porcelain dentures used the same porcelain for the base and teeth; they were fired as one unit. Archeological evidence confirms that complete porcelain dentures were available for the well-off people of the late 18th century (2); a porcelain denture set from this era had ivory-colored teeth and a gum/gingival base, with a pink glaze, that was designed to fit over the dental ridge – Figure 15.1. Porcelain dentures were far more sanitary than animal sources, with the added benefits of beauty, biocompatibility, insulation for food temperature changes, lower wear, durability, and avoiding metal allergies or exposure to lead.

The 18th century porcelain dentures and porcelain articles were generally primitive because they did not fit well; the impression materials were imprecise – beeswax was used, as noted in Chapter 14. The teeth were not articulated (separated) in the solid denture, so brown paint was used interproximally to suggest individual teeth. Making dentures was difficult in the available coke-fired ovens, which were large, hard to control, uneven in temperature, and expensive; the porcelain shrinkage was irreproducible, also contributing to poorer fit of the base. Many dentures were suitable for appearance but were unsuitable for eating because of their poor fit. In addition, the first porcelain dentures were easily chipped or broken if dropped or under mastication force. Duchateau worked with Dr. Nicholas De Chemant using Sevres and Wedgwood porcelains to improve

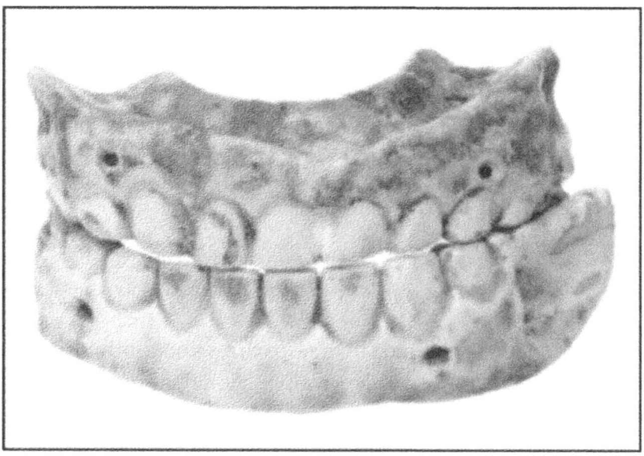

Figure 15.1 View of recovered porcelain denture interred in 1806 with its owner. *Source:* (2) / Springer Nature.

dentures' fit and coloring. Their porcelain was described as "hard," which may indicate it was in the high-fusing category of Chapter 10. The enhanced "mineral paste teeth" supposedly vitrified (formed glass during firing) but did not shrink; lack of shrinkage indicates that sintering was accompanied by formation of bubbles/pores.

In 1809, Dr. Guiseppangelo Fonzi invented a new approach, creating individual porcelain teeth called "terro metallic teeth", which were formed over an inserted platinum wire. After firing, the wires of each tooth were attached to a denture base made of another material. Early denture base materials, other than the porcelain of Duchateau, were diverse but expensive or technically challenging: gold or platinum alloys, silver alloys, aluminum, gold with porcelain enamel, gutta-percha, celluloid, and its related collodions (3). Soldering the porcelain teeth onto a metal base was costly but effective. Next, porcelain "tube teeth" were developed by Claudius Ash. These artificial teeth had a central cylindrical opening, formed around a gold or platinum alloy tube, which was used for attachment to the denture base. The tube teeth were adjusted for length to fit the base and the occlusion, then soldered or riveted to the metal denture base. Molten sulfur (~115 °C) was used in an interesting way: it was inserted through holes for the tube teeth in the metal denture base; when cooled, the teeth were secured (4) by the hardened sulfur. These methods were predecessors to the diatoric (pin less) attachment used today.

Denture manufacture was improving in this era, but it was the hard, rubber, "Vulcanite" denture base developed in the 1840s that significantly improved the durability and stability of the porcelain tooth denture. Vulcanite rubber revolutionized the acceptance and affordability of dentures, finally displacing the popular use of cadaver or animal materials combining the rubber base and porcelain teeth. A vulcanite denture base was made by heating latex fluid with sulfur powder to form rubber; the hardness of the rubber depended on the amount of sulfur and the heat treatment. The rubber was pigmented with zinc oxide and vermilion (mercury sulfide, HgS), and the latter was, thankfully, insoluble in water. Vulcanite was very versatile and came to be used for early orthodontic appliances.

Acrylic denture base supplanted "vulcanite" after 1937 because the acrylic polymer had better durability and attachment to teeth. Acrylic denture base (and teeth) is still in use today. Refer to ISO 20795-1 and ADA 139 for denture base polymer requirements, e.g., flexural strength, solubility, fracture toughness, color stability, bonding to artificial teeth, and residual monomer.

By the 20th century, artificial porcelain teeth were made – and patented – from minerals, including potassium feldspar and nepheline syenite; the latter is a mineral with sodium and potassium feldspar. Component minerals were crushed, blended, fused in an oven, and ground into −200 mesh (finer than 75 μm) powder. Several powders could be combined, molded into tooth shapes, and fired. In US Pat. 2,443,318, the artificial tooth powder composition consisted of 5% fritted (melted) feldspar and a glass. The glass was made from magnesium silicate, kaolin clay, and boron oxide; that is, the glass components were $MgO.XSiO_2$ $Al_2O_3.2SiO_2.2H_2O$, and B_2O_3. The value of X in the magnesium silicate was undisclosed, and Ca or Sr were alternatives to Mg. The glass was akin to Vycor®, a commercial silicate glass of low thermal expansion containing about 4% boron oxide, which was used in the patent's examples. The exact oxide compositions and presence of crystals in the porcelain artificial teeth are unclear. Formulas are vague, referencing "fritted feldspar," where the proportions of the alkali and alkaline earths in the feldspar were not specified. This was typical of traditional ceramics before the latter half of the 20th century when modern ceramic science blossomed. Microstructures of these denture porcelains were not available in references to identify the presence of crystals or pores in the ceramic artificial teeth.

Today, sophisticated polymeric binders are used to form high-tech ceramics, but starch flour and petrolatum have traditionally been mixed with the ceramic powders to make a dough for molding porcelain denture teeth. Several porcelains were combined, hand-filled into brass molds, unique to each of the permanent teeth. The first layer was the most transparent "incisal" dough, followed by "dentin" dough for most of the tooth, then a little "neck" or "cervical" dough, having a bit more pigment. Next, the packed molds were dried, and the nascent porcelain teeth removed. Many sizes and shapes of molds were required, and many shades of artificial teeth were offered.

Pigments included zirconia, vanadia, and iron oxide. Urania, ceria, and samaria (U_3O_8 or UO_2, CeO_2, Sm_2O_3) were combined in small amounts to achieve white fluorescence (US Pat. 2,895,050) in artificial porcelain teeth; urania alone had an unacceptable greenish-yellow fluorescence. Techniques were developed to frit (melt) the fluorescent oxides in high silica and boron oxide frits to make an effective and concentrated fluorescent glass powder that could be added to the feldspar powder and molded into teeth because adding the fluorescent oxides to feldspar powder was not as effective in creating fluorescence. This same technique of combining fluorescent components with other frits is used for making leucite-containing dental porcelains for enameling metals – Chapter 10.

Firing schedules were proprietary for such teeth but designed to avoid devitrification (crystallization) and possible cracking of the teeth during cooling. The first denture teeth were heated to burn off the starch binder, and then higher firing was performed in air until they were "vitrified"; that is, the teeth were sufficiently dense and translucent to be esthetic with some glass phase formed from the felspathic minerals.

By the 1950s, a two-step process was implemented to improve the strength and esthetics of artificial porcelain teeth. First the starch was burned out of the molded teeth in air, and then a separate vacuum firing (sintering) of the porcelain teeth was performed to cause densification and eliminate pores. Packing the molded teeth on trays for firing must be carefully recorded to ensure the sizes, shades, and the kinds of teeth are not confused.

Clever denture-making techniques were invented, such as forming a lower-fusing porcelain base over the higher-fusing porcelain teeth. To make such a denture, the porcelain teeth were set in wax in a mold, and the wax was burned off. Next, the wax was replaced by a dough of lower-fusing porcelain. The assembly was dried and removed from the mold, and the combined teeth and base were bonded by firing. A later invention used glass-ceramic denture teeth (5) mounted in an acrylic denture base.

Porcelain denture teeth continued to be used worldwide in the 20th century after the development of acrylic denture base materials, which gave an excellent fit to the alveolar ridges. Porcelain teeth were affixed to the acrylic with a combination of dovetailed shapes for diatoric retention, metal wires, and silane adhesives (US Pat. 3,369,297). Variations of artificial porcelain teeth have included filling a porcelain “shell” with polymer for improved adhesion to the base. Stronger artificial teeth were invented that used a core of fused steatite (magnesium silicate) porcelain, which was veneered with a more esthetic porcelain. One invention combined both the core and stronger porcelain concepts (US Pat. 3,423,829).

The first polymer teeth were too vulnerable to wear. Ceramic fillers were unsuccessfully used because ceramic powders’ adhesion to acrylic was not perfected in the 1960s. With the advent of silane coating, ceramic powders could be added to monomers for denture teeth (US Pat. 3,423,830). Acrylic denture teeth have been strengthened from the first versions and have deposed porcelain artificial teeth even though acrylic are softer and less durable. Acrylic teeth look natural, are less likely to fracture, do not make the clicking sound of porcelain teeth when occluding, and can be bonded to polymethacrylate denture base. In the 1970s, the bonding of denture teeth to natural teeth was tried, but only case reports were found with no widespread use. Modern dentures have a pink base to hold the teeth made of polymethyl methacrylate (PMMA). Three methods are used for setting denture teeth in a base resin: heating, milling, and three-dimensional (3D) printing. Heat-polymerization of PMMA has satisfactory mechanical properties, biocompatibility, esthetics, ease of processing, and repair but does shrink during processing and is time-consuming. Milling is an alternative method without shrinkage and is more accurate despite higher equipment costs and material waste for fabricating denture bases. 3D printing technology is the newest and offers rapidity, customized denture bases, and provisional teeth in the base with high accuracy and reduced material waste, although long-term durability is a concern (6).

One continuing problem is that the dentures may break when dropped, usually the base material. Many ideas for improving the strength have been tried, including embedding metal wires or silane-coated glass fibers (US Pat. 2,611,958) for reinforcement. Silica, titania, and zirconia nanoparticles have been tested for improving fracture toughness and impact strength, while decreasing water sorption and solubility (7) of denture teeth and denture base. Less than 1% of titania is used in some denture teeth for strengthening. Depending on the brand of denture base, graphene or fumed silica may be present (6). Research has been conducted on the beneficial effects of adding no more than 3% of boron compounds – borax, boric acid, and colemanite ($Na_2B_4O_7$, H_3BO_3, and $Ca_2B_6O_{11}.5H_2O$) – to denture base materials with some beneficial effects for fracture strength and surface hardness (8). Alumina additions have also been reviewed, with the complicated effects of particle size, shape, and coupling agent (silane) noted (9).

Technical excellence during prosthesis fabrication is essential for successful denture therapy. Poor-fitting and unstable dentures blight a patient's ability for normal daily activities. To stabilize an ill-fitting denture, a denture liner is used, commonly made of acrylic resin, polyvinyl siloxane, or a heat-cured acrylic (10); these liner materials are modifications of other dental impression or restorative materials. The "usual" ceramic fillers are included for pigmentation and creating a usable viscosity for their application to the denture base's intaglio.

A second method to help with fit is the use of denture adhesives (ISO 10873/ADA 135) placed on the denture base, a process that dates back to the 18th century. Adhesive is a confusing term, and here it means a paste or lining applied to the bottom of the denture to improve the fit and the security of the denture in the mouth, but it does not make the denture adhere to the gum tissue. Denture adhesive pastes expand with saliva to help stabilize the denture. Some denture adhesives may contain ceramic powders – sodium tetraborate or sodium borate – to improve their consistency for the application and add antimicrobial effects.

Partial Dentures

Partial dentures replace a few missing teeth rather than a full denture for an entire arch. Partial dentures also have artificial teeth, which began with porcelain teeth but now are primarily acrylic. The difference in partial and full dentures is the use of metal as the base of the material when strength is needed for mastication forces.

Summary of Chapter 15

Artificial teeth for removable prosthodontics were first manufactured from bone and natural teeth. Porcelain artificial teeth replaced animal materials beginning in the 17th century and were popular throughout the 18th through the first half of the 20th century. Porcelain teeth were surpassed by acrylic teeth in the 20th century due to the polymers' lower cost and resistance to fracture. Artificial teeth for full and partial dentures are "set" in a polymeric denture base often created by CAD-CAM machining. Polymeric temporary dentures can be entirely made by CAD-CAM and 3D printing.

Ceramics in Chapter 15

These ceramics and other inorganic materials were mentioned in this chapter.

- boron oxide
- ceria
- feldspar
- potassium feldspar
- nepheline syenite
- graphene
- kaolin clay
- magnesium silicate
- mercury sulfide
- porcelain, high-fusing
- silica, fumed
- samaria
- sulfur
- titania
- urania
- zirconia

References

1 Sproull, R. (1978). A history of porcelain in dentistry. *Bull Hist Dent* 26 (1): 3–10.
2 Powers, N. (2006). Archaeological evidence for dental innovation: an eighteenth century porcelain dental prosthesis belonging to Archbishop Arthur Richard Dillon. *Br Dent J* 201 (7): 459–463.
3 Ladha, L. and Mahesh, V. (2011). 19th century denture base materials revisited. *J Hist Dent* 59 (1): 1–11.
4 Hopwood, R. (2024). Sulphur cement. *Brit Dent J* 237 (8): 590.
5 Grossman, D.G. (1988). The science of castable glass ceramics. In: *Proceedings of the Fourth International Symposium on Ceramics Perspectives in dental ceramics* (ed. J.D. Preston), 117–133. Perspectives in Dental Ceramics: Quintessence.

6 Alhotan, A., Al-Johani, H., Altarazi, A. et al. (2025). Effect of uniaxial bending methods on the flexural strength and Weibull analysis of heat-polymerized, CAD/CAM milled, and 3D-printed denture base resins. *Dent Mater* 41 (3): e1–e7.

7 Azmy, E., Al-kholy, M.R.Z., Al-Thobity, A.M. et al. (2022). Comparative effect of incorporation of ZrO_2, TiO_2, and SiO_2 nanoparticles on the strength and surface properties of PMMA denture base material: an in vitro study. *Int J Biomater* 2022: 1–10.

8 Ozdemir, A.K., Ozdemir Dogan, D., Tugut, F. et al. (2021). Effects of boron on the mechanical properties of polymethylmethacrylate denture base material. *Eur Oral Res* 55 (1): 45–53.

9 Arora, P., Singh, S.P., and Arora, V. (2015). Effect of alumina addition on properties of poly-methyl methacrylate - a comprehensive review. *IJBTT* 5 (1): 7–12.

10 Abdul-Hussian, T.M., Shiyaa, S.A.J., Mohammed, W.I. et al. (2024). Denture lining materials. *Global J Res Dent Sci* 4 (1): 17–21.

16

Implanting in and Rebuilding the Jawbone

Teeth are extracted when they have root fractures, looseness, or incurable disease or are beyond repair by any dental treatment. This chapter is about the aftermath of extraction. In the 20th century, a bridge (fixed prosthodontic device) would have been common, with one or more pontics that span the missing teeth and attach to the remaining teeth. In the 21st century, a "bone-like" graft material is likely to be placed deep in the former root space, before the extraction site is sutured. After healing, a single dental implant may be prescribed, which is later topped with a crown. Both grafts and implants are "implanted materials", according to the definitions in ISO 10993-1 and ISO 7405 standards; that is, they principally contact tissue and bone and have long-term contact. These two medical devices must be tested to conform to more rigorous and extensive requirements by the FDA as "Dental Bone Grafts" and "Root-form Endosseous Dental Implants and Endosseous Dental Abutments" as "Class II devices with Special Controls"; these devices have more risk than the restoratives covered in Chapters 9 and 10.

Bone Grafts

After a tooth is extracted, the space in the alveolar bone formerly occupied by the tooth's roots will "collapse" as it heals; the faster-regenerating soft tissue fills the area that had been occupied by the hard root tissue, resulting in a narrower bony ridge. Over time, adjacent teeth may shift or tilt into the unoccupied space, causing various issues of esthetics or occlusion. These issues are especially problematic in the posterior, where the teeth are larger. Bone graft material can be immediately placed/implanted in the tooth socket – a socket graft – to minimize these problems. Grafted sockets heal in about four months as the cortical and cancellous particles gradually remodel (replace) the graft

Ceramics in Dentistry: Materials, Manufacturing, and Clinical Applications,
First Edition. Carolyn M. Primus.

material with native bone and revascularize the area. Graft materials are also used to augment a dental ridge that has already narrowed and to stabilize loose teeth by augmenting the surrounding bone as a consequence of periodontal disease. Sinus "lift" procedures require grafts to generate bone below the sinus while changing the position of the sinus floor's membrane to stimulate formation of more alveolar bone; more bone enables the placement of a stable implant. Bone graft materials are also used for complex maxillo-facial surgical uses – cranioplasty, repairing defects of the jaw such as congenital defects (e.g., cleft lip and palate), and replacement of bone after trauma or surgery to remove tumors. Graft materials are covered with sutures of soft tissue, membranes, and placement of "tenting screws" to minimize the washing out of particles.

Bone graft materials are microscopically designed to support the attachment of osteoblasts and chondroblasts – the precursor cells for bone and cartilage. The graft materials should be structurally similar to bone with comparable porosity and mechanical strength. Over time, the body responds to the graft by generating new bone cells on the ceramic particles. Eventually, the new bone cells supplant (resorb) the graft material as the bone undergoes "turnover" (remodeling). Bone remodeling is a lifelong process where mature bone tissue, or bone graft material, is removed from the skeleton (a process called bone resorption) and new mineralized tissue is formed and completely replaces the graft material. This is a remarkable dissolution and precipitation process for the calcium phosphate ceramics that occurs in vivo.

Bone graft materials come from sources categorized as autogenous, allogenic, xenogeneic, or alloplastic; that is, originating from oneself, another person, another species, or chemically made. The graft materials vary in their particle size, porosity size, and size distribution but are usually granular (0.5–2 mm) rather than the finer micro-sized powders mentioned in other chapters. Porosity is important for the osteogenic, osteoinductive, and osteoconductive properties of graft materials. "Block" autogenous grafts have been used for the rehabilitation of edentulous patients – the Khoury technique (1).

The autografts seem inherently preferable with their living cells and vascular channels; however, autografts require a second (source) surgical site, require more recovery time, and are less available. Surprisingly, autografts can cause painful donation sites, so usually alternatives are used. Autografts using an extracted tooth have been used as a block or powder, obviating the morbidity issue. These implants have been used for socket grafting and ridge augmentation (2).

Allografts are fresh, fresh frozen, or freeze-dried bone, which has been irradiated to avoid transferring infection from the other donor. Allogeneic bone grafts require irradiation as a precaution to prevent the potential of including infectious agents. Allogeneic materials are known as freeze-dried bone allograft (FDBA), demineralized freeze-dried bone allograft (DFDBA), or lyophilized bone.

Xenografts of bone are usually from bovine or porcine sources. The animal bone is heat-treated to remove the collagen, creating deproteinized bone that is osteoconductive (3). The elimination of the organic material in animal bones differentiates bone grafts from the historical use of animal tissues in prosthetic devices discussed in earlier chapters. Figure 16.1a shows the morphology of porcine, bovine and human graft particles, illustrating their similar porous "architecture." The autologous, allogenic, and xenografts originate from native bone, unlike the alloplastic synthetics.

A plethora (~90) of alloplastic (synthetic) bone grafts have been cleared by the FDA for filling periodontal defects, furcation defects, ridge augmentation or ridge preservation, sinus lift prior to implant placement, and peri-implantitis. Figure 16.1b illustrates the variations in morphology of a synthetic hydroxyapatite, a bovine graft, and a ß tricalcium phosphate graft materials. The ceramic alloplastic materials are available as granules, porous sections, moldable putties, pellets, injectable pastes, or customized 3D-printed shapes.

Calcia containing ceramic granules are used for grafts: tricalcium phosphate, biphasic calcium phosphate, calcium sulfate, calcium phosphate, bioglass, and carbonated apatite (3). Calcium sulfate was the first used as a bone graft in 1892, no doubt because it has a low cost and easy preparation, but this material is resorbed in 4–12 weeks, faster than native bone can regenerate to replace the sulfate. Calcium sulfate has been used creatively to reduce periodontal problems (6). Such grafts are slightly osteoconductive but lack appropriate porosity for bone ingrowth. A combination of calcium sulfate and calcium phosphate (2:1) material creates a self-setting ceramic indicated for maxillofacial and dental alveolar filling, augmenting and reconstructing bone defects.

The ß-tricalcium phosphate and the hydroxyapatite materials dominate the alloplastic bone graft materials. Tricalcium phosphate ($Ca_3[PO_4]_2$) was first used as a bone graft in 1920 and remains a popular synthetic bone graft because its chemical composition is most similar to human bone. It is osteoconductive and resorbed in 13–20 weeks after implantation, suitable for bone defects caused by trauma or tumors (7). Granules or a putty of ß-tricalcium phosphate particles have been used; the putty contained sodium hyaluronic acid (8). The granules vary from 150 to 1400 μm (0.15–1.4 mm), depending on the product. Biphasic calcium phosphate combines hydroxyapatite with tricalcium phosphate to allow a range of resorption times and mechanical properties for large defects in load-bearing areas, as well as resorption that synchronizes with the rate of bone growth (9).

Resorption of hydroxyapatite bone grafts is slower than tricalcium phosphate, with a speed that depends on the characteristics of the product. For instance, grafts with nanocrystalline hydroxyapatite crystals in the granules are resorbed faster. Some hydroxyapatite graft materials contain collagen (irradiated to eliminate potential contamination) from another natural source (e.g., demineralized dentin and bone matrices), which is primarily type I collagen (95%).

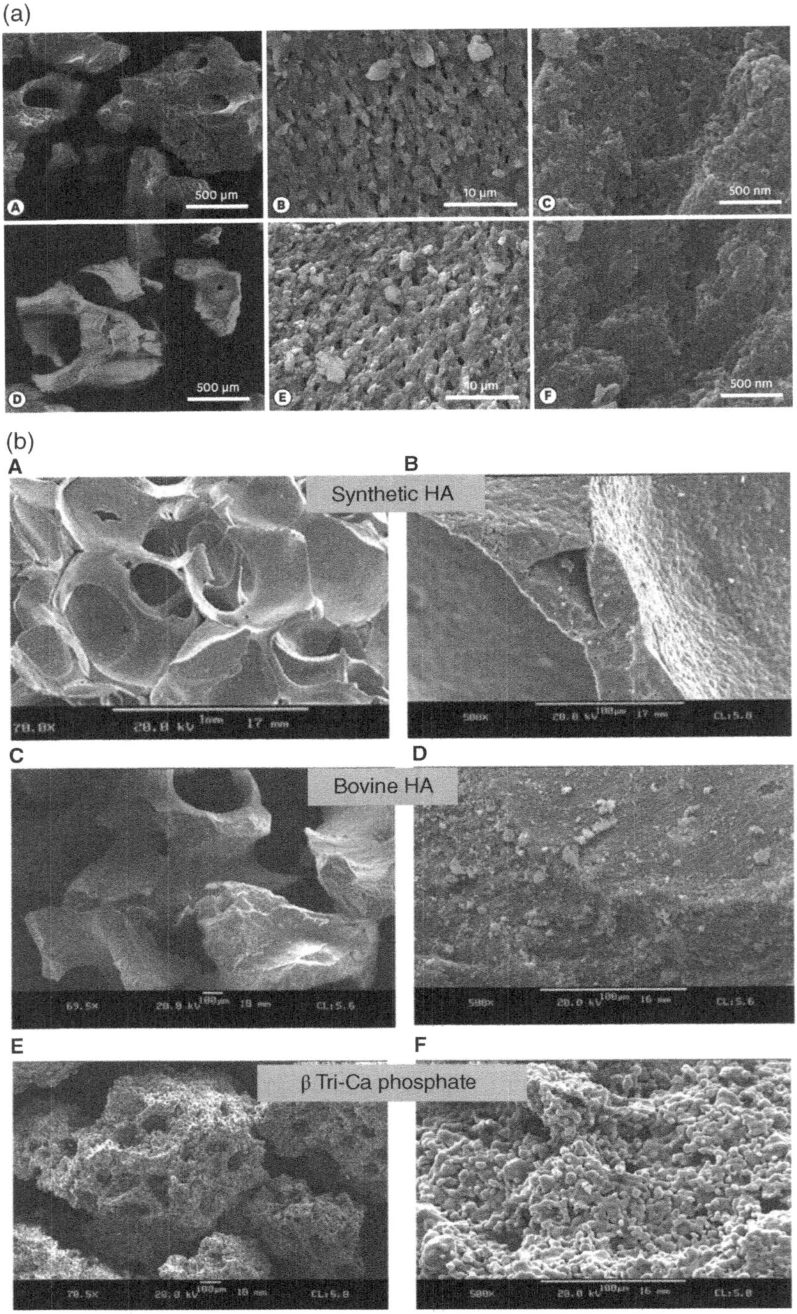

Figure 16.1 (a) SEM micrographs at three magnifications of porcine xenografts from SC Dental Supply / https://scdental.com.my/product/straumann-xenograft/ / Last Accessed on Sep 05, 2025. (b) SEM micrographs of three kinds of dental bone grafts, each at two magnifications, illustrating differences in morphology and porosity ISTI / https://koreascience.or.kr/article/JAKO201620853201189.page / Last Accessed on Sep 05, 2025.

Calcium phosphate cements (CPC) combine a calcium phosphate powder with a liquid that hardens in situ as described in Chapter 5. The cements rely on dissolution–precipitation reaction, first explored in the 1980s; see Eq. (5.9) for tetra calcium phosphate and dicalcium phosphate to form hydroxyapatite. CPC's hydroxyapatite crystals are gradually resorbed in vivo. Displacement (washout) of calcium phosphate cements has been a clinical problem (10); however, premixed putty-like pastes are beneficial (11). The most common uses of the calcium phosphates are synthetic hydroxyapatite and beta-tricalcium phosphate for bone grafting in the form of granules or pastes.

Bioactive glass granules are also used for bone grafts, including socket filling (12). Silica is released from the glass with some calcium and phosphate ions. The latter two form amorphous calcium phosphates on the surfaces of the particles, which crystallize into hydroxy-carbonate apatite and stimulate osteoblast formation. Gradually, the graft particles become more porous as they dissolve, and new bone replaces the graft material. Twelve stages have been proposed as the sequence of interfacial reactions for the bioactive glass integration (13). The bioactive glasses, first invented by Hench (14, 15), contained silica, calcia, and phosphorous pentoxide and some alkalis, which release ions that have inherently antibacterial properties in tissues (7). As described before, similar bioglasses contain other components, e.g., magnesia (16) and boron oxide (17). Bioactive glasses with 55–60 wt.% of silica (SiO_2) are considered to form bonds to bone. Alternative bioactive glasses have been evaluated for resorption, with the goal of matching the natural bone resorption/replacement rate, such as a bioglass having this composition: 38.8 SiO_2, 34 CaO, 13.4 P_2O_5, 13 MgO, and 0.8% CaF_2. The bioactive calcium silicate cements, mixed with gelatin or chitosan for suitable handling and resorption, have also been investigated for bone grafting in areas other than the head and neck (18–20). Strontium-substitution in calcium silicate cement has helped increase its resorption rate (21).

No consensus exists on the best bone graft product for clinical dental use. A variety of products are useful for the broad indications where bone grafts are needed (3). Manufacturers are obligated to create a technical file of the characteristics of their implantable materials, whether resorbable or non-resorbable, used for filling and augmenting bones in oral and maxillofacial surgery per ISO 22794/ADA 206. The documentation must include the chemical composition, physical properties, intended performance, preclinical and/or clinical evaluations, information on the manufacture, sterilization, packaging, and shelf-life. The ceramic phases need to be identified, both crystalline and non-crystalline, as determined by X-ray diffraction (XRD), Fourier transform infrared spectroscopy (FTIR), and/or differential scanning calorimetry (DSC), plus the cation-to-anion ratio (Ca/P, Ca/S) and the carbon/oxygen/nitrogen ratios (C/O/N) and all trace impurities. Furthermore, the surface features need to be disclosed, as well as the particle size, shape, porosity, and distribution. Handling characteristics, such as viscosity, extrusion force, temperature–water interactions, working time and setting time, and thermal behavior during setting, if it occurs, must be in the technical file. Other physical characteristics including compressive strength, elastic and shear moduli, the pH, and water solubility should be known. As for clinical features, the resorption rate should be identified from in vivo studies, stating a suitable time for an implant device to be placed after healing. Resorption can be estimated with acid dissolution tests or in clinical tests with x-rays and histology, the latter with animals.

The key to bone graft materials is low solubility and by concomitant replacement by native hydroxyapatite at the same rate, unlike other biomaterials that gradually dissolve (be resorbed) in vivo without bioactive benefits.

Periodontal pocket treatment is important to arrest the destruction of the gingiva, alveolar bone, periodontal ligament and cementum by bacteria invading the sulcular space. Mechanical processes are performed during hygiene treatments to remove dental plaque and calculus and from the surfaces of the roots and reduce inflammation. A myriad of treatments have been used to reduce pocket depth, among them antibiotics inserted in the periodontal pockets. Generally, ceramic materials are not a part of periodontal treatments although ceramic-organic particles (bioactive glass nanoparticles and pectin hydrogels) may be in future products.[i] Regeneration of the attachment of teeth to alveolar bone is the goal.

Bone Implants to Support Indirect Restoratives

Dentists perform restorative, periodontal, and endodontic treatments to save a tooth from extraction. After a tooth is extracted, a replacement is desired to maximize the comfort of daily living. An indirect, fixed or removable prosthodontic restoration may be constructed that spans the space between remaining teeth if the adjacent (abutment) teeth are healthy and can sustain the loading of a bridge. Less-common treatments to replace an extracted tooth have been intentional replantation and auto-transplantation, as mentioned in Chapter 8. A superseding need has existed for millennia for a dental implant in the alveolar bone – endosseous implant – that could support a crown, bridge, or denture.

Historical implant materials inserted in extracted tooth sockets were unsuccessful; these included seashells (calcium carbonate) carved into a tooth shape, bamboo pegs, animal or human teeth with roots, copper, gold, bone, and stone (22).

---

i Bioactive glass-laden ionically crosslinked pectin microspheres with pro-osteogenic and antibacterial activities for periodontal regeneration Qiu, S., Xu, X., Feng, Z., Li, L., Wang, X., Zheng, K. & Xu, Y. Ceramics International 2025 Issue 22 Pages 35323–35336 DOI: 10.1016/j.ceramint.2025.05.253

The prospects for endosseous dental implants changed when Prof. Per-Ingvar Brånemark investigated metals for orthopedic problems below the neck. He found that bone grew in apposition to titanium, which led to his pioneering work to develop dental implants in the 1960s. After 10 years of investigation, he reported 91% success for 4000 tooth implants (23). His keys to success were to use slow speed drilling of the implant socket, creating minimal trauma, by not raising the temperature of the surrounding tissue, and the use of uncontaminated, sterile, titanium implants. He allowed the surgical site to heal before loading the implant with a superstructure such as a crown. From his work, titanium implants have become accepted worldwide to support single crowns, bridges, full dentures, and partial dentures in multiple root forms, diameters and lengths.

Most endosseous (jawbone) implants are pure titanium. Titanium's success as a biomaterial is its inherent oxidation, forming a thin, tenacious, protective surface oxide (TiO_2) immediately on exposure to air, which prevents the leaching of titanium ions into the body. Commercially pure (cpTi) is usually used, and the common structural titanium alloys such as Ti6Al4V are avoided. However, some titanium–niobium alloys are possibly useful for their lower elastic modulus (140 vs. 90 GPa for Ti-30Nb) (24). A lower elastic modulus is more similar to enamel and dentin (54–120 and 11–28 GPa).

Titanium dental implants, like other orthopedic implants, have evolved over the decades with the goal to induce a tight fit in the bone. Many designs and surface treatments have been used; rougher surfaces are required, but not "too rough." Some designs had a stepped shape rather than the common screw design.

Ceramic implants and coatings on metal implants have also been exploited. In 1965, a screw-shaped dental implant fabricated from high alumina was used – the Tübingen-type (25) – and later a sapphire implant was commercialized (26). Alumina has been superseded by the stronger tetragonal zirconia, ZrO_2-$3Y_2O_3$ although ceria-doped zirconia with alumina has also been investigated. Zirconia endosseous implants are used for patients who are "metal phobic," have an allergic reaction to titanium, or to reduce metal "show through" where the tissue is thin or receding. All these implant materials are stiffer than cortical bone (~7–30 GPa), but a high modulus is not particularly desired. Zirconia has an even higher elastic modulus, about 230 GPa (27), than the titanium materials; however, the short-term performance of zirconia (1 year) versus titanium implants was equal (28). The ISO standard 13,356 "Implants for surgery – Ceramic materials based on yttria-stabilized tetragonal zirconia (Y-TZP)" is applicable to zirconia dental implants. Various ceramic implants have been cleared by the FDA since 2007; ceramic implants had been implemented in Europe before that.

Surface finish is key to any implant achieving intimate bone-to-implant contact on "moderately" rough surfaces. Nano-particle ink-jetting has been used to create a dense zirconia dental implant material with an outer, porous layer suitable for osteointegration (29). Plasma-sprayed hydroxyapatite (HA) coatings have been used on titanium dental implants as a rough biocompatible surface. The HA coatings are applied by entraining the HA powder in a noble gas (e.g., argon) that is injected into a plasma jet stream where the particles are melted and splattered on the surface of an implant. The difference in thermal expansion between the coating and the base materials must be considered for manufacture and use. Therefore, graded coatings, having layers of materials of different thermal expansions (4 vs. 10 ppm/K) have been designed to reduce the thermal stress from the Ti to the HA coating. Pre- or post-coating thermal treatments also reduce stresses to improve coating adhesion. Bioactive glasses have been used as coatings as well as wollastonite and diopside ($CaO.SiO_2$ and $MgO.CaO.2SiO_2$) (US Pat. 5,125,971). Additive printing parameters using the digital light processing method were comprehensively explored for a combination of zirconia and dicalcium silicate (30), for a potential dental implant. Selecting the printing parameters is complicated and interactive; the burn-off and sintering processes after printing are also challenging and have not achieved the same strength of tetragonal zirconia as with other methods as yet.

A completed single-tooth implant prosthesis is composed of three parts: the endosseous implant screwed (usually) into the bone, an abutment placed over the implant, which is the transition element providing inner support to the third component: a crown, bridge, or denture. Alumina implant abutments were FDA cleared beginning in 1991, and zirconia was first cleared in 1999. Abutments may be attached by a screw, cement, or friction fit. Crowns may be attached to the abutment with a screw or cement, the latter becoming less common. The attachments and screws for connections to the abutment vary with the manufacture, which can complicate placement and communication between the implant and prosthodontic dentists. The ISO 14801/ADA 127 standards specify a dynamic test method of single-post, endosseous transmucosal implants with their prosthetic components, enabling comparisons of different designs or sizes tested at a 10° tilt; however, the test is not a fatigue test. Dentures may be attached to the abutments with magnets.

An important aspect of dental implants is that they do not have the periodontal ligament that is present around natural teeth; therefore, implants do not have the sensory attributes of natural teeth. The result is less masticatory power (31) and no flexibility to absorb forces placed on the implant's restorative – forces are transmitted directly to the bone. Implants often suffer from peri-implantitis, analogous to periodontal pocketing (32, 33); hence, meticulous home care and specialized professional oral hygiene instruments are critical to avoid peri-implantitis and possible loss of the financial investment in the implant and the restorative. Both titanium and zirconia dental implants can fail via peri-implantitis. Figure 16.2 shows a titanium implant that loosened over time although bone remained partially attached. Dental implants do not have the characteristics of an individual tooth; they are not heterodonts; their

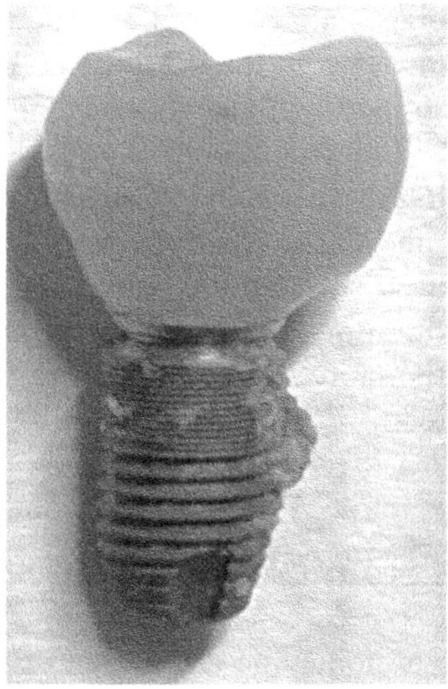

Figure 16.2 A failed titanium implant showing residual osseointegrated bone and cemented lithium disilicate crown.

diameter and length are not specific to a certain tooth number (Figure 2.1) implants are chosen based on what can be supported in the native bone.

The clinician must record all implant and grafting materials in the patient's case record as required by ISO 16498 and ADA 172 standards. Documentation must include the location and types of dental implant, connecting components, adjunctive devices, and grafting materials. The ISO 19429 and ADA 173 standards have a system for designating the location of an implant body within a jaw for the patient's case record.

Maxillary incisors and canines can be replaced by implants immediately after tooth extraction or trauma when all four walls of the socket are intact. Molar implants are placed after healing and resorption of the socket graft material rather than immediately. Placing any implant requires healing time, multiple procedures, specialized skills, and expense for patients, but a single implant can have an excellent esthetic result and eliminate problems a patient would have with flossing under a bridge or lesser esthetics.

Summary of Bone Grafts and Implants

Modern dentistry includes materials and methods to replace teeth using bone grafts and dental implants. Bone grafting materials are needed in dentistry when trauma, surgery, or tooth extraction create defects in the alveolar bone. Hydroxyapatite granules are frequently used, but the sources vary – from autogenous to allogenic to xenogeneic to alloplastic. Hydroxyapatite and other calcium phosphate compounds, calcium sulfate, and bioglass formulas have been used for bone grafting. All the grafting materials rely on ceramics serving as scaffolds supporting the body's healing bone regeneration.

Endosseous implants have been made of titanium since the 1980s and are highly successful because of their inherent, tenacious oxide surface coating. In the 21st century, tetragonal zirconia abutments and implant bodies began to be used successfully, with the advantage of their lighter color. Dental root-form titanium alloy implants are not ideal; peri-implantitis and occlusal issues occur; therefore, dentistry should emphasize preservation and retention of natural teeth.

Ceramics in Chapter 16

The following ceramics and other inorganic materials were mentioned in this chapter:

- calcium carbonate
- calcium sulfate
- carbonated apatite
- dicalcium phosphate
- diopside
- hydroxyapatite
- silica
  - bioactive glass
- tetracalcium phosphate
- titania
- tricalcium phosphate
- wollastonite

References

1 Sanchez-Sanchez, J., Pickert, F.N., Sanchez-Labrador, L. et al. (2021). Horizontal ridge augmentation: a comparison between khoury and urban Technique. *Biology (Basel)* 10 (8): 749.

2 Janjua, O.S., Qureshi, S.M., Shaikh, M.S. et al. (2022). Autogenous tooth bone grafts for repair and regeneration of maxillofacial defects: a narrative review. *Int J Environ Res Public Health* 19 (6): 1–14.

3 Fukuba, S., Okada, M., Nohara, K., and Iwata, T. (2021). Alloplastic bone substitutes for periodontal and bone regeneration in dentistry: current status and prospects. *Materials (Basel)* 14 (5): 1–24.

4 Lee, J.H., Yi, G.S., Lee, J.W., and Kim, D.J. (2017). Physicochemical characterization of porcine bone-derived grafting material and comparison with bovine xenografts for dental applications. *J Periodontal Implant Sci* 47 (6): 388–401.

5 Wuster, J., Neckel, N., Sterzik, F. et al. (2024). Effect of a synthetic hydroxyapatite-based bone grafting material compared to established bone substitute materials on regeneration of critical-size bone defects in the ovine scapula. *Regen Biomater* 11 (4): 1–33.

6 Gutmann, J.L., Sinjab, Y.H., Sinjab, K.H., and Navarrete-Bedoya, C. (2020). Calcium sulfate applications in dentistry: a literature review. *Endodontology* 32 (4): 167–174.

7 Gillman, C.E. and Jayasuriya, A.C. (2021). FDA-approved bone grafts and bone graft substitute devices in bone regeneration. *Mater Sci Eng C Mater Biol Appl* 130: 1–15.

8 Stiller, M., Kluk, E., Bohner, M. et al. (2014). Performance of beta-tricalcium phosphate granules and putty, bone grafting materials after bilateral sinus floor augmentation in humans. *Biomaterials* 35 (10): 3154–3163.

9 APN, H., Le, N.T.T., Truong, M.-D. et al. (2024). Alpha-calcium sulfate hemihydrate incorporated with tri-calcium phosphate and hydroxyapatite bioceramics as potential scaffold for bone regeneration. *Ceram Int* 50 (24): 54125–54133.

10 Ambard, A.J. and Mueninghoff, L. (2006). Calcium phosphate cement: review of mechanical and biological properties. *J Prosthodont* 15 (5): 321–328.

11 Kalagi, S., Feitosa, S.A., Munchow, E.A. et al. (2020). Chlorhexidine-modified nanotubes and their effects on the polymerization and bonding performance of a dental adhesive. *Dent Mater*: official publication of the Academy of Dental Materials 36 (5): 687–697.

12 Baskaran, P., Prakash, P.S.G., Appukuttan, D. et al. (2022). Clinical and radiological outcomes for guided implant placement in sites preserved with bioactive glass bone graft after tooth extraction: a controlled clinical trial. *Biomimetics (Basel)* 7 (2): 1–12.

13 Hench, L.L. (2016). Bioglass: 10 milestones from concept to commerce. *J Non-Cryst Solids* 432: 2–8.

14 Hench, L.L. (2013). Chronology of bioactive glass development and clinical applications. *New J Glass Cer* 3 (2): 67–73.

15 Bufersen, S., Jones, J., Shanmugham, J. et al. (2021). Survival of endodontically treated permanent teeth among children: a retrospective cohort study. *BMC Oral Health* 21 (1): 589–598.

16 Diba, M., Tapia, F., Boccaccini, A.R., and Strobel, L.A. (2012). Magnesium-containing bioactive glasses for biomedical applications. *Int J App Gl Sci* 3 (3): 221–253.

17 Rahaman, M.N., Day, D.E., Bal, B.S. et al. (2011). Bioactive glass in tissue engineering. *Acta Biomater* 7 (6): 2355–2373.

18 Ding, S.J., Shie, M.Y., and Wei, C.K. (2011). In vitro physicochemical properties, osteogenic activity, and immunocompatibility of calcium silicate-gelatin bone grafts for load-bearing applications. *ACS Appl Mater Interfaces* 3 (10): 4142–4153.

19 Ding, S.J., Shie, M.Y., Hoshiba, T. et al. (2010). Osteogenic differentiation and immune response of human bone-marrow-derived mesenchymal stem cells on injectable calcium-silicate-based bone grafts. *Tissue Eng A* 16 (7): 2343–2354.

20 Chen, C.C., Lai, M.H., Wang, W.C., and Ding, S.J. (2010). Properties of anti-washout-type calcium silicate bone cements containing gelatin. *J Mater Sci Mater Med* 21 (4): 1057–1068.

21 Huang, T.H., Kao, C.T., Shen, Y.F. et al. (2019). Substitutions of strontium in bioactive calcium silicate bone cements stimulate osteogenic differentiation in human mesenchymal stem cells. *J Mater Sci Mater Med* 30 (6): 68–81.

22 Addy, L.D. (2024). An introduction to dental implants. *Brit Dent J* 236 (10): 753–757.

23 Adell, R., Lekholm, U., Rockler, B., and Brånemark, P.I. (1981). A 15-year study of osseointegrated implants in the treatment of the edentulous jaw. *Int J Oral Surg* 10 (6): 387–416.

24 Marczewski, M., Wieczerzak, K., Maeder, X. et al. (2024). Microstructure and mechanical properties of Ti-Nb alloys: comparing conventional powder metallurgy, mechanical alloying, and high power impulse magnetron sputtering processes for supporting materials screening. *J Mater Sci* 59 (20): 9107–9125.

25 Giulio, M., Pierfrancesco Rossi, I., Luca, R., and Paolo Francesco, M. (2011). Alumina and zirconia ceramic for orthopaedic and dental devices. In: *Biomaterials* (ed. P. Rosario), Ch. 15. Rijeka: IntechOpen.

26 Al-Sanabani, F.A., Madfa, A.A., and Al-Qudaimi, N.H. (2014). Alumina ceramic for dental applications: a review article. *Am J Matl Res* 1 (1): 26–34.

27 Cordeiro, J.M. and Barao, V.A.R. (2017). Is there scientific evidence favoring the substitution of commercially pure titanium with titanium alloys for the manufacture of dental implants? *Mater Sci Eng C Mater Biol Appl* 71: 1201–1215.

28 Padhye, N.M., Calciolari, E., Zuercher, A.N. et al. (2023). Survival and success of zirconia compared with titanium implants: a systematic review and meta-analysis. *Clin Oral Investig* 27 (11): 6279–6290.

29 Cokic, S.M., Condor, M., Vleugels, J. et al. (2022). Mechanical properties-translucency-microstructure relationships in commercial monolayer and multilayer monolithic zirconia ceramics. *Dent Mater*: official publication of the Academy of Dental Materials 38 (5): 797–810.

30 Binobaid, A., De Lisi, M., Camilleri, J. et al. (2025). Zirconia-calcium silicate bioactive composites for dental applications using DLP additive manufacturing. *Bioprinting* 45: e00377.

31 Woodmansey, K.F., Ayik, M., Buschang, P.H. et al. (2009). Differences in masticatory function in patients with endodontically treated teeth and single-implant-supported prostheses: a pilot study. *J Endodont* 35 (1): 10–14.

32 Erduran, N.E., Guncu, G.N., Akman, A.C. et al. (2024). Evaluation of the effect of adjunctive diode laser application on peri-implant crevicular fluid biomarker levels: a randomized controlled trial. *Clin Oral Investig* 28 (8): 1–11.

33 El Sayed, N., Cosgarea, R., Rahim, S. et al. (2020). Patient-, tooth-, and dentist-related factors influencing long-term tooth retention after resective therapy in an academic setting-a retrospective study. *Clin Oral Investig* 24 (7): 2341–2349.

17

Drilling and Shaping Teeth

To treat a tooth with disease or other problems, some tooth structure is inevitably removed. For dental professionals, this is a conundrum because removing tooth anatomy begets more risk for treatment failure over time. Hand instruments, usually stainless steel, are used to remove tooth enamel and dentine softened by caries; rotating instruments are used for hard tissue removal and for shaping a tooth for the treatments described in Chapters 9 and 10. Grinding and polishing instruments are needed to prepare teeth and to customize the surface of a restorative material to an anatomically correct and interdigitated form. The equipment for tooth removal is referred to as drills; the handpiece of dental drilling equipment holds the drilling instrument – usually burrs.

The earliest drills were rotated by hand to remove hard enamel and create sites for the placement of a restorative material. Dental drilling equipment was mentioned by Fauchard, father of modern dentistry, in his 1728 book *Le Chirurgien Dentiste, ou Traité des Dents* (1); he used a bow drill on teeth, a device similar to those used to start a fire. George Harrington invented a motor-driven handpiece in 1864, and a foot pedal was added later for convenient operation (2). His invention evolved to include the belt and cord-driven equipment models of the early 20th century.

Turbines replaced the belt and cord motors in the 1960s. The first turbines were water-driven, but the faster, air-driven turbines (3) are now dominant. The faster handpieces were feared for their ability to cut teeth or soft tissues too quickly. However, the higher speed and low torque of the air-turbine handpieces have proved to be safer, with less vibration and heat, enabling dentists to make more precise cuts with smaller diameter instruments. Unfortunately, dentists may experience hearing loss from the noise of air turbines.

Ceramics in Dentistry: Materials, Manufacturing, and Clinical Applications,
First Edition. Carolyn M. Primus.

Air-turbine handpieces may be high-speed (300,000–800,000 RPM) or low-speed (below 40,000 RPM). The high-speed turbines cut hard tissue for procedures like cavity or crown preparation and crown finishing. The low-speed turbines are needed for cleaning teeth and for polishing and finishing restoratives requiring a speed of less than 5000 RPM for prophylaxis (Chapter 13).

Air-turbine handpieces require less than four bars (less than 60 psi) of air pressure to operate a contra-angle handpiece. Smaller head sizes and higher speeds of drill equipment have been achieved with miniaturized ceramic ball bearings in turbines. Silicon nitride (Si_3N_4) ceramic is the most common material for durable bearings; it is higher priced than steel bearings, but has benefits of higher hardness, corrosion resistance (for autoclaving), high-temperature tolerance with lower lubrication needs, lower friction, and less weight. The density of silicon nitride is about 3.20 g/cc, lower than steel (~7.8 g/cc). The minor components in silicon nitride ball bearings include alumina (2.0–3.5% Al_2O_3), yttria (4.0–5.0% Y_2O_3), titania (1.0–1.5% TiO_2), and carbon (0.3–0.8%) C. For the ceramic scientist reader, silicon nitride products are available that have a range of properties, as noted in Table 6.1. The 3-point bend strength and fracture toughness of some, but not all, silicon nitride products are high enough – more than 800 MPa and 6–10 MPa-m$^{-1/2}$; it has a high elastic modulus (300 GPa) and hardness (14.5–18.6 GPa). Only its gray color prevents silicon nitride from being considered for use as a restorative material. Ceramic ball bearings are also made of zirconia, alumina, or tungsten carbide, having Vickers hardness values of about similar hardness values to silicon nitride; hardness values of ceramics are influenced by minor constituents in the specific material formula and microstructure.

Electric motor handpieces are lighter, quieter, and deliver constant torque, unlike air turbines. Though slightly slower than air turbines (about 200,000 RPM), they can be used for high- or low-speed procedures and use the same burrs as an air turbine. Some electric handpieces are available uncorded with batteries for convenience. The role of ceramics in batteries is not discussed herein, but it is significant.

Specialized handpieces have been designed for surgery, root canal preparation, and implant placement (Chapters 8 and 16). The specialized procedures require slow speeds ($<$1000 RPM) to prevent excess heat in the tooth or bone and avoid endodontic instrument fracture. Reversibility of the rotational direction is essential for endodontics and implants. Some handpieces feature a watch-winding (unequal bidirectional clockwise/counterclockwise motion) for the preparation of root canals.

Today's dental drilling equipment is a combination of precision parts with various chucks to hold and rotate the intraoral burrs in air-turbine and electric drills. The gears, couplings for speed, and angles of the handpiece – straight or contra-angle – are important variations the clinician controls to perform the wide variety of procedures requiring precise access to the oral anatomy.

Seeing into the oral cavity has required optical glass fibers, halogen, and LED lights; these rely on ceramics and have been used to illuminate the oral cavity overhead and at the handpieces' tips. Water is a feature to cool and lubricate teeth.

Abrasives

Abrasives are fine powder particles, usually ceramic, that are harder than the item being ground, milled, or polished. Bonded abrasive instruments have the ceramic powders bound in a solid, such as rubber, metal, or polymer and mounted on a wheel or shaft. Coated abrasives denote a ceramic powder adhered to a flexible backing, like sandpaper or a polyethylene terephthalate (PET, polyethylene-type) sheet. Bonded and coated abrasives are designed to do the required shaping (material removal) before the matrix surrounding the abrasive particles fails. Loose abrasives are unbound powders; they are usually dispersed in a liquid that helps keep them in position before they are dispersed from the site they are polishing.

The primary abrasives for tooth anatomy and restoration removal are alumina, silicon carbide, tungsten carbide, and diamond. See Table 17.1 for a comparison of their Knoop hardnesses, which correlate with their dental applications; harder tissue and harder restorative materials require harder abrasives.

Several types of alumina abrasives are produced. High-purity (more than 99% Al_2O_3) powders create an aggressive, cool, fast-cutting action suitable for porcelain and metals. Alumina/chromia is a pink abrasive that is used with a bit more precision often for polishing. Brown alumina has iron oxide and 1–2% titania; also hard, tough, and lower cost. Silicon carbide (carborundum) was available for dentistry by 1907 (4); it is harder than alumina and is an everyday abrasive for tooth

Table 17.1 Comparative hardnesses of common abrasives.

Abrasive	Hardness (Knoop)
Nickel titanium alloy	100
Hardened steel	740
Tungsten carbide	1500–1900
Alumina	2000–2100
Silicon carbide	2300–2900
Cubic boron nitride	3500–4750
Diamond	7000–9500

anatomy drilling. Tungsten carbide burrs are made for cavity preparation, cutting metal, endodontic access to the canal system, sectioning teeth for extraction, cutting bone, finishing of crowns, and surgery. Tungsten carbide abrasive powder is manufactured by "cementing" it with cobalt via liquid phase sintering. Figure 17.1a compares the grain sizes of tungsten carbide available. Diamond is the hardest material known and is used for a multitude of grinding and polishing dental procedures. A vast array of designs and grits of diamond abrasives are used clinically and by dental laboratories. Diamond abrasives are essential for shaping zirconia crowns (Chapter 10). An example of a coarse grit diamond burr is shown in Figure 17.1b. Zirconia–alumina abrasives are reported to stay sharp longer and may find increasing dental use.

The size, particle shape, grain size in the particles, heat dissipation, and fracture resistance (friability) of the abrasive grains influence the cutting ability of any material. Generally, faster and greater material removal is achieved with coarser particles, higher speed, higher hardness material, sharper angles of the particles, more pressure, higher concentration, and a more durable matrix for bonded or coated abrasives. With all removals, finer abrasives are successively used. The lubricant also affects removal by reducing friction and cooling the matrix.

Burrs

Each dental practice needs at least a high-speed, slow-speed air turbine, and usually an electric handpiece having a wide assortment of dental burrs for excavating caries and other tooth anatomy removal, shaping restoratives, polishing teeth or restoratives, and root canal procedures. The current best practice is for these burrs, or endodontic instruments, to be "single-use" to avoid the communication of disease. Autoclaving for sterilization is considered adequate for the handpieces but incomplete for instruments (7). Single-use instruments ensure the most efficient cutting rather than a used, duller burr.

The most common dental burr contains tungsten carbide (WC) ceramic particles, an abrasive that revolutionized wood cutting since 1925 and was introduced to dentistry in the 1940s (3). Such instruments contain fine, tungsten carbide (ceramic) grains cemented (bound) to the metal shaft of an instrument by sintering 6% Co with 94% WC. The liquid phase sintering binds the high-melting carbide grains, usually 1–3 μm, onto the shaft; the combination is sintered at less than 1300 °C in hydrogen to avoid cobalt oxidation. Carbide cutting instruments are available with various numbers of cutting blades, shank sizes and styles, shapes, diameters, and head lengths. Examples are shown in Figure 17.2. The shanks are standardized in ISO 1979 and ADA 179.

Diamond rotary burrs are used to refine the final shape of tooth restorations, especially for hard ceramics such as alumina or zirconia. Diamond grit can be

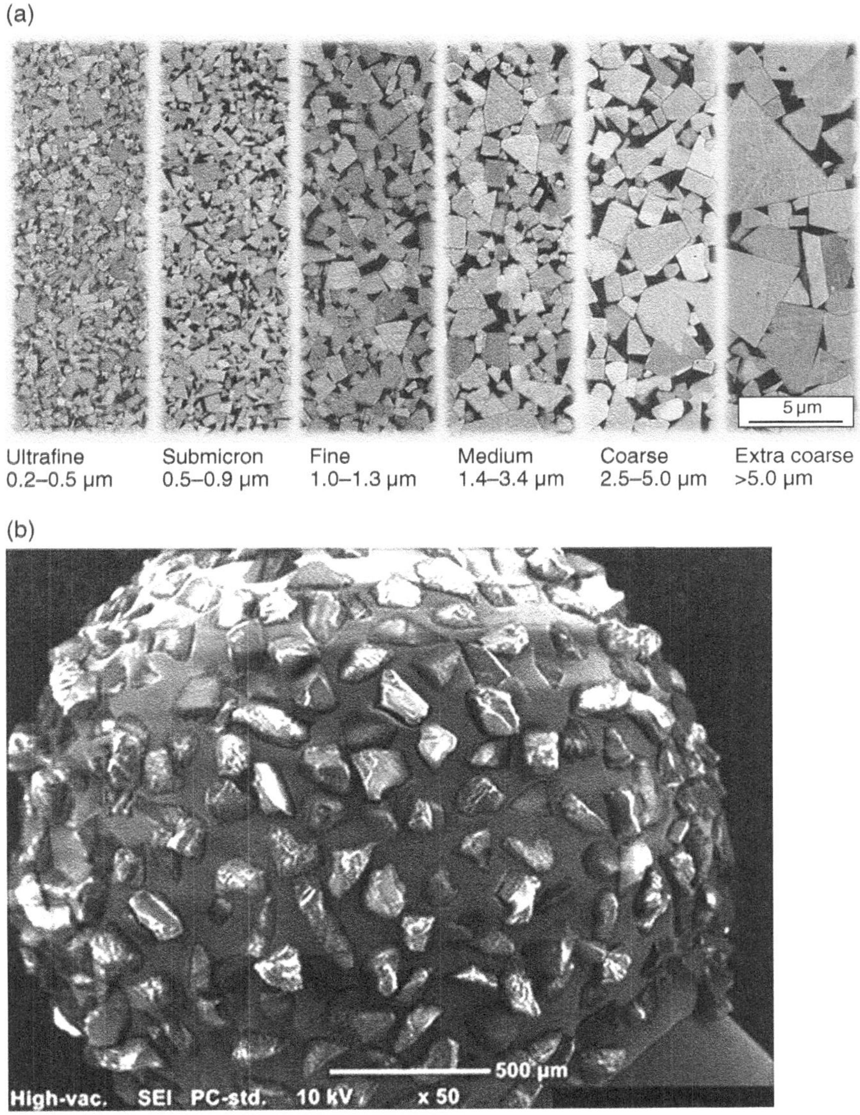

Figure 17.1 (a) Microstructures of WC-Co. *Source:* (5)/Elsevier. (b) SEM image of a spherical diamond bur, showing coarse diamond particles cemented onto the head of the round bur. *Source:* (6) / Elsevier / CC BY 4.0.

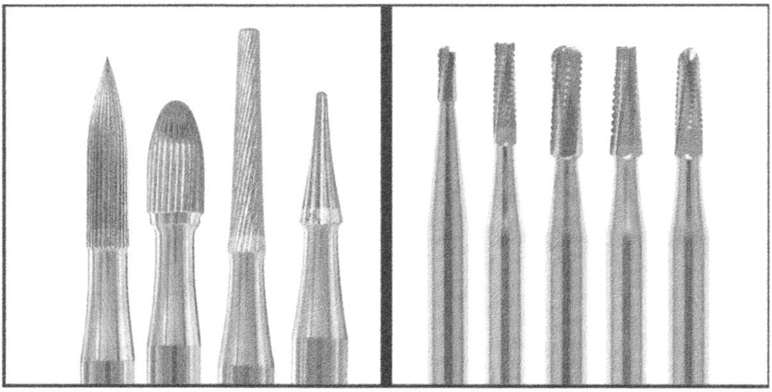

Figure 17.2 Various tungsten carbide instrument shapes for dentistry.

Table 17.2 Designation, color-code, and grit sizes for diamond grits per ISO 7711-1.

Designation	Abbreviation	Color code	Grit designation	Mean grit size (μm)
Ultrafine	UF	White	M 4–M 14	8
Extra fine	EF	Yellow	M 10–M 36	25
Fine	F	Red	M 27–D 76	46
Medium	M	Blue	D 64–D 126	107
Coarse	C	Green	D 107–D 181	151
Very coarse	VC	Black	D 151–D 213	181

bonded to the shaft via any number of methods and matrices. Early diamond rotary instruments were manufactured by hammering the diamond powder into soft copper or iron. Modern diamond instruments have diamond particles on stainless steel created by powder-metal sintering, bonding with polymer, electroplating the particles in place with nickel, brazing with a metal, or diffusion welding. Diamond rotary instruments have a stainless-steel shank 18–34 mm long with a working head. The diamond particles may be from natural or synthetic sources, and such instruments are classified by grit in ISO 7711-1, as in Table 17.2. The diamond heads are available in several shapes (shown in Figure 17.3) to facilitate access to the desired area of a tooth: round, egg, football, pear, torpedo, cylinders (straight or tapered, of various angles and tips), or flame (of multiple lengths and diameters and tip shapes). Other diamond tools are wheels of various cross-section sizes, depth markers (to help with crown preparation), and end-cutting

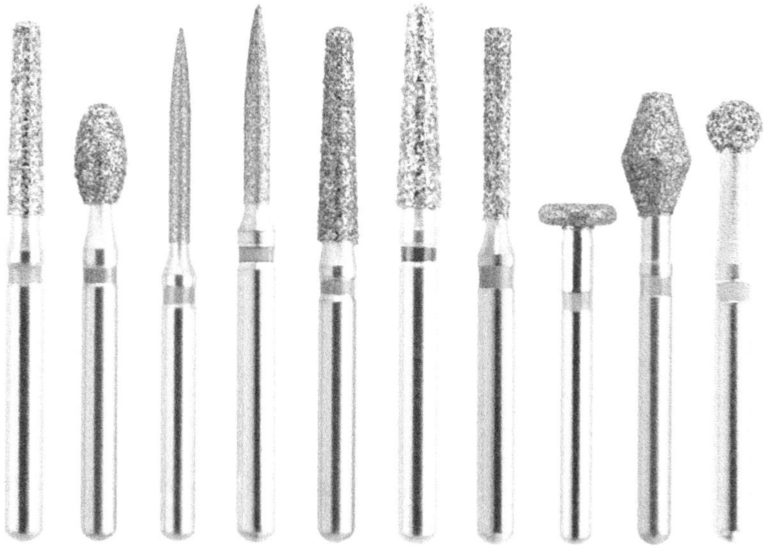

Figure 17.3 Various diamond bur shapes for dentistry.

burrs that only cut on their tip. Some instruments for ultrasonic, endodontic uses have diamond coatings made by chemical vapor deposition (8).

Some abrasive powders are "bound" into a matrix. Alumina, silicon carbide and diamond powders are molded into rubber wheels, points, or harder matrices and used to adjust enamel or metals (see the variety in Figure 17.4). Diamonds (C) and cubic boron nitride (cBN) grains are also bound to instruments with resins (such as polyimide or phenolic), glass (vitrified), or metals (such as bronze). Manufacturers have not advertised cBN on specific dental tools, but industrial cBN is used for the harder metals such as nickel alloys and titanium.

Zircon, diamond, and alumina are bonded to thin abrasive disks or interproximal strips on polymer film. Zircon-embedded glass fibers in instruments have also been featured for removing excess cement and some stains without the abrasiveness that would damage the enamel or soft tissue (see Figure 17.5).

Some burrs have thin, ceramic coatings, commonly titanium nitride and chromium nitride, to create harder surfaces for better durability, efficiency, and cooling compared to uncoated steel burrs. Coatings may be applied by chemical vapor deposition, reactive sputtering, or ion implantation. Adhesion of coatings is critical to providing the benefits of less friction and durability. A multilayer coating is sometimes needed to accommodate thermal expansion differences from the instrument to the coating, as noted for hydroxyapatite on titanium. Such tailored

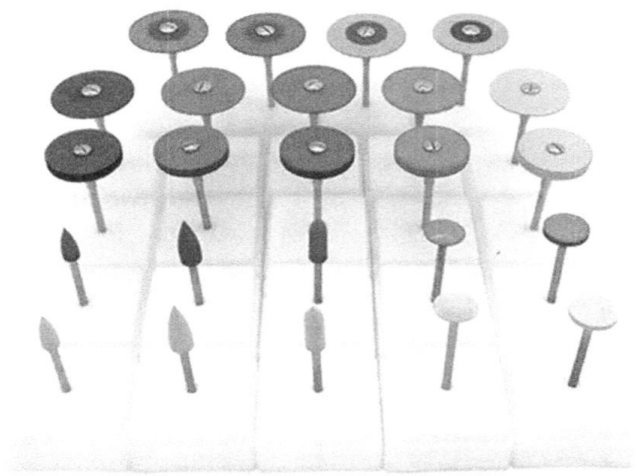

Figure 17.4 Bound abrasive shapes for dentistry.

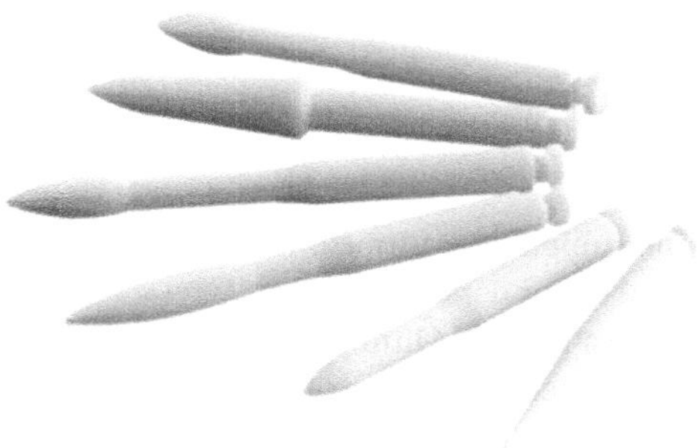

Figure 17.5 Glass fiber instruments embedded with zircon ($ZrSiO_4$) for cement removal near soft tissue or scaling.

coatings may include chromium-aluminum-nitride (CrAlN) to reduce stress between the alloy and the top coating. A titanium silicium nitride (TiSiN) coating – Figure 17.6 has a microstructure image – includes nano-sized TiN grains embedded in amorphous alpha-silicon nitride. cBN thin films are of interest because of their diamond-like structure, high thermal conductivity, and chemical inertness against ferrous metals, even at high temperatures.

Restorative materials placed in the interproximal area of teeth must have a smooth transition from the restorative to the tooth to facilitate flossing and plaque removal. Abrasive strips with ceramic powder embedded in a thin polyethylene film are helpful in finishing the shaping of resin-based composites in interproximal spaces. See Figure 17.7 for examples of the strips, which are available with various grit sizes so that the interproximal area can be finished smoothly by hand

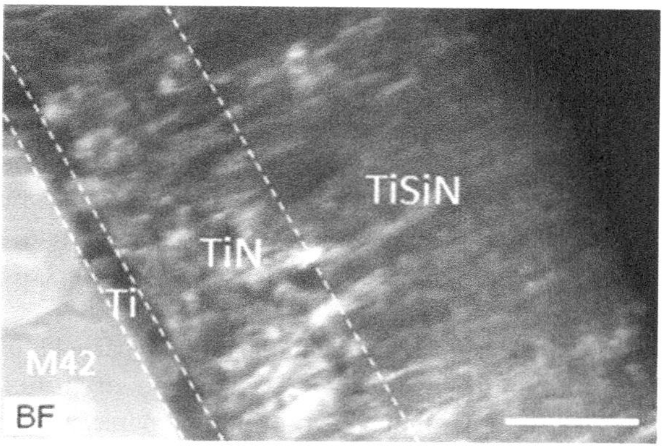

Figure 17.6 Microstructure seen in bright-field transmission electron microscopy of a TiSiN coating on steel (M42). The scale bar is 700 nm. *Source:* (9) / Elsevier.

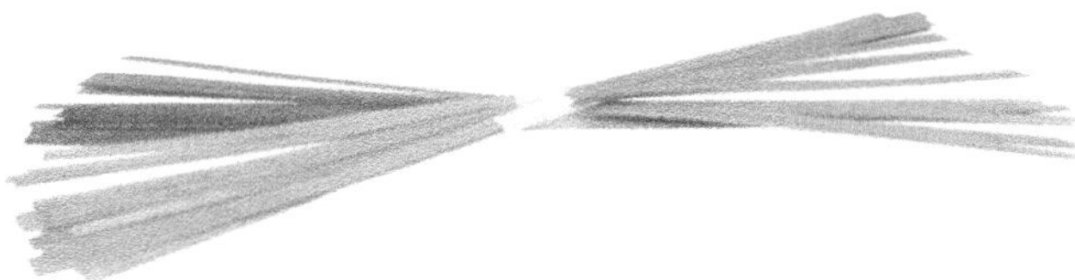

Figure 17.7 Interproximal strips (coated abrasives) for interproximal use.

by a dentist drawing the thin abrasive strip between the teeth. The abrasives vary from silicon carbide to diamond.

Loose Abrasives – Abrasive Powders

Abrasive powders are extensively used for dental prophylaxes, polishing or adjustment of cemented fixed prosthodontics, and extraoral finishing of dental prostheses. The loose abrasive powders are suspended with liquid agents and applied with brushes, rubber cups, felt cones, and felt or cloth wheels. The powders standardized in ISO 20608/ADA 37 mention pumice, quartz, zircon, and feldspar powders for stain removal and polishing but exclude prophylaxis powders and sandblasting media used for the intaglio of restorations. Loose abrasives have been used for "finishing" (the final polish) of dental restorations, especially resin-based composite materials (Chapter 9). Alumina pastes are especially popular;

their fineness is presumed to be less than 1 µm. Whether the softer gamma or the harder alpha phase is supplied is not clear. Ceria powder has also been used as a loose abrasive, sometimes with alumina. Polishing pastes may contain desensitizers (potassium nitrate, KNO_3) or flavorings because they are used intraorally. Diamond pastes, nominally 1 or 3 µm particles, are used for polishing crowns; the paste is applied to rubber and felt wheels or brushes and cups (Figure 17.8) by dental laboratories and dentists. Loose abrasive powders are also used to refine and polish native tooth anatomy. The common liquids mixed with powders are water, alcohol, or glycerin.

As described in Chapter 13, prophylaxis powders are loose abrasive particles of pumice, sodium bicarbonate, aluminum hydroxide, glycine, and erythritol. Pumice powder ranges in coarseness from "flour" (extra fine) to coarse. Today, pumice is used less frequently for prophylaxis than in the past.

Intraoral air abrasion, which uses loose abrasives, came into use after 1945 (10) with concurrent use of air pressure and abrasive powder for caries removal and cavity preparation, periodontal surgery, orthodontic pretreatment of enamel, and roughening resin composites for bonding more resin-based composite. Air abrasion minimizes treatment time and patient discomfort. Skill is needed because the effects depend on the hardness of the abrasive and its particle size, air pressure, distance to the tooth, angle of impact, and nozzle design. Whether air abrasion increases or decreases the bond strength of resin-based composites is debatable (11) and may relate to a tooth's surface roughness or if particles became

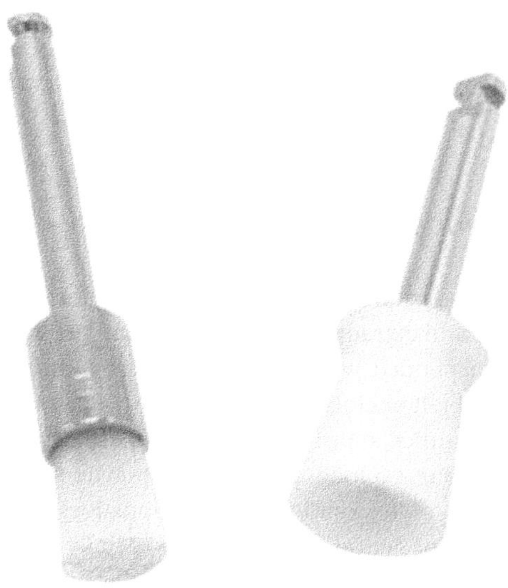

Figure 17.8 Brush and cup for applying loose abrasives with a latch handpiece.

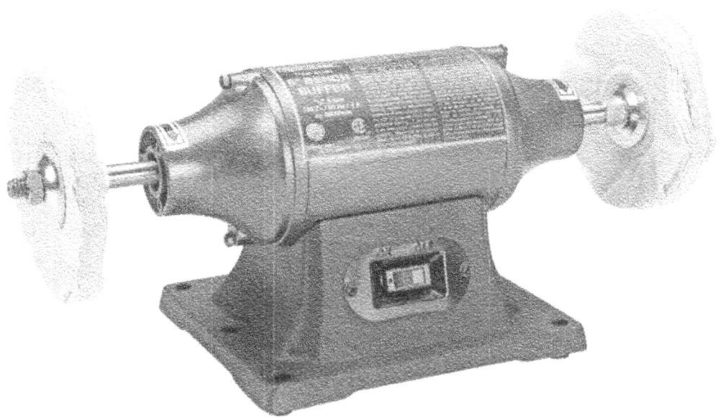

Figure 17.9 Dental laboratory buffing wheel on which abrasives may be used, including pumice.

embedded. Alumina is commonly used, but glass particles have also been tested; usually, the particles are 25–100 μm.

Extraoral air abrasion is important and common for making dental restoratives. Other chapters have mentioned sandblasting for preparing metal before porcelain enameling or polymer veneering, and the preparation of the intaglio of some indirect restorations. Coarser (> 25 μm) silica and alumina powders are used.

Dentures may be polished extra-orally on a dental laboratory lathe with loose abrasives such as pumice on felt or muslin buffing wheels, as shown in Figure 17.9.

CAD-CAM Mills

Milling and grinding are the machining processes performed with the CAM equipment to shape ceramic fixed prosthodontics, among other items, according to a CAD design. These rotating abrasive tools use carbide or diamond abrasives but have unique designs for CAD, not interoral, machining.

Metal Instruments for Tooth Anatomy Removal

Metal instruments are used on teeth and their success as medical devices is their protective oxide surface. The inherent oxide surface layer on stainless steels, attributed to their chromium content, makes these metals so useful. Stainless steel hand instruments are used in dentistry for tooth excavation and prophylaxis for their corrosion resistance, toughness, tensile strength, fatigue strength, hardness, and sterilizability. Standard instruments are made with austenitic 316 steel, also referred to as surgical steel, although 304 and some 400 series stainless steels are used depending on the application. The same grades of stainless are used for pediatric crowns and orthodontic brackets and bands.

Endodontic instruments are spiral or helicoidal-shaped metal instruments available in various sizes, tapers, pitches, cross-sections, shapes of the cutting edges, and axes of rotation. They maximize the removal of pulpal tissue and create a pathway for filling with sealer and gutta-percha, functioning like specialized internal burrs. At first, only stainless steel instruments were used, twisted by hand, in a watch-winding motion. Now, the more flexible nickel–titanium (NiTi) alloy instruments are popular for use in a slow-speed handpiece, having either continuous rotating or reciprocating rotation. The Ni–Ti alloys, usually equimolar nickel and titanium or 56Ni–44Ti, have three phases: austenite, premartensitic, and martensite. Proprietary heat treatments are performed to achieve the flexural and elastic requirements needed for preparing root canals for obturation. These heat treatments change the phases and enhance the oxide layer, primarily titania, which is less than 150 nm thick. Nano-sized diamonds are also being considered for removing debris within a root canal during root canal therapy (12).

Summary of Ceramic Tools

Teeth and dental restorative materials often require precise custom tailoring of the surfaces to complete a procedure or alleviate an occlusion problem. Shaping and polishing of teeth and restorative materials is done with materials harder than the teeth or the restorative material. Silicon carbide, tungsten carbide, alumina, and diamond are the common materials used in the tooling for these processes. Future abrasives may include carbon nitrides, three-dimensional frameworks of CN_4 tetrahedra made under high pressure and high temperatures. These C_3N_4 polymorphs are considered "superhard," comparable to diamond. The abrasives may be bound to rotating instruments, coated on polymer strips, embedded in rubber, or used as loose pastes. No one material or method is used because results depend on the location, the material being shaped, the abrasive material, the speed of rotating instruments, the force used, and the time available (11). At least one text (12) is devoted to dental tools. Restorations are desired to be smoother than 0.2 μm in average roughness on the occlusal surfaces. Abrasives are also dispensed by sandblasting with silica or alumina powder, to roughen a surface, either intra- or extraoral, e.g., a rough surface is required on the intaglio of crowns to increase the surface area for adhesion.

Ceramics in Chapter 17

The following ceramics and other inorganic materials were mentioned in this chapter:

- alumina
- aluminum chromium nitride
- aluminum hydroxide
- boron nitride
- carbon
- carbon nitrides
- ceria
- chromia
- chromium nitride
- diamond
- potassium nitrate
- silica
- pumice
- silicon carbide
- silicon nitride
- sodium bicarbonate
- titania
- titanium nitride
- titanium silicium nitride
- tungsten carbide
- yttria
- zircon

References

1 Andrew, I., Spielman, J.K., Lepor, A., and Shaner, A. (2007). The birth of the most important 18th century dental text: Pierre Fauchard's Le Chirurgien Dentist. *J Dent Res* 86 (10): 922–926.
2 Sproull, R. (1978). A history of porcelain in dentistry. *Bull Hist Dent* 26 (1): 3–10.
3 Eshleman, J.R. and Sarrett, D.C. (2013). How the development of the high-speed turbine handpiece changed the practice of dentistry. *J Am Dent Assoc* 144 (5): 474–477.
4 Land CH. Porcelain dental art. *Dent Cosm.* 1903;45(6):437–44 and 615–20.

5 García, J., Collado Ciprés, V., Blomqvist, A., and Kaplan, B. (2019). Cemented carbide microstructures: a review. *Int J Refract Met Hard Mater* 80: 40–68.
6 Gopal, P., Claussen, E., Azzolin, K., and Megremis, S. (2022). Validating cleanability of dental rotary diamond instruments soiled with 2 clinically relevant dental test soil components. *J Am Dent Assoc* 153 (3): 221–232.
7 Kohn, W.G., Collins, A.S., Cleveland, J.L. et al. (2003). Guidelines for infection control in dental health-care settings – 2003. *MMWR Recomm Rep* 52 (Rr-17): 1–61.
8 Rajnekar, R., Mankar, N., Chandak, P.N. et al. (2021). Dental burs in restorative dentistry and endodontics – past and present: a review. *J Res Med Dent Sci* 9 (8): 163–170.
9 Akhter, R., Zhou, Z., Xie, Z., and Munroe, P. (2021). TiN versus TiSiN coatings in indentation, scratch and wear setting. *Appl Surf Sci* 563: 1–14.
10 Eram, A., Vinay Kr, R., Chethan, K.N. et al. (2024). Air-abrasion in dentistry: a short review of the materials and performance parameters. *J Biomed Phys Eng* 14 (1): 99–110.
11 Huang, C.T., Kim, J., Arce, C., and Lawson, N.C. (2019). Intraoral air abrasion: a review of devices, materials, evidence, and clinical applications in restorative dentistry. *Compendium* 40 (8): 508–514.
12 Huang, C.S., Hsiao, C.H., Chang, Y.C. et al. (2023). A novel endodontic approach in removing smear layer using nano and submicron diamonds with intracanal oscillation irrigation. *Nanomaterials (Basel)* 13 (10): 1646.

18

Miscellaneous Ceramics for Dentistry

Incidental dental uses of ceramics are described in this chapter, including investment materials, ceramics for electronic purposes, and lasers.

Investment Materials

Ceramic materials are, usually, insulating and refractory (they withstand higher temperatures) Investment materials are ceramic powders that are mixed with a liquid product to form a customized container for processing a metal or ceramic at elevated temperature. These refractory ceramics are common in dental laboratories who construct the metal or ceramic restorative devices via high-temperature processes. For example, a refractory ceramic investment material is essential for the lost-wax, metal casting process that was pioneered in the early 20th century. Refractory investment materials are also required for sintering porcelain veneers, casting glass-ceramic crowns, hot-pressing of porcelain or glass-ceramics, and brazing or soldering metals. Important considerations for selecting a material are the investment's expansion to compensate for casting/forming shrinkage, ease of removing the investments, and the ability to obtain complete nonporous metals or ceramics with minimal defects (1). An investment material should have a thermal expansion similar to the material being formed, a higher melting or deformation temperature and be unreactive with the material being cast or supported. ISO 15912 and ADA 126 are dental standards with requirements for ceramic investment materials: gypsum-bonded casting; phosphate-bonded casting; refractory die materials; ethyl silicate bonded casting; and soldering investments. The dental standard specifies four types of investment materials: (1) for the construction of inlays, crowns, and other fixed restorations; (2) for the construction of complete or partial dentures or other removable appliances; (3) for the construction of casts

Ceramics in Dentistry: Materials, Manufacturing, and Clinical Applications,
First Edition. Carolyn M. Primus.

used in brazing procedures; and (4) for the construction of refractory dies. Two classes of such materials are included; those requiring slow or step-wise heating, and others needing quick-heating; heating decomposes (burns out) any organic materials. These standards have methods for measuring some handling properties and for measuring the linear thermal dimensional change; the latter is critical to creating a dental restoration that will fit the tooth preparation.

Investment powders are usually mixed with water-based liquids to harden and form a mold for casting. A few exceptions exist where the powders are mixed with polymers. Many refractory materials are based on quartz (crystalline SiO_2) and plaster of Paris ($CaSO_4$. ½H_2O, dental stone). As the investment mold is heated, the water is driven off, and hexagonal anhydrite ($CaSO_4$) is formed. At about 350 °C, the hexagonal $CaSO_4$ transforms into the orthorhombic crystal having a higher density causing about 4.3% linear shrinkage. The quartz component (crystalline silica) counters this shrinkage by expanding as it transforms α to ß crystalline quartz at 573 °C. The resulting investment material has no net dimensional change; ideally this calcium sulfate/quartz investment has a thermal expansion similar to the material being formed such as a metal or ceramic. The conventional method used to compensate for shrinkage inherent in the solidification of alloys is to change the investment's liquid-to-powder ratio. Minor constituents are boric acid (BH_3O_3), sodium chloride, and sometimes calcium fluoride. Such investments are limited to 1250 °C because at higher temperature the sulfate decomposes to calcia and releases sulfur dioxide gas, which is hazardous to the lungs.

Phosphate-bonded investment materials rely on ceramic setting reactions with magnesia. When magnesia powder is mixed with an ammonium dihydrogen phosphate solution, the reaction precipitates struvite ($MgNH_4PO_4.6H_2O$), magnesium phosphate ($Mg_3[PO_4]_2$) and newberyite ($MgHPO_4.3H_2O$) (2). See Equations 18.1 to 18.3. Silica powder is used as a filler:

$$\mathrm{MgO + NH_4H_2PO_4 + 5H_2O \rightarrow NH_4MgPO_4.6H_2O\,(struvite)} \tag{18.1}$$

$$\mathrm{NH_4H_2PO_4 + 3MgO + \rightarrow Mg_3\left(PO_4\right)_2 + 2NH_4^{+} + H_2O + 2OH^{-}\,(Mg\,phosphate)} \tag{18.2}$$

$$\mathrm{NH_4H_2PO_4 + MgO + 3H_2O \rightarrow MgHPO_4.3H_2O + NH_4^{+} + OH^{-}\,(newberyite)} \tag{18.3}$$

Ethyl silicate-based (TEOS, organic $Si[OC_2H_5]_4$) investments contain quartz and less than 10% magnesia. The powder is mixed with two liquids, ethyl silicate in ethanol (about 67/33 ratio) and an acidic HCl solution; ethylene glycol may also be present. The ethyl silica is hydrolyzed when mixed with the water solution, forming orthosilicic acid gel ($Si[OH]_4$) on the powder and binding the particles.

When the set investment material is heated, the alcohol evaporates and the gel releases water becoming silica. Other ceramic powders may be included in investment powders: magnesia/alumina phosphate, alumina/gypsum, magnesia/silica, magnesia/calcium aluminate cement, magnesia/alumina/spinel, or calcia/resin (2). The alumina/gypsum investment materials are usable at higher temperatures than silica because they form calcium aluminate compounds ($CaO.6Al_2O_3$ or $CaO.2Al_2O_3$). Magnesia/silicate investment materials form enstatite ($MgSiO_3$, $MgO.SiO_2$) above 830 °C, releasing heat and expanding. Magnesia and calcium aluminate cement investments are combined in a ratio of about 85/15 and include about 3% zirconium metal powder for expansion – Zr oxidizes during heating. The calcia/resin investment materials contain, for instance, calcia (78%), calcium fluoride (2%), and methylmethacrylate monomer (20%). The polymer causes unwanted shrinkage as it sets but decomposes at about 400 °C. Unreactive fillers, e.g., silica and magnesia, are often present in the investment powders.

The magnesia/alumina/spinel investments were designed for casting titanium metal; such investment powders contained 70% MgO, 25% Al_2O_3, and 5% ZrO_2/ZrN and were mixed with a magnesium acetate ($Mg[CH_3COO]_2$) solution to form spinel ($MgAl_2O_4$, $MgO.Al_2O_3$) during setting. Calcium zirconate investment material was also developed for casting titanium metal copings; it contained primarily rather coarse (up to 3 mm) calcium zirconate ($CaZrO_3$), calcium carbonate, monoclinic zirconia, and calcium aluminate cement. Another material was cleverly used to cast titanium; a magnesia/alumina/silica powder releases aluminum into the molten titanium to create a protective oxide layer (case) on the titanium casting.

As noted in Chapter 10, a unique investment material was patented for the ceramming process of the Dicor glass-ceramic. The investment material was mixed with water and inserted within the intaglio of the glass crown to provide support and avoid its distortion during the ceramming heat treatment. The patented ceramic composition for the investment composition (US Pat. 4,478,641) was 5–30% plaster of Paris and 70–95% leucite frit. An alternative composition was 45–60% Al_2O_3, 25–35% cristobalite, 5–20% plaster of Paris, and 0–15% leucite. The leucite was developed by heat treatment of potassium feldspar, but the proportions of the glass and leucite crystals were not clearly specified.

A crushable crucible investment material was noted in Chapter 10 (US Pat. 6,818,573 B2) for lithium disilicate crown forming. Cups were slip-cast of the patented glass composition (US Pat. 6,346,306B1) containing 78% silica, 15% boric oxide, 4.5% sodium oxide, and 2.5% alumina. The cups were removed from the plaster of Paris molds and partially sintered. The cup held the lithium disilicate ingots; when inserted in the uniaxial dental furnace for pressing and filling the investment mold of the restoration, one end of the investment was sealed as the cup was crushed and the ingot was pressed into the mold.

Ceramic fiber insulating materials are also needed for investment casting. Fibrous, wool-like or felt-like ceramic products surround the cast investment within a metal ring; the fibers are compressed as the investment expands during heating and casting. The ceramic fibers are not asbestos (fibers of $Mg_3Si_2O_5(OH)_4$) but are commonly derived from kaolin clay ($Al_2O_3.2SiO_2.2H_2O$). This clay is dried and then "fiberized" from the molten condition using a stream of air at about 2000 °C into a glass with about 50% silica, 45 % alumina, plus minor amounts of iron and titanium. The fibers are then formed into insulating fabrics for use at temperatures less than 1200 °C; tradenames include Kaowool® and Kaoliner®. Fibers of an alumina-silica-zirconia composition are suitable for up to 1430 °C. Fiber insulation is essential for any dental furnace or oven.

Ceramics in Electronics

In 1952, Geoffrey W.A. Dummer presented the first integrated circuit concept – the microchip – which is the basis for all modern electronic equipment. The integrated circuit is an advanced form of the electrical circuit, composed of a transistor (invented in 1947), a resistor, a capacitor, and a diode, linked together on a silicon (ceramic) substrate; this invention reduced the distance between components to speed up the electronic signal. The transistor was a significant advancement over vacuum tubes although both rely on ceramics to function. Microchips are used in virtually every electrical device – battery-operated or plugged in – and depend on ceramics to function. We rely on integrated circuits for our computers, phones, watches, calculators, screens, microwaves, screens, stereos, cars, refrigerators, toys, musical greeting cards, and dental equipment.

Electronic ceramic components also serve unique roles as electrical insulation or semiconductors, and some have thermal stability and mechanical strength. Components include electronic substrates and packaging, insulators or encapsulants, capacitors, resistors, piezoelectric devices, sensors, radio frequency and microwave filters, resonators, and antennas.

Alumina and aluminum nitride (AlN) have high thermal conductivity and are used as substrates in circuit boards to dissipate heat generated by electronics with electrical insulation and to physically support the circuitry. Silicon nitride (Si_3N_4) and alumina are used in electronic packaging to enhance heat dissipation. Other ceramic materials, having thermal and electrical insulation, serve as hermetic electronic packaging, arc tubes, and insulate wires, and protect electronic components from environmental factors, such as moisture, dust, and chemicals. Other examples of ceramics for electronics are insulators (steatite), dielectrics (silica and tantalite [SiO_2, Ta_2O_5]), piezoelectrics (lead zirconate titanate, $Pb[Zr_xTi_{1-x}]O_3$), optical materials (lithium niobate, $LiNbO_3$), and transparent semiconductors (indium tin oxide (ITO, In_2O_5Sn)). These examples are a sampling of the large class of metal oxides with current and potential electronic applications.

Thick-film pastes of specialized glass powder are used for the metallization of electronic components to seal and protect electronic devices from the environment. Radiofrequency and microwave filters, resonators, and antennae contain ceramic materials with high dielectric constants to minimize signal loss and enhance the signals. Diverse and unique glass formulas are needed for the display panels of equipment, computers, and mobile devices.

Multilayer ceramic capacitors can be microscopic to macroscopic and are ubiquitous in electronics. The capacitors use the insulating properties of a ceramics (dielectrics) when placed between two or more metal layers to store electrical charges. Capacitors are valued for their stability, high capacitance density, and low losses. Ceramic fixed and variable resistors dissipate energy. Inductors use magnetically permeable ceramics to create a magnetic field. Circuit protection devices use semiconducting ceramics to protect the circuit against transient voltage surges.

Piezoelectric materials, discovered by Pierre Curie in the 1880s, expand or contract when an electric charge is applied, generating force and linear displacement. Piezoelectric ceramics generate an electrical charge when pressure is applied or change size under an electric field – transforming mechanical energy into electric energy or vice versa. Certain ceramic crystals and polymers have this property, such as lead zirconate titanate ($Pb[Zr,Ti]O_3$), barium titanate ($BaTiO_3$), lead titanate ($PbTiO_3$), sodium potassium niobate ($[K,Na]NbO_3$), gallium nitride (GaN), and zinc oxide (ZnO). These components are used in electronic filters, resonators, transducers, acoustic elements, actuators, and components for pressure sensors. When multiple piezo elements are stacked, the device is capable of mechanical work and produces movement from the combined effect of each element's expansion; displacement is proportional to the height of the stack.

Ultrasonic scalers are based on magnetostrictive or piezoelectric materials; the latter rely on piezoelectric ceramics. Ultrasonics also have endodontic uses, vibrating diamond-coated tips, circulating irrigants in the canal, condensing gutta-percha, removing obstructions (silver points, broken instruments, or posts), creating root-end access through bone during surgery, or polishing the dentin apices reached surgically (3, 4). "Stacked" piezoelectric ceramics can be devised to actuate (vibrate) a nickel–titanium root canal file and augment or abbreviate the shaping (dentin removal) step of root canal therapy.

Electronic technology is transforming dental practices (5). Digital cameras are used by most practices to record cases before and after a procedure and during healing. Electronic health records, including images, intra-oral scanners, digital models, computer-aided design, computer-aided manufacture, virtual reality simulators, and dental informatics cannot happen without the ceramics in the electronics. The unseen ceramics in insulators, screens, capacitors, insulators, and semiconductors of electronics enable the smooth operations of the modern dental office. Table 18.1 has a summary of ceramics in electronics.

Table 18.1 Ceramic in electronics.

Application	Ceramic	Comments, uses
Non-conductive substrates	Alumina	Common in resistors having high thermal conductivity
	Steatite	Good insulator and dimensionally stable for high-voltage resistors
	Beryllia	High thermal conductivity for high-power resistors
Resistors	Mixed oxides	Mixtures of zirconia or alumina with ruthenia or tin oxide
	Metal oxides Zinc oxide	For varistors (voltage-dependent resistors for surge protection)
	Silicon carbide	High temperature or high voltage resistors
Capacitors	Barium titanate Calcium niobate Strontium titanate	Common in multilayer ceramic capacitors with higher permittivity but more variations with temperature and voltage
	Magnesium titanate	Tunable
	Titanium dioxide	For radio frequency & microwave devices
	Zirconium titanate	Low loss, low dielectric constant
	Niobates with Sr, and Na	
Piezoelectrics	Lead zirconate titanate	Most common, high piezoelectric coefficients for actuators, sensors, ultrasound devices
	Barium titanate	1st piezoelectric, lead-free
	Potassium sodium niobate	Lead-free
	Lithium niobates and Lithium tantalate	Surface acoustic wave filters, optical modulators
	Zinc oxide	

Ceramics for X-ray Detection

Film has been used to record X-ray images for over 100 years, but digital x-rays are now common, with the benefit of lower X-ray exposure for the patient, captured with photostimulable phosphor plates (PSPs) or solid-state detectors.

PSPs are flexible plates inserted into a plastic sleeve, or "barrier envelope," and then into the patient's mouth. X-ray exposure excites electrons in the phosphor material that remain "trapped" in its crystal lattice. After X-ray exposure, the phosphor plate is inserted in a scanning unit and the laser beam of the scanning unit stimulates the phosphor's crystals, releasing the trapped electrons. Light is emitted in proportion to the amount of radiation absorbed by the phosphor crystals, which is converted into a digital image. This image file may be displayed on a video monitor for interpretation or electronically saved. The phosphors on these plates are alkaline-earth halide powders, $BaFBr{:}Eu^{2+}$or $BaFCl{:}Eu^{2+}$, created by coprecipitation of an acidic solution of barium chloride, sodium fluoride, and europium fluoride ($BaCl_2$, NaF, and EuF_3) (6). The powders are mixed with an organic binder and applied to a polymeric film. The plates can be erased and reused; however, artifacts and incomplete "erasure" of the prior image gradually reduce image quality (7).

Solid-state detectors (sensors, direct digital radiography) have eclipsed using X-ray film use in developed countries. The key clinical feature of these detectors is the rapid availability of the image on a computer screen after exposure via a cable connected to the detector – a thin-film transistor array of silicon, charge-coupled detector (CCD), or a complementary metal oxide semiconductor (CMOS) detector. CCD detectors are light-sensitive arrays of silicon, silicon-germanium, silicon-gallium arsenide-based capacitors; silicon nitride and silicon oxynitride provide an insulating layer as part of the circuit. CMOS detectors also rely on silicon transistors. These sensors lower patient X-ray exposure, have higher contrast, greater resolution of the images versus film, and are durable. X-ray equipment has also evolved: hand-held equipment is available, and the need for a lead shield for patients has diminished although for older patients it is a well-recognized safety accessory.

Other Uses of Glass in Dentistry

The fundamental instrument of dental professionals is a glass mirror; ISO 9873/ADA 191 documents have requirements and test methods for reusable intra-oral mirrors with a coated-glass reflecting surface, both magnifying and planar. Soda-lime silica glass may be used for metallizing. Other glasses are integral and ubiquitous in dentistry and our electronics, both seen and unseen: optical fibers for communication or illumination, magnifying lenses (loupes), and microscopes. As mentioned in Chapter 5, van Leeuwenhoek ground lenses for microscopes (over four hundred), becoming the first person to observe bacteria, protozoa, and blood cells. Now, the use of magnifying lenses is standard for dentists to perform the highest level of dental treatment. Headband magnifiers and lights enable improved adaptation of direct dental restorative materials into prepared teeth; operating microscopes are de rigeur for endodontic treatment, where vision into the root canal system is crucial.

Glass vials are needed for anesthetic carpules/cartridges; carpules are made from borosilicate glass because it is non-reactive and can be sterilized. The ISO 11419/ADA 190 standards specify tests for leakage, plunger movement, extractable volume, and underfilling, including overall dimensions to ensure they fit into dental cartridge syringes, which are subject to the ADA 34 standard for syringes. Dental operating lights, the subject of ISO 9680/ADA 89 standards, provide the dental staff with visual ease and comfort without adversely affecting their perception of color or causing excessive fatigue. These fixtures may include glass shields and glass-enclosed bulbs.

Artificial Intelligence

Artificial Intelligence (AI) is now "rampant" in the field of dentistry. Every dental specialty publishes articles on AI, from pediatric dentistry (8, 9) to endodontic education (10). The reader is referred to other resources for an in-depth understanding (10–15) including texts (16), although it is evolving faster than can be captured in this text. Presently, AI is not entirely imitative of human intelligence, lacking the reasoning, planning, or ability to interact with the surrounding world or dental maladies. The skills are currently narrow but useful in education (17), behavior management for pediatrics, and diagnostics (18).

Unlike computer programs that use a set of rules to produce the same output each time for the same input, generative AI finds patterns in data sets to produce multiple possible answers from the same input. AI is "weak" or "strong." Weak AI – *artificial narrow intelligence* (ANI) – is coding that focuses on performing specific tasks; strong AI is *artificial general intelligence* (AGI) and *artificial super intelligence* (ASI). AGI is coding such that a machine would have to become self-aware with a consciousness and have the ability to solve problems, learn, and plan for the future, and ASI will surpass the intelligence and ability of the human brain. Figure 18.1 summarizes the hierarchy of computations and software.

Machine learning is a sub-discipline of AI, and deep learning is a sub-discipline of machine learning. Both machine learning and deep learning algorithms "learn" from data and programs modeled after humans' decision-making processes to enable predictions of what new data represents. Deep learning algorithms use automated, multiple data set to extract features from large, unlabeled, and information; for instance, deep learning is used in the analysis of cone-beam CT images. Generative AI refers to deep-learning models that can take data sets and generate statistically probable outputs when prompted.

The "intelligence" generated in chatbots, intraoral scanners, CAD/CAM software, and CT scans assists dental practices with patients, supporting decisions by the practitioner in an ever-increasing stream of information and analysis of anatomical data. Machine learning is used to understand root morphology and

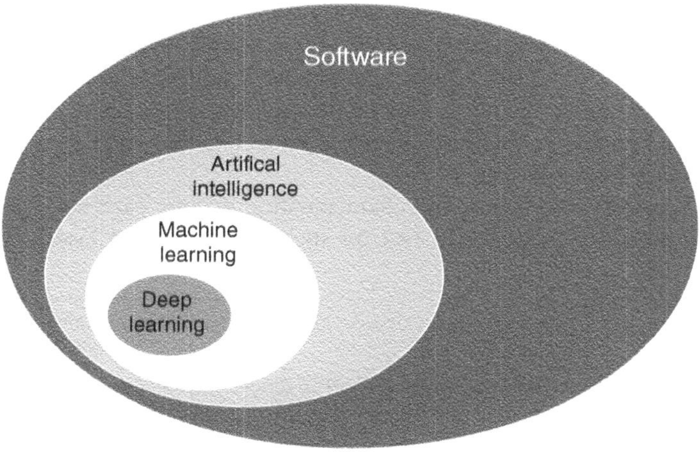

Figure 18.1 The hierarchy of software for the future.

fracture, diagnose apical lesions, consider the ideal placement of implants, detect caries, select a shade, design restorations, diagnose oral cancer, select irradiation protocols for cancer, and perform cephalometric or histological analyses. Deep learning may enhance the detection and diagnosis of oral lesions (19), ultimately improving patient care and predicting treatment outcomes. Critically, AI is not possible without the ceramics used in electronics described above.

Lasers

The first lasers for dentistry were slower than drills for tissue removal, but contemporary dental lasers are versatile and have been indicated for over 80 dental procedures. Laser light can heat the target (tissue) or stimulate a photochemical response. They offer precise targeting of tissue for treatment, reduce bleeding, minimize discomfort, use less anesthesia, and create post-operative pain more than traditional surgical instruments. The primary dental laser uses are to incise, excise, or ablate (vaporize) the hard and soft tissues in the oral cavity. Lasers are used in periodontal curettage or tissue cutting, endodontic surgery or disinfection, bone cutting, and removal of crowns. Low-level laser therapy is being investigated for osseointegration of implants because in peri-implant tissues, the laser stimulates bone activity and the number of viable osteoclasts by promoting local blood flow, increasing the area of bone that contacts the implant, to accelerate bone maturation around the implant (20, 21). Lasers' use and effectiveness vary with the individual case and the dentist's expertise using the laser technology.

High-power laser can have deleterious effects – charring tissue, causing coagulation necrosis in the pulp, degenerating the odontoblastic layer (pulp-generating cells), or melting dentin (22). The safety goals with dental lasers are to avoid damaging tissues by overheating, fracturing hard tissue, or generating a smear layer. High-power output has driven the development of lasers for industry; however, dentistry does not need much power.

Each laser has its own wavelength and characteristics, making each suitable for only specific procedures. See Table 18.2 for the commonly used lasers in dentistry.

Table 18.2 Ceramic laser materials (roughly from short to longer wavelengths and by type).

Laser type	Wavelength range (nm)	Applications
Excited dimer (excimer, gas):		
Ar & Fe	193	
Kr & NF_3,	248	Dentin removal
Xe & Cl_2	308	
Argon (Ar gas)	351, 458, 488, 514.5 & 528.7	Photopolymerization
Diode laser	810–980	Soft tissue procedures, teeth whitening
Semiconductors:		
InGaAs, GaN, GaAs,	780–1,550	
GaAlAs	820–930	Soft tissue removal
Erbium-YAG laser	2940	OH & apatite absorption: Hard and soft tissue removal; desensitization. Removing cements (GIC) and resin-based composites.
Solid state:		
Nd:YAG	532	Soft tissue procedures, periodontal therapy
1% Nd:YAG	1064	
Er:YAG	1550	
Er,Cr:YSGG laser	2780	Hard and soft tissue procedures
Alexandrite laser	720–810	Soft tissue procedures
KTP potassium titanyl phosphate ($KTiOPO_4$)	532	Soft tissue procedures; "power bleaching"
Carbon dioxide (CO_2)	9300–10,600	Soft tissue procedures, oral surgery; hard tissue ablation. Low depth of penetration

- Neodymium-doped yttrium aluminum garnet (Nd:YAG): Used for soft tissue procedures, including periodontal treatment and lesion removal.
- Erbium or Erbium–chromium-doped yttrium aluminum garnet (Er:YAG and Er,Cr:YSGG): Used for hard and soft tissue removal, including periodontal treatment, gum contouring, cavity preparation (decayed tooth removal), and bone surgery.
- Carbon dioxide (CO_2): Used for procedures involving soft and hard tissues, including cavity preparation, oral surgery, and reshaping bone.
- Argon (Ar): Two power levels are beneficial: 200–300 mW for curing light-activated restorative materials in a shorter time; 1.5 W for soft tissue cutting (23).
- Semiconductors or diodes: Commonly used for soft tissue surgery, including gum contouring, gingivectomy (removing gum tissue), treating gum disease, and managing lesions in the mouth.
  - Common materials for semiconductor lasers are gallium arsenide, aluminum gallium arsenide, gallium phosphide, indium gallium phosphide, gallium nitride, indium gallium arsenide, indium gallium arsenide nitride, indium phosphide, and gallium indium phosphide – GaAs, AlGaAs, GaP, InGaP, GaN, InGaAs, GaInNAs, InP, and GaInP.
  - Low-level laser therapy (LLLT, cold laser therapy or photobiomodulation): Low-power (<150 mW), infrared (~820 nm) lasers are used for reducing pain, inflammation, promoting tissue healing, and managing conditions such as temporomandibular joint (TMJ) disorders. Gallium aluminum arsenide is an infrared semiconductor used for LLLT (21).

Lasers have been used to remove the smear layer on root canal walls after biomechanical instrumentation with CO_2, argon, Nd:YAG, Er, Cr:YSGG, and Er:YAG lasers (24). Lasers are under evaluation to more completely disinfect the canals, an important goal of root canal therapy. Laser light can be transmitted through a glass fiber placed in the root canals; however, the emission of laser light from a glass fiber tip will not uniformly treat the root canal walls; a radiating circumference is needed. Lasers may also be used to heat and soften gutta percha during the obturation step of root canal therapy to gain better conformity in the anatomy. Thermal damage to the periapical tissues is possible, and laser irradiation beyond the apical foramen of a tooth injures the supporting tissues, including nerves, the periodontal ligament, and adjacent teeth.

Soft tissues have been cut with blue wavelength lasers; blue light is absorbed by hemoglobin and melanin. Soft tissue laser procedures include removal of granulation tissue, sulcular debridement and sterilization, pulpotomies, gingivectomy, operculectomy, frenectomy, gingival contouring, implant uncovering, lesion removal, troughing for an impression, removing aphthous ulcers or herpetic lesions, and tooth desensitization (25).

The diode lasers are precise for cutting and removing soft tissue, with slight damage to the surrounding tissue, excellent coagulation and hemostasis, maintaining a clear view of the operative field, low scarification, less post-operative or post-surgical discomfort, and faster healing. Often, local anesthesia is not required for treatment. For instance, the SIRO diode laser, with a wavelength of 970 nm and a power range of 0.5–7 W, can operate in three modes: continuous wave (CW), pulsated, and chopped. The continuous wave (CW) mode is an uninterrupted laser beam with good power control. Pulsed power output is a very short treatment at higher power (1000–20,000 W). The chopped mode interrupts the laser, for instance, for 50% ON and 50% OFF, to avoid tissue overheating.

Laser applications abound and will continue to grow; this brief section only highlights their variety and uses. For more discussion of laser and light therapies, the reader is referred to ADA Technical Report 133.

Summary of Miscellaneous Ceramics for Dentistry

Diverse ceramics covertly contribute to dental procedures. Ceramic investment materials are especially important to dental laboratories making indirect restorations using ovens/furnaces. Ordinary glasses are essential for anesthetic vials, microscopes, and loupes.

Ceramics are integral to electronics in the dental office from x-ray machines to handpieces, and all software, including phones. Ultrasonic scalers rely on piezoelectric ceramics, which are present in many other electronic devices. X-ray detection and recording uses ceramic detectors. Lasers are increasingly necessary for specialty procedures and will continue to expand their utility.

Chat GPT was used to search for "ceramics in dentistry." The result was a single page giving broad restorative indications, four advantages, and four ceramics. AI missed all the ceramics recounted in this tome, which are integrated into every part of dentistry; however, it's future in education and dental diagnostics is soaring.

Ceramics in Chapter 18

These ceramics and other inorganic materials were mentioned in this chapter.

- alumina
- aluminum nitride
- ammonium dihydrogen phosphate
- barium titanate

- barium fluoride chloride/bromide
- boric acid
- calcium mono- and dialuminate
- calcium fluoride
- calcium sulfate and hydrates
- enstatite
- feldspar
- gallium nitride
- gallium indium phosphide
- gallium phosphide
- hydrochloric acid
- indium gallium arsenide nitride
- indium gallium phosphide
- indium phosphide
- indium tin oxide
- kaolin clay
- lead titanate
- lead zirconium titanate
- leucite
- lithium niobate
- magnesia
- magnesium phosphate
- newberyite
- silica
- cristobalite
- glass fibers
- silicon
- silicon-germanium
- silicon-gallium arsenide
- silicon nitride
- silicon oxynitride
- soda
- sodium chloride
- spinel
- struvite
- yttrium aluminum garnet
- erbium doped
- erbium-chromium doped
- neodymium doped
- zinc oxide
- zirconia

References

1 Hutton, J.E. and Marshall, G.W. (1993). The expansion of phosphate bonded investments: part I-setting expansion. *J Prosth Dent* 70 (2): 121–125.

2 Khurana, P., Singhal, R., Agarwal, S.K. et al. (2020). Investment materials. A review. *Eur J Pharm Med Res* 7 (7): 457–461.

3 Balakrishnan, P., Sreekala, S.M., and Thomas, S. (ed.) (2018). *Fundamental biomaterials: metals*. Duxford: Woodhead Publishing.

4 Plotino, G., Pameijer, C.H., Grande, N.M., and Somma, F. (2007). Ultrasonics in endodontics: a review of the literature. *J Endodont* 33 (2): 81–95.

5 Wright, J.T. (2022). Transforming dentistry with technology. *J Am Dent Assoc* 153 (1): 1–2.

6 Ozasir, T., Ozasir, B., Aribal, N. et al. (2024). In vitro comparison of fracture strength of maxillary incisors with the simulated external root resorption cavities repaired with BioMTA or Biodentine. *J Dent Sci*.

7 Caliskan, A. and Sumer, A.P. (2017). Definition, classification and retrospective analysis of photostimulable phosphor image artefacts and errors in intraoral dental radiography. *Dentomaxillofac Radiol* 46 (3): 20160188.

8 Acharya, S., Godhi, B.S., Saxena, V. et al. (2024). Role of artificial intelligence in behavior management of pediatric dental patients-a mini review. *J Clin Pediatr Dent* 48 (3): 24–30.

9 Hartman, H., Nurdin, D., Akbar, S. et al. (2024). Exploring the potential of artificial intelligence in paediatric dentistry: a systematic review on deep learning algorithms for dental anomaly detection. *Int J Paediatr Dent* / the British Paedodontic Society [and] the International Association of Dentistry for Children 34 (5): 639–652.

10 Ding, H., Wu, J., Zhao, W. et al. (2023). Artificial intelligence in dentistry – a review. *Front Dent Med* 4: 1–14.

11 Zulfiqar, R., Khuwaja, I.G., Hussain, S.S. et al. (2023). Artificial intelligence as a diagnostic tool in medicine and community dentistry: a systematic literature review. *Chin J Otorhinolaryn-Head and Neck Surge* 54 (9): 1253–1264.

12 Agrawal, P. and Nikhade, P. (2022). Artificial intelligence in dentistry: past, present, and future. *Cureus* 14 (7): 1–10.

13 Schwendicke, F., Samek, W., and Krois, J. (2020). Artificial intelligence in dentistry: chances and challenges. *J Dent Res* 99 (7): 769–774.

14 Grischke, J., Johannsmeier, L., Eich, L. et al. (2020). Dentronics: towards robotics and artificial intelligence in dentistry. *Dent Mater*: official publication of the Academy of Dental Materials 36 (6): 765–778.

15 Khanagar, S.B., Al-Ehaideb, A., Maganur, P.C. et al. (2021). Developments, application, and performance of artificial intelligence in dentistry – a systematic review. *J Dent Sci* 16 (1): 508–522.

16 Orhan K, Jagtap R, SpringerLink (Online service). Artificial intelligence in dentistry. 2023. Available from: https://yale.idm.oclc.org/login?URL=https://doi.org/10.1007/978-3-031-43827-1.

17 Aminoshariae, A., Nosrat, A., Nagendrababu, V. et al. (2024). Artificial intelligence in endodontic education. *J Endodont* 50 (5): 562–578.

18 Allihaibi, M., Koller, G., and Mannocci, F. (2025). The detection of apical radiolucencies in periapical radiographs: a comparison between an artificial intelligence platform and expert endodontists with CBCT serving as the diagnostic benchmark. *Int Endod J* 58: 1146–1157.

19 Ye, Y.J., Han, Y., Liu, Y. et al. (2024). Utilizing deep learning for automated detection of oral lesions: a multicenter study. *Oral Oncol* 155: 1–8.

20 Convissar, R.A. (2011). *Principles and practice of laser dentistry*, 328. St. Louis, MO: Mosby Elsevier.

21 Rathod, A., Jaiswal, P., Bajaj, P. et al. (2022). Implementation of low-level laser therapy in dentistry: a review. *Cureus* 14 (9): 1–7.

22 Hargreaves, K. and Cohen, S. (ed.) (2011). *Cohens Pathways of the Pulp*, 10the. Elsevier.

23 Powell, G.L. and Blankenau, R.J. (2000). Laser curing of dental materials. *Dent Clin N Am* 44 (4): 923–930.

24 Sanghera, J., Kim, W., Villalobos, G. et al. (2012). Ceramic laser materials. *Materials (Basel)* 5 (2): 258–277.

25 Zandparsa, R. (2014). Latest biomaterials and technology in dentistry. *Dent Clin N Am* 58 (1): 113–134.

19

Summary and Future

The teeth of historical figures such as Buddha and St. Apollonia are treasured as relics (1) in temples around the world. Parents sometimes save their precious children's primary teeth, but it is our permanent teeth that are precious organs and are often underappreciated as they serve us under the adverse circumstances of pounding and grinding in a milieu of bacteria, fungus, and mild acids. Our teeth require care. The corollary is: ignore your teeth, and they will go away ... and you will need the magic of ceramics!

The essence of dentistry is to protect and preserve our beleaguered natural teeth, eliminate pain or restore their function using procedures that are as comfortable, conservative, durable, and natural-looking as possible. Over the centuries, ceramic materials have been instrumental in approaching these goals in a wide variety of dental substances. Materials scientists/engineers specializing in ceramics have innovated a broad spectrum of ceramic and inorganic items – glasses, polycrystalline and single crystals, plus various inorganic solutions – for every branch of dentistry. Some of these dental materials are used temporarily, from minutes to months; others are intended to last a lifetime.

The previous chapters shared how many of the same ceramics are used for varied dental procedures. The most frequently mentioned are silica, alumina, fluoride, calcium phosphates, calcium sulfate, zinc oxide, and zirconia.

Every chapter has highlighted the versatility of silica crystals and glasses for dentistry; silica powder has been used as a fossil, crystalline, fumed nanoparticles, and as the amorphous matrix for a multiplicity of glasses and glass-ceramics. Sundry silicate glass powders are used for creating dental ceramic restoratives – especially for the ubiquitous resin-based composites and glass ionomers. Crystalline forms of silica are also a component of various restorative materials as well as some products used on a temporary basis. Many silicate glasses contain boron oxide, sometimes for its enhanced durability, anti-caries effects, or contribution to bioactivity

Ceramics in Dentistry: Materials, Manufacturing, and Clinical Applications,
First Edition. Carolyn M. Primus.

and resorption. Other alkaline and alkaline earth oxides are also glass components. The bioactive glasses, interact in vivo for repair and healing in an active research area with ever-evolving formulas.

Silicate glass ceramics are an important restoratives especially lithium disilicate (Li_2SiO_5). Over the past two decades, beautiful anterior restorations of Li_2SiO_2 have been made for teeth and supplanted porcelain-fused-to-metal. The laboratory techniques for glass-ceramics have evolved from uniaxial hot-pressing in refractory investment to computer-aided design and manufacture (CAD-CAM), followed by ceramming. This sequence fits with a modern dental laboratory's workflow and enables higher-strength (more crystalline) materials to be made.

Alumina is also common as a component of dental glasses as well as a minor component in zirconia restoratives; it is essential for the glasses used with ionomers and in lithium disilicate. Plus, alumina has wide-ranging uses as a pigment, an abrasive, a polishing compound, an orthodontic bracket, and formerly as a fixed prosthodontic restorative.

Fluoride has been recognized for its anti-caries potential since the first silicate restoratives (Chapter 9). The fluoride compounds and glasses have broad-based utility in dentistry to enhance the chemical durability of our enamel with fluoropatite. Fluoride compounds are used as raw materials for melting many dental glasses to create powders or cements that inhibit caries by sparingly releasing fluoride ions to the surrounding enamel. The fluoride salts are used topically for ion exchange into enamel in many preventive products. Despite the denigration of community fluoridation, fluoride compounds will remain in the dental armamentarium, and professional fluoride treatments may become more critical in preventing caries if community fluoridation is abandoned.

Hydroxyapatite (a calcium phosphate) is the fundamental mineral of vertebrates, including dental enamel and alveolar bone; it is mentioned in most chapters. Related calcium phosphate compounds (Table 5.3) have been used in dentistry to enhance the bone or pulpal healing of diseased or injured teeth, implant coatings, and limited cementation products; their broader biomedical utility is expected to increase (2). Calcium phosphate compounds similar to those of hydroxyapatite but have not yet been successfully used as a restorative material (3). However alveolar bone preservation/augmentation is enhanced by the granular calcium phosphate grafting products – from animal or synthetic sources – a benefit for patients' restorative choices including dentures and implants. The porous phosphate compounds, such as octacalcium phosphate, may be enhanced with drug delivery into a grafting site (4). Undoubtedly, calcium phosphate compounds will continue to have utility in dentistry.

Calcium sulfate has made versatile contributions to dentistry. It has been used for impressions, as a material for models, in endodontic sealing materials, in some grafting materials, and as a component in impression materials. Its easy hydration, setting control, and calcium release properties, coupled with its low cost, are key to the use of calcium sulfate in many dental materials.

Likewise, zinc oxide has had remarkably broad dental uses: impression material, pulp medicament, temporary restorations, and cementation of fixed prosthodontics. Zinc oxide chemically sets with several liquids – chlorides, eugenol, phosphoric acid, and polyacrylic acid – is antibacterial, reduces enamel solubility, neutralizes sulfur compounds, and is useful in some dental glasses – it is a remarkable ceramic!

Tetragonal zirconia was uncommon until the late 20th century; today, no stronger, ceramic is currently known for a crown/bridge material for the posterior teeth. Multilayered tetragonal-and-partially stabilized zirconia products, containing tetragonal and cubic crystals, are also available for CAD-CAM processing having good strength and better esthetics than fully tetragonal ZrO_2. Other zirconia manufacturing methods – such as spark or microwave sintering – and modified stabilizers may provide improved esthetics, reduce the potential for low-temperature degradation, and enhance digital dentistry workflow in the future.

Many other supplemental glass components, ceramic crystals, or inorganic salt solutions were mentioned in this text as part of the interim steps for dental treatment or for creating a lasting, permanent dental device. The components have spanned the entire periodic table, with exceptions for some of the higher atomic number elements.

Dental materials have broadly borrowed from industrial and medical fields. The industrial methods of producing solid and powdered and ceramics into useful products were partially described. As yet, undiscovered properties of ceramic powders – nanoparticle's features, bioactivity or antimicrobial effects – may be discovered, developed, and commercialized to deliver better dental treatment, perhaps invented by biomedical engineers or dental researchers.

Several leitmotifs were woven throughout this book that may be helpful for engineers and dentists to retain:

- Ceramics for dental use (bioceramics) have been adapted and adopted from industrial applications and methods.
- Bioceramics encompasses all the ceramics used in medical devices, including dental.
- Many bioceramics are oxides, but not all.
- Most bioceramics are inert; a few are bioactive in the sense that biomineralization (hydroxyapatite precipitation) occurs on the surface of the bioceramic.
- Silica, alumina, calcium compounds, zinc oxide, and zirconia are the most common materials used; however, many alkalis and alkaline earth compounds are essential in dental glasses.
- Silicate glasses with specialized compositions are essential components of many dental materials, including both temporary and permanent ones.
- Fumed silica is ubiquitous in dental materials for all kinds for thickening pastes, including toothpaste, and creating smooth composite surfaces.

- Fluoride ions have essential uses for the hardening of enamel, deterring bacterial attack and are present in many dental products.
- Ceramic powders for dentistry may be naturally occurring mined minerals or specially manufactured by a wide variety of intricate methods. The morphology and particle size distribution determine their performance.
- Fine particles are especially useful in dental products, but coarser particles or granules are needed for bone grafting. Nanoparticles are already broadly used in dentistry, especially silica. Nanoparticles are not inherently beneficial but are used to advantage in nano-ionomers, for example.
- Strength is essential for direct and indirect restorative materials. Zirconia has been the strongest but not the most esthetic restorative material. Lithium disilicate glass-ceramic materials are less strong but more esthetic and have superseded porcelain enamel-based leucite glasses fused to metal substructures.
- Heat treatments matter for zirconia and the glass-ceramics; they are individualized by the manufacturer.
- Hard ceramic particles are needed as abrasives for all kinds of dental restorations; prominent are alumina, silicon, or tungsten carbide, and diamond powders of various grades, either on burrs, bound to a substrate, or as a loose polishing powder.
  - Softer and finer materials may play a part in polishing surfaces.
  - Wear-resistant ceramics are needed in dental equipment.
- Ceramics cements have varied setting reactions. No setting reaction goes to completion; residual starting components always remain, which may or may not be consequential for biocompatibility or durability.
- High atomic number elements are necessary for radiopacity; not all high atomic number compounds are hazardous.
- Metals used in dentistry are biocompatible because they are inert (noble) or form a protective ceramic oxide surface layer.
- Polycrystalline ceramic lasers are gaining popularity for many oral tissue treatments.

Ceramics are used in every electronic device in the dental office and operatory. Although unseen and unrecognized, these ceramics make modern dentistry possible.

Future Uses of Ceramics in Dentistry

These key issues remain for all dental materials: their ability to prevent disease, alleviate pain, and ensure any treatment with restorative materials will adhere, seal, and endure with esthetic appeal as needed. Any new developments must also ensure the biocompatibility, safety, and affordability of the treatment in the United States and worldwide. Future dental ceramics will likely include new unique formulas and powders for their integration into dental products, either alone, in combination with polymers, or in liquid solutions, providing benefits to further the goals above.

Better resin-based composites will certainly be invented with superior bonding systems. New bonding/adhesive systems may be the key to avoid recurrent caries at their margins, better combat oral biofilms, reduce mineral loss adjacent to the material, increase remineralization of the adjacent collagen, or be "self-healing" to avoid fracture. Researchers for manufacturers and in academia will continue to strive for monomers with less shrinkage, composite resins that have a higher depth of cure, and related products that are more biomimetic and durable. Future restorative materials may include ceramic fibers (5) or more effective bioactive ceramics (6) that elute ions to reduce caries and create hydroxyapatite where needed. For the foreseeable future, direct dental restorative materials containing ceramic powders will continue to be essential, barring the elimination of dental caries as a disease or the ability to regrow dental hard tissue.

Future indirect ceramic restorations will offer improvements, including better durability of surface porcelains or coatings, reduced fracture in the posterior region of the mouth, and easy and secure adhesion with dental cements. Indirect restorations may become more life-like in appearance but must have appropriate wear and durability with opposing teeth. Yttria-stabilized zirconia is now the top-ranked material for posterior restorations or bridges but new, stronger ceramics may emerge for restoratives, potentially offering greater translucency for improved esthetics, perhaps via improved glass-ceramics. Implant placements, including those made of zirconia, will blossom and hopefully, more effective treatments for peri-implantitis will be developed.

CAD-CAM processing of restorative materials will undoubtedly continue, perhaps with greater heat-treatment speed and lower-cost equipment.

The 3D printing methods based on digital dentistry will certainly be used for constructing polymeric and all-ceramic restorations via digital workflow in dental laboratories. Using 3D printing and post-printing processing may lead to more reliable and perhaps lower-cost indirect ceramics. 3D printing of could lead to the production of indirect resin-based composites, replacing the direct compaction and curing processes typically performed by dentists. Instead, scanning, laboratory printing, and curing may be integrated into the dental office workflow with only preparation of the cavity and cementing performed by the dentist.

CAD-CAM and 3D printing of dental devices, many including ceramics, will be combined with optical scanning equipment and artificial intelligence for diagnostics and treatment planning. Spark, microwave, or combustion sintering may be adopted by dental laboratories or manufacturers for zirconia to create implants, abutments, or indirect restoratives. These techniques may impart unusual and perhaps improved properties for appearance and suitability for intraoral uses.

Abrasive ceramic tools will always be needed for perfecting the shape of restorations via intraoral "adjustments," which is where cubic boron nitride or carbon nitrides may contribute to dentistry. The CN_4 or related C-N compounds could make it easier to adjust zirconia crowns or have other piezoelectric properties for equipment (7). Nanoparticles will continue to thrive and may impart special therapeutic effects, including via silica and its glasses (8). Thin films of graphene, diamond-like carbon, and borophene will become more common and may impart unique, unforeseen benefits for instruments, implants, or in other treatments (9).

The use of lasers will continue to rise, enabling more precise treatments with less pain and ideally, faster and easier healing. The lasing equipment is likely to be based on ceramic compounds. Lasers will become more common for even the general practitioners; very dentist will likely be using a laser for their everyday procedures.

New diagnostic equipment will certainly become available including higher resolution CT scans emitting lower radiation; more sensitive X-ray detectors may be presaged. The diagnostic capabilities of artificial intelligence and deep learning will assist dentists with diagnosis and treatment planning for the complexities of root canal treatments, implants, and other surgeries (10). More equipment will be battery-operated for convenience and may benefit "field" work.

Tissue engineering and regenerative medicine (TERM) research is focused on using biocompatible scaffolds, cells, and growth factors to create functional, living replacement teeth. Remineralization of enamel or revitalization of a pulp will progress, and ceramics may be combined with tissue engineering concepts. Remineralizing enamel to a depth of more than a few nanometers to replace enamel or dentin destroyed by caries remains an elusive but not hopeless goal. Pulp regeneration via tissue engineering is an important research effort in endodontics. No doubt, bioactive ceramic powders will be combined with drugs, proteins, or growth factors for improved periodontic and pulp regeneration to forestall tooth loss.

Nanoparticles and finer grain sizes will continue to be developed to enhance properties of the spectrum of ceramic powders and ceramic solids in diverse applications from restoratives to prophylaxis. Glass formula innovations – inert, ion-releasing, or biomineralizing – will continue to contribute to dentistry, perhaps in restoratives, and likely in bone grafting. Oral cancers were not discussed herein, but a gallium-doped bioactive glass is being developed to treat osteosarcoma, which does occur in the jaw (11). Osteonecrosis of the jaw and cervical resorption need new treatments; ceramic materials may contribute, perhaps with biomineralizing cements or bioactive glasses.

In the more distant future, dental-related electronic devices may include qubits and ceramic superconductors, which allow the passage of electrical current with zero resistance below a certain critical temperature (T_c). The majority of "high-temperature" superconductors are ceramics. However, the highest critical temperature is for $HgBa_2Ca_2Cu_3O_8$ at 134 K, which is about 90 °C below room temperature and is still impractical. The first ceramics with superconductivity were from the lanthanum–barium copper oxide (La–Ba–Cu–O) system (1986), at 28 K; this was followed by superconductivity in $Bi_2Sr_2CuO_6$, among other ceramics (12). Lab-grown samples of a few minerals display superconductivity: covellite (copper sulfide, CuS), parkerite ($Ni_3Bi_2S_2$), miassite ($Rh_{17}S_{15}$), and palladseite ($Pd_{17}Se_{15}$) (13). If new superconductive compounds functioned closer to ambient temperatures and pressures, significantly smaller and more efficient electronic circuits could be created for dental and office equipment, and support artificial intelligence.

Artificial intelligence will proliferate from dental education to diagnosis and may be integrated with robotic procedures. Its performance cannot match that of humans in licensing exams ... yet (14). A dentist's life will change well before they retire!

Summary of Ceramics for Dentistry

This text canvassed the breadth of the peer-reviewed and patent literature regarding the uses of ceramics in dentistry. It serves as an introduction to the diverse range of applications that ceramics have satisfied for numerous successful dental treatments. A rough timeline for the introduction of certain key ceramics in dentistry is in Figure 19.1. A multitude of prosaic and uncommon ceramics and inorganic materials are used in dentistry for routine and specialized procedures. The most common ones are silica, alumina, calcium phosphates, calcium silicate/aluminate cements, calcium sulfate, lithium disilicate, zinc oxide, and zirconia. However, ceramics containing most of the elements of the periodic table have been mentioned.

Ceramic materials are needed in restoratives, both direct and indirect, but are also key to dental practice of dentistry in temporary-use liquids and pastes, in refractory uses in dental laboratories, as abrasives for technicians, hygienists, and clinicians, and for wear-resistant components of instruments and equipment. Supplementary ceramic powders are ubiquitous as pigments and for other specialized features such as radiopacity. Many fluoride compounds and a plethora of glass formulas containing fluoride are used.

Every dental practice and specialty relies on ceramics. Generalizations about dental ceramics are below:

- Zinc oxide-eugenol containing materials are useful for their obtundent and antimicrobial properties in pulp medicaments, temporary cements, and endodontic sealers.
- Calcium silicate/aluminate cements are a very wonderful bioactive cement for pulp and endodontic therapy performed by general and pediatric dentists, and especially endodontists.

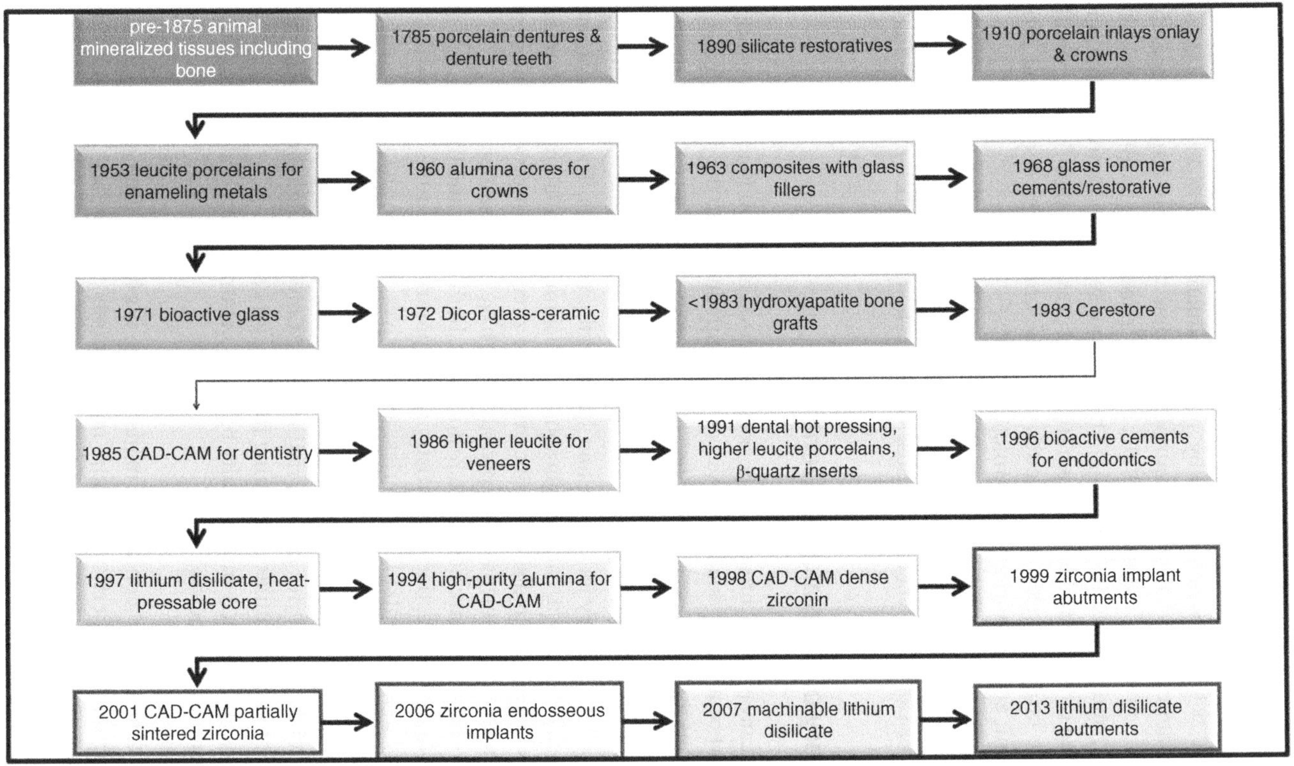

Figure 19.1 Rough timeline of the uses of ceramics in dentistry based on publication dates and 510(k) clearances. Core refers to coping in this figure.

- Glass ionomer cements are useful for their adhesion and fluoride release, especially for pediatric dentistry, orthodontic cements, and for situations where light curing equipment is unavailable, e.g., mission work.
  - Calcium aluminate cement has been combined with glass ionomer cements for use as a crown cement.
- Every dentist relies on composite restoratives and cements. Composites are primarily composed of glass powders of various particle size distributions.
- Lithium disilicate glass-ceramics are a very popular indirect restorative for anterior teeth.
- Tetragonal zirconia is the current reigning indirect restorative for its strength and is also used for endosseous implants and abutments.

Materials science and engineering will be at the heart of the success of every dental material for the future, borrowing new ideas, methods, and materials from industrial applications. Ceramic materials, primarily ceramic powders, will continue to make major contributions to ~~the~~ clinical dental practices often because of their inherent biocompatibiliity and beauty.

Ceramics in Chapter 19

The following ceramics and other inorganic materials were mentioned in this chapter:

- calcium silicate/aluminate cements
- covellite
- glass ionomer
- lanthanum-barium copper oxide
- lithium disilicate glass-ceramic
- miassite
- parkerite
- silica glasses, including bioactive glasses
- zinc oxide
- zirconia

References

1 Cheng, F.-C. and Chiang, C.-P. (2024). The tooth relic of the Buddha: The viewpoint from paleodontology and modern dentistry. *J Dent Sci* 19: 729–731.
2 Dorozhkin, S.V. (2017). A history of calcium orthophosphates (CaPO4) and their biomedical applications. *Morphologie* 101 (334): 143–153.

3 Pereira, L.F., de Azevedo-Silva, L.J., Minim, P.R. et al. (2024). Are we approaching the development of a novel calcium phosphate-based bioceramic dental material? *Dent Mater: Official Publication of the Academy of Dental Materials* 40 (11): 1843–1853.

4 Kovrlija, I., Locs, J., and Loca, D. (2021). Octacalcium phosphate: Innovative vehicle for the local biologically active substance delivery in bone regeneration. *Acta Biomater* 135: 27–47.

5 Liu, J., Zhang, H., Sun, H. et al. (2021). The Development of Filler Morphology in Dental Resin Composites: A Review. *Materials (Basel)* 14 (19): 1–21.

6 Tiskaya, M., Shahid, S., Gillam, D., and Hill, R. (2021). The use of bioactive glass (BAG) in dental composites: A critical review. *Dent Mater: Official Publication of the Academy of Dental Materials* 37 (2): 296–310.

7 Laniel, D., Trybel, F., Aslandukov, A. et al. (2024). Synthesis of Ultra-Incompressible and Recoverable Carbon Nitrides Featuring CN(4) Tetrahedra. *Adv Mater* 36 (3): 1–12.

8 Mbitta Akoa, D., Avril, A., Helary, C. et al. (2025). Evaluation of Silica and Bioglass Nanomaterials in Pulp-like Living Materials. *ACS Biomater Sci Eng* 11 (2): 891–902.

9 Li, G., Zhou, T., Lin, S. et al. (2017). Nanomaterials for Craniofacial and Dental Tissue Engineering. *J Dent Res* 96 (7): 725–732.

10 Khanagar, S.B., Al-Ehaideb, A., Maganur, P.C. et al. (2021). Developments, application, and performance of artificial intelligence in dentistry - A systematic review. *J Dent Sci* 16 (1): 508–522.

11 Hanaei, S.B., Murugesan, R.C., Souza, L.P. et al. (2024). Multifunctional gallium doped bioactive glasses: a targeted delivery for antineoplastic agents and tissue repair against osteosarcoma. *Biomed Mater* 19 (6): 1–16.

12 Cava, R.J. (2008). Oxide Superconductors. *J Amer Ceram Soc* 83 (1): 5–28.

13 Kim, H., Tanatar, M.A., Kończykowski, M. et al. (2024). Nodal superconductivity in miassite Rh17S15. *Commun Mater* 5 (17): 1–7.

14 Chan-Chia Lin, C., Sun, J.-S., Chang, C.-H. et al. (2025). Performance of artificial intelligence chatbots in National dental licensing examination. *J Dent Sci* 20: (in press).

Index

Ceramics in Dentistry: Materials, Manufacturing, and Clinical Applications,
First Edition. Carolyn M. Primus.

Printed and bound by CPI Group (UK) Ltd, Croydon, CR0 4YY
17/09/2026
14964241-0006